PATHOLOGY OF PULMONARY HYPERTENSION

PATHOLOGY OF PULMONARY HYPERTENSION

C. A. WAGENVOORT, M.D.

Professor of Pathology
Chairman of the Department of Pathological Anatomy
Wilhelmina Gasthuis, University of Amsterdam, The Netherlands

and

NOEKE WAGENVOORT

Foreword by

JESSE E. EDWARDS, M.D.

Clinical Professor of Pathology
University of Minnesota Medical School
Minneapolis, Minnesota

A Wiley Medical Publication

JOHN WILEY & SONS   New York • London • Sydney • Toronto

Library of Congress Cataloging in Publication Data:

Wagenvoort, Cornelis Adriaan.
  Pathology of pulmonary hypertension.

(A Wiley medical publication)
  Includes bibliographies and index.
  1. Pulmonary hypertension. I. Wagenvoort, Noeke, joint author. II. Title. [DNLM: 1. Hypertension, Pulmonary—Pathology. 2. Pulmonary artery—Pathology. 3. Pulmonary veins—Pathology. WF600 W131p]

RC776.P87W33   616.2′4   76-39782
ISBN 0-471-91355-3

Printed in the United States of America

10 9 8 7 6 5 4 3 2 1

to Donald Heath
in friendship

Foreword

The pulmonary vascular bed is now generally recognized as a compartment that has strong influences upon the circulation, either as it is involved in intrinsic disease or in relation to pulmonary parenchymal and cardiac diseases.

Broad as the influence of the pulmonary vascular bed is on the circulation, it is significant that much of the work done in this field has been done principally during the past twenty-five years. It was through the availability of pressures and flow determinations, by the introduction of cardiac catheterization, that the pathology of the pulmonary vascular bed obtained a firm footing in relating structural patterns to functional states.

In the early years of what might be called "the modern era," the authors of this book entered the field. From their early days, they have contributed significantly in many ways, including quantitation of structural changes, delineation of the hitherto poorly understood entity of primary pulmonary hypertension, and identification of qualitative patterns of change among the various types of pulmonary hypertension. In a word, the authors have consistently and significantly fed into the reservoir of accumulating knowledge concerning the pulmonary vascular bed.

From this reservoir, the Wagenvoorts have come up with a clear distillate concerning the normal and the many disease states affecting the pulmonary vascular bed. This book represents a composite of information—information that now rests on a secure foundation. While work is yet to be done with regard to mechanisms leading to abnormalities, this book serves as a valuable reference, both as to what has been done and as to the now existing wealth of information concerning the relationship between structure and function and its inevitable meaning to the afflicted.

By clarity of expression, both in word and illustration, coupled with generous and appropriate references, this book will serve as a classic, both to the student and to practitioners of many facets of medicine.

Jesse E. Edwards, M.D.

vii

Preface

The study of the pulmonary circulation has a long history, even though most of our present knowledge has accumulated in the last twenty-five years. The ancient Egyptians, having acquired some insight in human anatomy from their custom to preserve the bodies of their dead, had a rough concept of blood vessels emerging from the heart and reaching the various organs including the lungs.

It was Galen who in the second century A.D. demonstrated that blood is moving from the right ventricle through the pulmonary artery to the lungs and from there by way of the pulmonary veins to the left side of the heart. Nevertheless he believed, as Vesalius still did fourteen centuries later, that part of the blood seeped through invisible pores in the interventricular septum from the right to the left side of the heart.

The concept of an unidirectional blood flow through the lungs was gradually amplified by others but it was only after the work of Harvey and Malpighi that the interaction of blood flow and respiration became accepted.

Even so, it was a long road to the understanding of the hemodynamic and physiologic principles of the pulmonary circulation and their response to pathologic conditions, and this road has certainly not yet reached its end.

The share the pathologist has had in increasing our knowledge of the pulmonary circulation and the reactions of the pulmonary vasculature, modest as it may be, is not without significance. However, few pathologists are familiar with the various pulmonary vascular lesions and know how to interpret them in terms of hemodynamic alterations or clinical significance. This also applies to the clinician, even though he may be regularly involved with the problems concerning the circulation of the lungs and of pulmonary hypertension in particular.

The aim of this book is to provide a survey of the pulmonary vascular alterations in the various forms of pulmonary hypertension. The publishers have allowed us a liberal use of illustrations. In addition, vignettes with a schematic representation of the lesions, characteristic for each form of pulmonary hypertension, have been placed at the end of the respective chapters. If the simplistic nature of these vignettes is appreciated, they may be of help to the reader as a summary of the essential features.

The clinical, physiologic, and hemodynamic implications have been covered briefly particularly for the benefit of morphologists, since only when related to such data will knowledge of the pathology of the lungs and their blood vessels become meaningful. On the other hand, we hope that this book also will serve its purpose for clinicians and physiologists dealing with the cardiologic and pulmonologic sides of pulmonary hypertension.

We are greatly indebted to those who, by their criticism and help, have contributed to this monograph. In this respect we would like to mention particularly with gratitude Dr. A. S. Groen, Amsterdam, and Dr. H. W. H. Weeda, Leiden, for their comments on some of the chapters. We also gratefully acknowledge the expert photographic assistance of Mr. R. E. Verhoeven, the excellent technical help of Mrs. H. J. Dijk, and the competent secretarial assistance of Mrs. M. de Vries.

Finally we would like to thank the publishers, John Wiley and Sons, New York, for their help and understanding during the production of this book.

C. A. WAGENVOORT, M.D.
NOEKE WAGENVOORT

Contents

PATHOLOGY OF PULMONARY HYPERTENSION

CHAPTER ONE

Normal Circulation
of the Lungs

The lungs possess a double source of blood supply. As part of the systemic circulation, the bronchial or "private" circulation takes care of the nutrition of part of the lung tissue. The pulmonary or "public" circulation, on the other hand, serves the body as a whole, since its primary function is gas exchange.

This gas exchange takes place only in the alveolar capillaries of the lung; but from the right ventricle, serving as a pump, to the pulmonary arteries and veins with their conduction and resistance and various regulatory mechanisms, the whole pulmonary circulation is subservient to this primary function. This does not mean that with respiration the functional possibilities of the lungs are exhausted. It is now known that the lungs, with their strategic location within total body circulation, are involved in a wide variety of metabolic processes and that many substances that occur naturally in the blood are formed, stored, metabolized, or destroyed in the lungs (Fishman and Pietra, 1974). Moreover, the lungs serve as a filter that may intercept some particulate matter from the blood.

The pulmonary circulation is not a "lesser" circulation since it has a blood flow greater than that of any other organ. Also, the pulmonary vasculature in many respects differs from the systemic vasculature, and these differences are recognizable in virtually all segments of the vascular tree.

PULMONARY CIRCULATION

The adult pulmonary circulation is a low resistance-high reserve circulatory system (Edwards, 1957), carrying the whole cardiac output. Under normal circumstances, apart from the first postnatal weeks, the resting pulmonary arterial pressure in man is fairly constant throughout life. It is much lower than in the systemic circulation as the mean pulmonary arterial pressure is in the range of 15 mmHg, while the systolic and diastolic pressures are about 22 and 10 mmHg, respectively (Harris and Heath, 1962).

Measurement of pulmonary arterial pressures has been possible since Cournand and his coworkers (1944) introduced cardiac catheterization, thus making accessible the cavities of the right ventricle and pulmonary artery. The cardiac catheter may be moved up distally in the pulmonary arterial bed until it becomes impacted in a branch. Since this branch must admit the tip of the catheter, the external diameter of which is usually over one millimeter, it must be an elastic pulmonary artery. Pulmonary arterial branches of this size are all of the elastic type (p. 25).

Functionally, pulmonary arteries are "end-arteries," thus the pressure recorded, when the catheter is wedged in this position, gives a rough estimate of the pulmonary venous or left atrial pressure. This pulmonary arterial wedge pressure is of practical value, although its interpretation has given rise to some controversies (Harris and Heath, 1962). Under normal circumstances the wedge pressure in man has been reported to be in the range of 7 to 15 mmHg (Hellems et al., 1949), with about 9 mmHg as an average. If blood samples are taken from the wedged catheter, an oxygen saturation of 100 percent usually is found, indicating that the blood has been drawn from the alveolar capillaries.

In normal individuals there is a variability in resting pulmonary arterial pressures. Therefore, the borderline between a normal and an abnormally elevated pressure is not sharp. Pulmonary hypertension generally is accepted when mean and systolic pulmonary arterial pressures exceed 25 and 30 mmHg, respectively.

Pulmonary arterial pressure depends on the pulmonary blood flow and the resistance within the pulmonary vascular bed. The circulation through the lungs, however, is a complex mechanism, since it is influenced by many factors, particularly by various cardiorespiratory events, and predominantly in a passive way. Obviously, the function of the right ventricle and that of the left atrium have a close bearing on the circulation in the lung.

The effect of respiration is noticeable for instance in the relatively small alterations in pressure and flow during inspiration and expiration. Pulmonary arterial pressure is slightly higher during expiration than during inspiration, as a result of the increased intrathoracic pressure. A deep inspiration may cause a sudden, although transient, increase in the flow through the lungs (Armitage and Arnott, 1949), since the intrathoracic pressure falls while the intra-abdominal pressure rises, so the blood is forced from the abdominal veins.

Blood viscosity potentially influences pulmonary circulation, but normally it is hardly of any significance. If there is an increased hematocrit, it may have some effect on the resistance, but even then this is often only moderate.

In a normal individual, in the upright position, hydrostatic pressure due to gravity causes the flow in the upper parts of the lungs to be less than in the lower parts. At rest the flow in the top of the lung may come close to nil (West and Dollery, 1960).

The pulmonary vessels are not rigid tubes but are distensible, and their distensibility influences the pressure-flow relationship, particularly since we are dealing with a pulsatile system. Arteries with an elastic wall structure, as we will see, are more prominent in the pulmonary than in the systemic circulation, since the elastic structure is retained from the pulmonary trunk down to small vessels of a caliber of one millimeter (p. 25), whereas in the systemic circulation only the walls of the aorta and its largest branches are of the elastic type.

Distensibility of elastic pulmonary arteries is enhanced by their relatively thin walls. During exercise the output of the right ventricle may increase by a factor of two to three. But as a result of the vascular distensibility and also since previously nonfunctioning channels may open up, there is little rise in pulmonary arterial pressure. A high distensibility of the pulmonary arterial system also is suggested by the observation that generally in patients with a congenital pretricuspid shunt, who may have a very large pulmonary blood-flow, pulmonary arterial pressures are only moderately elevated. Similarly, when one lung is surgically removed or one main pulmonary artery is obstructed by a balloon catheter, thus doubling the flow through the other lung, the rise in pressure, if any, is usually disproportionately mild. Conduction and storage of blood are likely to be the main functions of the elastic pulmonary arteries.

Active vasomotor regulation may contribute to the changes in pulmonary vascular resistance. This regulation, in principle, may be of a nervous, chemical, or humoral nature.

Little is known about a nervous regulation of the pulmonary vasculature. By morphologic methods a rich supply of nerve fibers has been demonstrated in the walls and particularly in the adventitia of the large elastic pulmonary arteries and the large pulmonary veins. In animals, at least, these fibers probably stiffen these large vessels, thus influencing the distensibility of the so-called capacitance vessels (Szidon and Fishman, 1969).

Nervous regulation of the pulmonary vascular resistance, although it has been demonstrated (Kadowitz et al., 1974a), is probably of less significance. In the resistance vessels of the lung, nerve fibers are much more difficult to demonstrate than in the larger arteries (Mitchell, 1956).

The resistance vessels are formed by the muscular pulmonary arteries with an external diameter of less than one millimeter, particularly those with a diameter of less than half a millimeter. They have a media consisting of circularly arranged smooth muscle cells. Their function is different from that of the elastic arteries and is closely related to the fact that they have a vascular tone and are capable of active constriction and dilatation.

Such an active vasomotion of pulmonary arteries has long been doubted. Various drugs, active in the systemic circulation, apparently failed to have any effect on the pulmonary circulation. It must, however, be taken into account that normal pressures in the lung circulation are low as compared to those in the systemic circulation and that the variations in pressure under normal circumstances are extremely small. In this situation a considerable change in resistance may result in only very small changes in pressure or flow, which may be difficult to detect.

Now it is clear that active changes in pulmonary vascular resistance do occur, not only in experimental animals but also in man. The most potent pulmonary vasoconstrictive agent known is alveolar hypoxia. How the constriction of the vessels is mediated in the presence of a low oxygen pressure is unknown, although it is likely that there is a direct effect on the smooth muscle cells of the small muscular pulmonary arteries and arterioles. The subject is dealt with more extensively in a discussion of hypoxic pulmonary hypertension in Chapter Eleven.

Conversely, oxygen may produce dilatation of the same vessels. The role of hypoxia on the one hand and oxygen on the other again indicates the close connection between gas exchange and circulatory regulation within the lungs, particularly since it has appeared that both have a local and direct effect on the lung vessels. By the same token, acidosis enhances the vasoconstrictive effect of hypoxia.

Various substances, occurring naturally in the body, have an effect on the pulmonary circulation. A characteristic example, which is also one of the most active substances in this respect, is acetylcholine. Acetylcholine dilates pulmonary arteries and arterioles, particularly in patients with pulmonary hypertension in whom the vascular tone is higher than in normal individuals, so its effect becomes more noticeable (Harris, 1957; Fritts et al., 1958). Its action, however, is transient, since acetylcholine is rapidly destroyed by the lungs. More important is that the dose needed for an appreciable lowering of the pulmonary arterial pressure is so far from the physiologic range that it is doubtful whether the substance is effective in humoral regulation.

Epinephrine, norepinephrine, angiotensin, and bradykinin have no, or at best a dubious or variable, effect on the pulmonary circulation. These and many other substances often act predominantly on the systemic circulation, on the heart, or on ventilation. Therefore an eventual effect on the lung circulation often does not indicate a direct action on the pulmonary vasculature but a change secondary to other hemodynamic or respiratory alterations.

Serotonin or 5-hydroxytryptamine is very effective as a vasoconstrictive agent in experimental animals (Shepherd et al., 1959), but it has little or no effect in man (Harris et al., 1960). Patients with malignant carcinoid of the bowel, who produce large quantities of serotonin, do not develop pulmonary hypertension. In the fully developed carcinoid syndrome, endocardial and valvular changes in the right side of the heart are commonly found, but even then, as we could demonstrate in several cases, there is no appreciable increase in the thickness of the media of muscular pulmonary arteries nor are there other changes of the lung vessels.

Histamine, finally, has produced contradictory results (Storstein et al., 1959; Harris and Heath, 1962; Colebatch, 1970). It has, however, been suggested that it may be locally released by mast cells and that in this way it may mediate hypoxic pulmonary vasoconstriction (Kay et al., 1974).

Prostaglandins have been the subject of much recent investigation. Prostaglandins are fatty acids of which four series have been recognized according to their chemical composition. These are indicated as E, F, A, and B and within each series further identified by a number. They occur in almost all tissues and have a great variety of biological activities. Lung tissue is particularly active in the synthesis, metabolism, and release of prostaglandins, and some of them have a specific effect on the pulmonary circulation. Prostaglandin E_1 is a moderately active vasodilator, while prostaglandins $F_{2\alpha}$ and A_2 are known as vasoconstrictors of the pulmonary vasculature in various animals (Kadowitz et al., 1974b; Kadowitz and Hyman, 1975). The role of the prostaglandins in the regulation of the human pulmonary circulation may well be significant but awaits further clarification.

Many of these naturally occurring agents can be taken up actively by lung tissue, particularly by endothelial cells (Cross et al., 1974; Fishman and Pietra, 1974), to be subsequently metabolized and destroyed even during a single passage through the lung circulation (Junod, 1972; Nicholas et al., 1974).

It also has been shown that these substances when injected in the bronchial circulation may reach, either by way of vasa vasorum or by diffusion, the pulmonary vessels and thus influence their vascular tone (Hyman et al., 1975).

From this very condensed and incomplete survey, it may appear that the evidence for a humoral regulation of the human pulmonary circulation is still fragmentary. So far there is no firm basis for the assumption that the part played by humoral factors in this regulation is a predominant one.

Chemical substances that do not occur naturally in the body, such as various drugs, may also affect the pulmonary vasculature. In most instances, however, this effect is small or variable and often results from an indirect action of the substances on the lung vessels.

Tolazoline (Priscoline) has been reported to bring about a fall in pulmonary arterial pressure and an increase of flow in patients with various forms of pulmonary hypertension (Dresdale et al., 1951, 1954).

The same effect has been attributed to isoproterenol (Kaufman et al., 1951) and to aminophylline, although this dilates systemic arteries and veins as well (Aviado, 1965). For a more detailed discussion of the action of these and other drugs, the reader is referred to the work of Aviado since it does not fall within the scope of the present book.

BRONCHIAL CIRCULATION

The bronchial circulation contributes to the blood supply of the lungs but under normal circumstances its consequences for the hemodynamics of the pulmonary circulation are very limited. The flow through the bronchial arteries, insofar as it brings blood to the lungs, represents approximately one percent of the cardiac output. The pressure in these arteries depends on the pressure in the aorta from which they arise, directly or indirectly.

Bronchopulmonary arterial anastomoses do occur but in the normal individual their functional significance is probably limited (p. 48). Bronchopulmonary venous anastomoses, on the other hand, have a more important function (p. 20).

Under pathologic conditions, such as severe obstruction to the blood flow through the pulmonary arteries and particularly in bronchiectasis, the bronchial circulation may increase considerably and even may have a distinct effect on pulmonary circulatory hemodynamics which may contribute to pulmonary hypertension (Liebow et al., 1949). We will discuss this in Chapter Twelve.

PERINATAL PULMONARY CIRCULATION

Pulmonary circulation in fetal life differs essentially from that in the postnatal period. In the fetus the source of oxygen is the placenta. From the placenta oxygenated blood is directed by the ductus venosus and the inferior vena cava to the right atrium. From here the greater part of the blood passes through the patent foramen ovale to the left atrium and from there to the left ventricle and the aorta. A much smaller portion of the blood from the inferior vena cava and almost all the blood from the superior vena cava enters the right ventricle and the pulmonary artery (Lind and Wegelius, 1954). But since most of this blood flows through the patent ductus arteriosus to the aorta, only 10 to 15 percent of the right ventricular stroke volume streams through the lungs (Rudolph, 1970).

Since the left ventricle receives blood that is considerably better oxygenated than that entering the right ventricle, the blood supplied to the fetal coronary and cerebral arteries has a higher oxygen pressure than that supplying the lower part of the body. Distal from the ductus arteriosus the aorta will contain a mixture of left and right ventricular blood.

The diversion of blood flow through the ductus arteriosus is enhanced by the high resistance in the lung vessels. This finds its morphologic expression in the thick media and the narrow lumen of the muscular pulmonary arteries and arterioles (p. 38), which resemble systemic arteries. Also, the walls of right and left ventricles have approximately the same thickness. The pressure in the pulmonary artery equals that in the aorta and the elastic configuration of the wall of the pulmonary trunk resembles that of the aorta (p. 23). The fetal pulmonary veins, on the other hand, are thin-walled.

At the time of birth there is a complete change in the type of circulation. The supply from the placenta stops and oxygenation of the blood is taken over by the lungs. When the lungs expand following the first respiratory movements of the thorax, the pulmonary arteries and arterioles dilate as a consequence of the pull provided by the distending lung tissue combined with the effect of the alveolar surface tension.

It has been demonstrated in fetal lambs (Dawes et al., 1953a) that the fall in vascular resistance in the lungs follows immediately, within a few minutes, after birth. Although this fall in resistance may be less dramatic in the human infant (Adams and Lind, 1957), the morphologic picture of the pulmonary arteries initially does not reflect any decrease of resistance at all. In newborns dying within the first 3 days of life, the pulmonary arteries have narrow lumina and a medial thickness in the same range as in the stillborn infant (Wagenvoort et al., 1961). In this very early period of postnatal life the lungs have a marked tendency to collapse completely, after having been removed from the thorax, and possibly, since the outward pulling effect of the lung tissue is lost, the arteries resume their preventilation state.

Soon after, and particularly during the first 6 weeks of life, the lumina of the arteries and arterioles become rapidly wider while the media becomes thinner (p. 38).

In principle, the fetal and early postnatal pulmonary vessels react essentially in the same way as those in the adult. They respond, however, more vigorously to various stimuli, which may well be related to the relatively greater amount of smooth muscle in their pulmonary vascular walls. Vasoconstriction of fetal pulmonary arteries in response to hypoxia and hypercapnia has been demonstrated repeatedly (Cassin et al., 1964; Campbell et al., 1967). The effect of various vasoactive substances on fetal pulmonary arteries in principle is also very much like that in the adult. It must be borne in mind that inactivation of these substances in the newborn is probably considerably less than in the adult (Friedli et al., 1973).

The postnatal fall in pulmonary vascular resistance is accompanied by the closure of the ductus arteriosus, so that eventually the whole right ventricular output flows through the lungs. Due to this pronounced increase in pulmonary blood flow and consequent increase of the pulmonary venous return, there is a rise in left atrial pressure leading to closure of the foramen ovale (Dawes et al., 1953b).

Closure of the ductus arteriosus is presumably brought about mainly by contraction of the thick and irregularly arranged bundles of smooth muscle tissue in its wall. In the human newborn this happens usually within 12 hours (Moss et al., 1963) but physiologic patency of the ductus arteriosus may remain demonstrable for up to 3 days after birth (Harris and Heath, 1962). Oxygen-saturated blood thus may shunt to the pulmonary circulation during this period.

The functional closure of the ductus is followed much later by anatomic closure with obliteration of the lumen. In the majority of the cases the ductus is obliterated within 4 weeks after birth but in some cases the process may take several months (Mitchell, 1957).

REFERENCES

Adams, F. H., and Lind, J.: Physiologic studies on the cardiovascular status of normal newborn infants (with special reference to the ductus arteriosus). *Pediatrics* **19**: 431, 1957.

Armitage, G. H., and Arnott, W. M.: Effect of voluntary hyperpnoea on pulmonary blood flow. *J. Physiol.* **109**: 64, 1949.

Aviado, D. M.: *The Lung Circulation.* Pergamon Press, Oxford, 1965, vol. 2, p. 595.

Campbell, A. G. M., Dawes, G. S., and Milligan, J. E.: Neural control of pulmonary circulation in the fetal lamb as studied by a cross-circulation technique. *Circulation* **34** (suppl. 2): 80, 1967.

Cassin, S., Dawes, G. S., Mott, J. S., Ross, B. B., and Strang, L. B.: The vascular resistance of the foetal and newly ventilated lung of the lamb. *J. Physiol.* **171**: 61, 1964.

Colebatch, H. J. H.: Adrenergic mechanisms in the effects of histamine in the pulmonary circulation of the cat. *Circulation Res.* **26**, 379, 1970.

Cournand, A., Lauson, H. D., Bloomfield, R. A., Breed, E. S., and Baldwin, E. deF.: Recording of right heart pressures in man. *Proc. Soc. Exper. Biol. Med.* **55**: 34, 1944.

Cross, S. A. M., Alabaster, V. A., Bakhle, Y. S., and Vane, J. R.: Sites of uptake of ^{3}H-5-hydroxytryptamine in rat isolated lung. *Histochemistry* **39**: 83, 1974.

Dawes, G. S., Mott, J. C., Widdicombe, J. G., and Wyatt, D. G.: Changes in the lungs of the new-born lamb. *J. Physiol.* **121**: 141, 1953a.

Dawes, G. S., Milne, E. D. F., Mott, J. C., and Widdicombe, J. G.: The closure of the foramen ovale after birth. *J. Physiol.* **122**: 38P, 1953b.

Dresdale, D. T., Schultz, M., and Michtom, R. J.: Primary pulmonary hypertension. I. Clinical and hemodynamic study. *Amer. J. Med.* **11**: 686, 1951.

Dresdale, D. T., Michton, R. J., and Schultz, M.: Recent studies in primary pulmonary hypertension including pharmacodynamic observations on pulmonary vascular resistance. *Bull. N. Y. Acad. Med.* **30**: 195, 1954.

Edwards, J. E.: Functional pathology of the pulmonary vascular tree in congenital cardiac disease. *Circulation* **15**:164, 1957.

Fishman, A. P., and Pietra, G. G.: Handling of bioactive materials by the lung. *New Engl. J. Med.* **291**: 884, 953, 1974.

Friedli, B., Kent, G., and Olley, P. M.: Inactivation of bradykinin in the pulmonary vascular bed in newborn and fetal lambs. *Circulation Res.* **33**: 421, 1973.

Fritts, H. W., Harris, P., Clauss, R. H., Odell, J. E., and Cournand, A.: The effect of acetylcholine on the human pulmonary circulation under normal and hypoxic conditions. *J. Clin. Invest.* **37**: 99, 1958.

Harris, P.: Influence of acetylcholine on the pulmonary arterial pressure. *Brit. Heart J.* **29**: 272, 1957.

Harris, P., Fritts, H. W., and Cournand, A.: Some circulatory effect of 5-hydroxytryptamine in man. *Circulation* **21**: 1134, 1960.

Harris, P., and Heath, D.: *The Human Pulmonary Circulation. Its Form and Function in Health and Disease.* E. & S. Livingstone Ltd., Edinburgh and London, 1962.

Hellems, H. K., Haynes, F. W., and Dexter, L.: Pulmonary "capillary" pressure in man. *J. Appl. Physiol.* **2**: 24, 1949.

Hyman, A. L., Knight, D. S., Joiner, P. D., and Kadowitz, P. J.: Bronchopulmonary arterial shunting without anatomic anastomosis in the dog. *Circulation Res.* **37**: 285, 1975.

Junod, A. F.: Uptake, metabolism and efflux of ^{14}C-5-hydroxytryptamine in isolated perfused rat lungs. *J. Pharmacol. Exp. Ther.* **183**: 341, 1972.

Kadowitz, P. J., Joiner, P. D., and Hyman, A. L.: Effect of sympathetic nerve stimulation on pulmonary vascular resistance in the intact spontaneously breathing dog. *Proc. Soc. Exper. Biol. Med.* **147**: 68, 1974a.

Kadowitz, P. J., Joiner, P. D., and Hyman, A. L.: Effects of prostaglandins E_1 and $F_{2\alpha}$ on the swine pulmonary circulation. *Proc. Soc. Exp. Biol. Med.* **145**: 53, 1974b.

Kadowitz, P. J., and Hyman, A. L.: Differential effects of prostaglandins A_1 and A_2 on pulmonary vascular resistance in the dog. *Proc. Soc. Exp. Biol. Med.* **149**: 282, 1975.

Kaufman, J., Iglauer, A., and Herwitz, G. K.: Effect of Isuprel (isopropylepinephrine) on circulation of normal man. *Amer. J. Med.* **11**: 442, 1951.

Kay, J. M., Waymire, J. C., and Grover, R. F.: Lung mast cell hyperplasia and pulmonary histamine-forming capacity in hypoxic rats. *Amer. J. Physiol.* **226**: 178, 1974.

Liebow, A. A., Hales, M. R., and Lindskog, G. E.: Enlargement of the bronchial arteries and their anastomoses with the pulmonary arteries in bronchiectasis. *Amer. J. Path.* **25**: 211, 1949.

Lind, J., and Wegelius, C.: Human fetal circulation: changes in the cardiovascular system at birth and disturbances in the postnatal closure of the foramen ovale and ductus arteriosus. *Cold Spring Harbor Symposia on Quantitative Biology* **19**: 109, 1954.

Mitchell, G. A. G.: *Cardiovascular Innervation.* E. & S. Livingstone, London and Edinburgh, 1956, p. 229.

Mitchell, S. C.: The ductus arteriosus in the neonatal period. *J. Pediatrics* **51**: 12, 1957.

Moss, A. J., Emmanouilides, G., and Duffie, E. R.: Closure of the ductus arteriosus in the newborn infant. *Pediatrics* **32**: 25, 1963.

Nicholas, T. E., Strum, J. M., Angelo, L. S., and Junod, A. F.: Site and mechanism of uptake of ^{3}H-/-norepinephrine by isolated perfused rat lungs. *Circulation Res.* **35**: 670, 1974.

Rudolph, A. M.: The changes in the circulation after birth. Their importance in congenital heart disease. *Circulation* **41**: 343, 1970.

Shepherd, J. T., Donald, D. E., Linder, E., and Swan, H. J. C.: Effect of small doses of 5-hydroxytryptamine (serotonin) on pulmonary circulation in the closed-chest dog. *Amer. J. Physiol.* **197**: 963, 1959.

Storstein, O., Cudkowicz, L., and Attwood, H. D.: Effect of histamine on the pulmonary circulation in dogs. *Circulation Res.* **7**: 360, 1959.

Szidon, J. P., and Fishman, A. P.: Autonomic control of the pulmonary circulation. In A. P. Fishman and H. Hecht (eds.), *Pulmonary Circulation and Interstitial Space.* University of Chicago Press, Chicago, 1969, p. 239.

Wagenvoort, C. A., Neufeld, H. N., and Edwards, J. E.: The structure of the pulmonary arterial tree in fetal and early postnatal life. *Lab. Invest.* **10**: 751, 1961.

West, J. B., and Dollery, C. T.: Distribution of blood flow and ventilation-perfusion ratio in the lung, measured with radioactive CO_2. *J. Appl. Physiol.* **15**: 405, 1960.

CHAPTER TWO

Pulmonary Hypertension: General Remarks

Pulmonary hypertension is considered to be present when at rest the systolic-diastolic pressure in the pulmonary artery exceeds 30/15 mmHg or when the mean pressure exceeds 25 mmHg. It is clear, however, that since the upper limits of normal pressures are not strictly defined, the same is true for the lowest pressures at which the term pulmonary hypertension is applicable.

In principle, pulmonary hypertension could result from an increased pulmonary vascular resistance or from an increased pulmonary flow. But as we have seen (p. 3), an increased pulmonary blood flow alone, even if it is very high, does not usually lead to more than a mild elevation of the pressure as long as there are no vascular alterations. The pulmonary vessels will dilate, causing the resistance to fall. Due to the high distensibility of the pulmonary vasculature, a large flow can be accommodated by the vessels of the lung without a marked rise in pressure.

Following pneumonectomy, when the flow to the remaining lung is doubled, the pressure is hardly raised as long as the pulmonary vasculature in this lung is normal. It has been shown that up to 60 percent of the total lung tissue may be removed in experimental animals without significant elevation of pulmonary arterial pressures. If more lung tissue is resected, pulmonary hypertension, which over the years may gradually abate, becomes manifest (Carlson et al., 1951; Harrison et al., 1957).

If, after resection of lung tissue, the maximal distensibility of the remaining vessels is approached or if the distensibility of the vascular bed is impaired by vascular lesions, increase of pulmonary flow, as for instance during exercise, may cause a severe increase in the pulmonary arterial pressure.

Pulmonary hypertension usually is due either to an increased resistance in the pre-capillary vessels or to an impediment to the pulmonary venous outflow. Changes in the pulmonary arteries and arterioles leading to increased resistance may be either functional or organic. Functional changes based on vasoconstriction are seen, for instance, in hypoxic pulmonary hypertension. Examples of organic changes are occlusive thromboemboli and obliterative intimal fibrosis as observed in congenital heart disease with a shunt (Edwards, 1957).

For the effect of various pulmonary vasoconstrictive and vasodilatory agents we may refer to what has been discussed in Chapter One. It may be added here that an eventual effect of these agents is usually more marked in patients with pulmonary hypertension than in normal individuals. If, however, vascular changes have progressed to a degree in which they have become largely irreversible and in which the vessels have lost their reactivity, the effect as a rule abates or disappears (Harvey et al., 1971).

In some conditions, pulmonary arterial pressures may become very high and may equal those in the systemic circulation. If there is a congenital cardiac shunt, the direction of the shunt may become reversed. The wedge pressure in these cases is unaffected. When there is pulmonary venous hypertension, as in mitral stenosis, the left atrial pressure and the wedge pressure are increased. The pulmonary arterial pressure rises proportionally with the wedge pressure until the latter has attained a value in the range of 25 mmHg. Thereafter, in some cases the pulmonary arterial pressure rises disproportionally, while the rise in wedge pressure lags far behind (Dexter et al., 1950; Harris and Heath, 1962).

In the presence of pulmonary hypertension, the right ventricle is exposed to an increased pressure load. This will result in right ventricular hypertrophy or eventually in right cardiac failure.

The elevated pressure has its effect not only on the right side of the heart but also on the pulmonary vasculature, causing the development of vascular alterations. Conversely, pulmonary vascular lesions may, by narrowing or obstructing the lumen of the vessels, bring about an increase of vascular resistance and pressure. Although in many instances it is impossible to decide how exactly the increase of pressure started, it is clear that there is often a circulus vitiosus in which pulmonary hypertension causes vascular lesions, which in turn result in further elevation of pressure.

Although it has been claimed (East, 1940; McKeown, 1952) that the pulmonary vasculature may be normal in the presence of pulmonary hypertension, in our experience the muscular coat of the pulmonary arteries and/or arterioles is always thickened when there is a significant elevation of pulmonary arterial pressure. Even when an increased medial thickness is not immediately apparent in the histologic sections, morphometric appraisal (p. 31) will reveal that the pulmonary arteries are abnormal.

In some conditions with pulmonary hypertension, the severity of the pulmonary vascular lesions is roughly proportional to the degree of elevation of pressure in the pulmonary circulation (p. 200), although there are exceptions to this rule. On the other hand, it must be realized that pronounced vascular alteration and particularly intimal fibrosis based on organization of thrombi, may occur, for instance, in patients with tetralogy of Fallot, in whom the pulmonary arterial pressures are normal or even subnormal (Wagenvoort et al., 1964).

There is a wide variation in conditions associated with pulmonary hypertension. Some of these conditions, although they may be very different in nature, have a similar effect on the hemodynamics of the pulmonary circulation and lead to the same form of pulmonary vascular disease. Other conditions with their own type of hemodynamic disturbance are associated with other patterns of pulmonary vascular lesions.

Since it appears that the pattern of pulmonary vascular disease is more or less characteristic for the form of pulmonary hypertension and thus for a certain group of diseases a classification can be made (Wagenvoort, 1973; 1974). The pathologist, in examining lung tissue derived from autopsy or lung biopsy and in studying the vessels therein, may identify the form of pulmonary hypertension, the type of hemodynamic disturbance, and thus the underlying disease or group of underlying diseases.

Such a statement cannot be made without certain reservations. The expression "group of underlying diseases" already indicates a certain limitation. As we have just seen, conditions vastly different in nature may produce the same form of pulmonary vascular disease.

One example may suffice here. A frequent form of pulmonary hypertension, associated with a characteristic pattern of vascular lesions, is based on an impeded outflow of the pulmonary venous blood (Chapter Nine). This may be caused not only by rheumatic mitral stenosis or incompetence of the mitral valve but also by chronic left ventricular failure, a left atrial myxoma, or an inflammatory process in the mediastinum obstructing the major pulmonary veins. While these underlying diseases are totally different, they all have the same hemodynamic effect on the pulmonary circulation—they produce the same type of pulmonary venous hypertension and the same pattern of lesions in the lung and in the pulmonary vasculature. All one can say from a study of the lung vessels in these instances is that there is obstruction of the pulmonary venous outflow.

A technical limitation may be the amount of the lung tissue available for study. Many vascular lesions in the lung tend to be diffuse or so widespread that they usually can be recognized in a single histologic section. Others are scattered over the lung tissue and can be missed easily if the examination is limited to one or two blocks of lung tissue. If, at autopsy, whole lungs are available, it is preferable to study at least four blocks of each lung.

In examining lung biopsies the risk of the histologic section not being representative is of course much greater, since it will contain only a limited number of lung vessels. It may be helpful to study various sections at different levels within the biopsy. Even so, interpretation of the histologic findings should be done with caution.

There are other pitfalls in the study of the pulmonary vasculature and several will be discussed in the appropriate chapters. Two more may be mentioned here. In the early stages of pulmonary hypertension the pattern may be incomplete. It is even likely that in some instances it takes considerable time before the pattern is fully developed. Sometimes this may hamper an adequate classification. The implications, however, will be discussed later.

Another problem may arise when more than one pattern of pulmonary vascular disease is present in the same patient. For instance, this may happen when a patient with a ventricular septal defect develops chronic left ventricular failure or when mitral stenosis is combined with chronic pulmonary thromboembolism. In these more complicated cases, much experience in the interpretation of the pulmonary vascular lesions is necessary, and sometimes even then one may fail to arrive at a correct conclusion.

On the whole, however, it can be said that the study of the pulmonary vasculature in cases of pulmonary hypertension may be carried out with much profit when the pathologist is aware of the various causes of pulmonary hypertension and of the accompanying patterns of pulmonary vascular lesions.

CAUSES OF PULMONARY HYPERTENSION

In cases of pulmonary hypertension there is usually an underlying condition, such as cardiac disease, responsible for the elevated pressure in the pulmonary circulation. Such a condition is considered the cause of the pulmonary hypertension because it induces changes in the hemodynamics of the pulmonary circulation which clearly result in increased pressures. Even though we classify a case like this as pulmonary hypertension of known cause, this generally does not mean that we understand the mechanisms by which the pulmonary hypertension is produced. To the contrary, in most cases the actual mechanism is obscure or speculative.

Much more rare are cases in which the cause of the pulmonary hypertension is unknown. Some patients develop pulmonary hypertension in the absence of any associated condition that can be held responsible. Occasionally, there is an associated condition, but it is not clear why this should lead to pulmonary hypertension. The cause in such cases may be suspected but at best is usually doubtful.

It is obvious from the above survey of causes that it is not possible to arrive at a clear-cut etiologic classification of pulmonary hypertension. The best approach may be to form a number of broad etiologic groups by bringing together those conditions that produce elevated pressure in the pulmonary circulation by similar hemodynamic principles, resulting in the same pattern of pulmonary vascular lesions. Here we will refer briefly to these groups, which will be discussed more extensively in the following chapters.

Patients with *congenital heart disease with a shunt* between systemic and pulmonary circulations are likely to develop pulmonary hypertension when the shunt is large enough and when there is no concomitant pulmonic stenosis to protect the lung vessels. The risk to the pulmonary circulation is not the same, however, in the various types of shunts.

If there is a left-to-right shunt at the level of the atria, as in the various forms of atrial septal defect, or if there is an anomalous pulmonary venous drainage to the right atrium, the pulmonary blood flow will be increased considerably. This, as we have seen before (p. 3), usually does not lead to pulmonary hypertension since the lung vessels to a very marked degree are adaptable to this increased flow. It appears, however, that sometimes between the ages 15 and 20, but much more often at ages around 40, a certain number of patients with atrial septal defects may develop pulmonary hypertension. In this group of so-called pretricuspid shunts (Harris and Heath, 1962), pulmonary hypertension is a late phenomenon, if it occurs at all. This is in contrast to those congenital cardiovascular defects in which a large flow is shunted to the pulmonary circulation from an area where a systemic arterial pressure prevails. A large ventricular septal defect, a widely patent ductus arteriosus, a truncus arteriosus persistens, or a communication between aorta and pulmonary trunk are the most common examples of these post-tricuspid shunts.

In these instances there is generally pulmonary hypertension from birth, and changes in the pulmonary arteries and arterioles are usually present very soon after birth. These changes therefore tend to become severe at a much earlier period of life, with all the consequences this may have for the pulmonary circulation and the right side of the heart (Harris and Heath, 1962).

Post-tricuspid shunts are sometimes acquired in later life. Perforation of a ventricular septum as a result of myocardial infarction or rupture of an aneurysm of the ascending aorta in the pulmonary trunk may cause pulmonary hypertension and in principle the same pattern of pulmonary vascular alterations. Advanced alterations in the lung vessels under these circumstances are uncommon, however, since a patient will rarely survive such disastrous events long enough to permit their development.

In all patients with large cardiac shunts who develop pulmonary hypertension, the pulmonary vascular alterations are in principle the same, irrespective of whether the shunt was pre- or post-tricuspid, congenital, or acquired in later life. The pattern of these lesions, for reasons to be discussed later (p. 85), has been termed "plexogenic pulmonary arteriopathy."

In the rare cases of *cirrhosis of the liver associated with pulmonary hypertension* and in so-called *unexplained plexogenic pulmonary arteriopathy* or primary pulmonary hypertension, the changes in the pulmonary vasculature are essentially the same as in cardiac disease with a shunt. In the first group the cirrhosis of the liver has been suspected to be the cause of the elevated pulmonary arterial pressure, although it is not clear how this is brought about. In the second condition, the cause of the pulmonary hypertension is completely obscure. Many possibilities have been suggested. These will be reviewed in the discussion of this subject in Chapter Seven.

Pulmonary thromboembolism is a common disease, but sustained *embolic pulmonary hypertension* is fairly rare. It may be appropriate to discuss it immediately following unexplained or primary pulmonary hypertension, since the two have often been confused and clinically may be indistinguishable from each other. Moreover, there are some forms of nonthrombotic embolism that may give rise to pulmonary hypertension, although such cases are very uncommon except for schistosomiasis.

In a great proportion of all patients with pulmonary hypertension, there is obstruction to the pulmonary venous outflow. The cause of *pulmonary venous hypertension* is almost always to be found in the left side of the heart, with mitral valve disease as the most common cardiac lesion. Cardiac diseases that cause pulmonary venous hypertension include mitral stenosis, usually of rheumatic origin, sometimes on a congenital basis, and mitral incompetence due to rheumatic disease or to bacterial endocarditis or eventually as part of congenital cardiac malformations. In these instances, left atrial pressure always will be raised.

It appears, however, that also in patients with previous myocardial infarction or healed myocarditis (Heath et al., 1957) and furthermore in patients with aortic stenosis or aortic incompetence (Smith et al., 1954), there are very often distinct pulmonary vascular alterations, even if cardiac catheterization showed that patients exhibited no pulmonary hypertension at rest. It must be assumed that in these cases there is a significant increase of pulmonary arterial pressure during exercise, and that this intermittent elevation of pressure in the long run has a similar effect as a sustained pulmonary hypertension.

Left atrial myxoma's may simulate rheumatic mitral stenosis by obstructing the mitral orifice and causing pulmonary hypertension.

Uncommonly the cause of pulmonary venous hypertension rests outside the heart. Compression of major pulmonary veins by processes in the mediastinum or hilar region with subsequent pulmonary hypertension are reported occasionally (Edwards and Burchell, 1951; Inkley and Abbott, 1961; Yacoub and Thompson, 1971).

In all these conditions the pulmonary venous pressure is elevated and, unless the obstruction is at pulmonary venous level, the left atrial pressure is elevated as well. It is understandable that this will cause a proportional rise in alveolar capillary and in pulmonary arterial pressure in order to guarantee an adequate blood flow through the lungs. When there is pronounced and sustained pulmonary venous hypertension it appears, however, that the pressure in the pulmonary artery rises disproportionally and may even become very high. The mechanisms involved are obscure. The various hypotheses regarding this phenomenon will be discussed in Chapter Nine.

The pulmonary vascular changes in pulmonary venous hypertension are essentially the same, irrespective of the underlying disease. They differ from those in other forms of pulmonary hypertension notably because pulmonary veins as well as pulmonary arteries are affected.

Pulmonary veno-occlusive disease is a rare condition characterized by fibrous obstruction of pulmonary veins and particularly of pulmonary venules. The cause is unknown, although it is suspected that infection, particularly viral, may be responsible for its development. It is questionable, however, whether the cause is always the same in various patients.

An important cause for pulmonary hypertension and one that has attracted much interest is hypoxia. *Hypoxic pulmonary hypertension* may be found in patients with lung diseases such as chronic bronchitis and obstruction of airways and also in individuals living at high altitudes where, as a result of low barometric pressures, hypoxia prevails.

From this it is clear that sometimes in patients with *lung diseases* hypoxia may play an important part in the production of the associated pulmonary hypertension. On the other hand, hypoxia is certainly not the only factor responsible for an increased pulmonary arterial pressure in these instances. Fibrosis with destruction of alveolar capillaries, concomitant intravascular thrombosis and other mechanisms, have to be taken into account. Therefore, this heterogeneous group of diseases will be discussed in Chapter Twelve.

Rarely *malformations of the pulmonary vasculature* are responsible for pulmonary hypertension. Also very uncommon is *postoperative pulmonary hypertension* following palliative or corrective surgery in tetralogy of Fallot or other forms of congenital cardiac disease, which are not primarily associated with pulmonary hypertension.

For an insight into the causes of pulmonary hypertension and into the way they affect the pulmonary vasculature, it obviously is of importance to observe what happens when the cause is removed. The tendency for *regression of pulmonary vascular lesions* under these circumstances has been demonstrated. This reversibility of vascular changes is discussed in Chapter Fifteen.

Various forms of pulmonary hypertension can be produced experimentally in animals. In this way our knowledge of the effect of *experimental pulmonary hypertension* on the pulmonary vasculature has increased considerably. It must be realized, however, that the pulmonary vasculature differs greatly in various species and that in most animal species the relative thickness of the vascular wall of the pulmonary arteries is much greater than in humans. Even in those animals, such as the dog and the pig, in which the lung vessels resemble those in man, there is reason to believe that their reaction to abnormal hemodynamic circumstances differs from that in patients with similar conditions. The results of these experiments have been discussed in the relevant chapters dealing with the various forms of pulmonary hypertension.

VARIABILITY

The same cause for pulmonary hypertension may be present in various individuals, even to the same extent, and yet the degree of elevation of pressure and of pulmonary vascular disease may be widely different. In some residents of high altitudes the response to hypoxia is much more pronounced than in others living in the same area, and the lung vessels exhibit marked changes in some, while they are normal in others.

Sometimes, a patient with a fairly large ventricular septal defect may have no more than mild pulmonary hypertension, while another patient with a smaller defect has much more elevated pressures and more severe vascular lesions.

This variability suggests that the mechanisms underlying pulmonary hypertension are complicated, and that more than one, and probably multiple factors, are involved in its development.

Grover et al. (1963) described a species variability with regard to pulmonary vascular reactivity. This is particularly observed in chronic hypoxia. Cattle are prone to develop pulmonary hypertension at high altitudes, whereas sheep are little sensitive to such conditions. Grover used the terms hyperreactors and hyporeactors for these categories.

Variability according to race is not with any certainty known in man. As far as we know, there is no race particularly susceptible to the development of pulmonary hypertension nor does it appear that any race is exempt. It has been suggested that some races of cattle are more susceptible to chronic hypoxia (chronic mountain disease) than others (Astrup et al., 1968).

An individual variability also has been observed in cattle (Grover et al., 1963). Some animals, under similar circumstances, react with much greater elevation of pulmonary arterial pressure than others. It is likely that such an individual reactivity of the pulmonary vascular bed may also play an important part in the development of pulmonary hypertension in other animals and in man. Individual variability, as Grover has pointed out, occurs with regard to every biologic system and every type of stimulus. It seems likely, however, that this variability is particularly great when the reactivity of lung vessels is concerned.

There is strong evidence that individual reactivity in cattle is genetically determined since it could be shown that the trend to hyperreactivity, respectively to hyporeactivity, could be transmitted to progeny for at least three generations (Weir et al., 1974). In man this could be an important factor in the rare familial occurrence of primary pulmonary hypertension (p. 121).

Variability according to sex is evident in several forms of pulmonary hypertension in the human. The most striking example is primary pulmonary hypertension in which there is marked female preponderance. This, however, is limited to adults. In children the sex ratio is equal (p. 121).

In young female rats, hypoxia induced pulmonary vascular changes. On the other hand in old male rats hypoxia had no effect on the pulmonary arteries (Kay and

Smith, 1973). The factor, or factors, responsible for these sex differences are unknown.

Variability according to blood groups was recently suggested by Daoud and Reeves (1973). They found that the pulmonary arterial pressure response to hypoxia was particularly great in individuals with blood group A. They also thought it significant that the original residents of the high altitude area in the Andes have predominantly blood group O.

REFERENCES

Astrup, T., Glas, P., and Kok, P.: Lung fibrinolytic activity and bovine high mountain disease. *Proc. Soc. Exper. Biol. & Med.* **127**: 373, 1968.

Carlson, R. F., Charbon, B. C., Charbon, H. G. A., and Adams, W. E.: The effect of decreasing the amount of lung tissue on the right ventricular pressures in animals. *J. Thorac. Surg.* **21**: 621, 1951.

Daoud, F. S., and Reeves, J. T.: Increased hypoxic pulmonary pressor response in patients with blood type A. *Circulation* suppl. IV, 134, 1973.

Dexter, L., Dow, J. W., Haynes, F. W., Whittenberger, J. L., Ferris, B. G., Goodale, W. T., and Hellems, H. K.: Studies of the pulmonary circulation in man at rest. Normal variations and the interrelations between increased pulmonary blood flow, elevated pulmonary arterial pressure, and high pulmonary "capillary" pressures. *J. Clin. Invest.* **29**: 602, 1950.

East, T.: Pulmonary hypertension. *Brit. Heart J.* **2**: 189, 1940.

Edwards, J. E.: Functional pathology of the pulmonary vascular tree in congenital cardiac disease. *Circulation* **15**: 164, 1957.

Edwards, J. E., and Burchell, H. B.: Multilobar pulmonary venous obstruction with pulmonary hypertension. *Arch. Int. Med.* **87**: 372, 1951.

Grover, R. F., Vogel, J. H. K., Averill, K. H., and Blount, S. G.: Pulmonary hypertension. Individual and species variability relative to vascular reactivity. *Amer. Heart J.* **66**: 1, 1963.

Harris, P., and Heath, D.: *The Human Pulmonary Circulation: Its Form and Function in Health and Disease.* E. & S. Livingstone, Ltd., Edinburgh and London, 1962.

Harrison, R. W., Adams, W. E., Beuhler, W., and Long, E. T.: Effects of acute and chronic reduction of lung volumes on cardiopulmonary reserve. *Arch. Surg.* **75**: 546, 1957.

Harvey, R. M., Enson, Y., and Ferrer, M. I.: A reconsideration of the origins of pulmonary hypertension. *Chest* **59**: 82, 1971.

Heath, D., Cox, E. V., and Harris-Jones, J. N.: The clinico-pathological syndrome produced by co-existing pulmonary arterial and venous hypertension. *Thorax* **12**: 321, 1957.

Inkley, S. R. and Abbott, G. R.: Unilateral pulmonary arteriosclerosis. *Arch. Int. Med.* **108**: 903, 1961.

Kay, J. M., and Smith, P.: The small pulmonary arteries in rats at simulated high altitude. *Path. & Microbiol.* **39**: 270, 1973.

McKeown, F.: The pathology of pulmonary heart disease. *Brit. Heart J.* **14**: 25, 1952.

Smith, R. C., Burchell, H. B., and Edwards, J. E.: Pathology of the pulmonary vascular tree. IV. Structural changes in the pulmonary vessels in chronic left ventricular failure. *Circulation* **10**: 801, 1954.

Wagenvoort, C. A., Heath, D., and Edwards, J. E.: *The Pathology of the Pulmonary Vasculature.* Charles C Thomas, Springfield, Ill., 1964.

Wagenvoort, C. A.: Classifying pulmonary vascular disease. *Chest* **64**: 503, 1973.

Wagenvoort, C. A.: Classification of pulmonary vascular lesions in congenital and acquired heart disease. *Adv. Cardiol.* **11**: 48, 1974.

Weir, E. K., Tucker, A., Reeves, J. T., Will, D. H., and Grover, R. F.: The genetic factor influencing pulmonary hypertension in cattle at high altitude. *Cardiovasc. Res.* **8**: 745, 1974.

Yacoub, M. H., and Thompson, V. C.: Chronic idiopathic pulmonary hilar fibrosis. *Thorax* **26**: 365, 1971.

CHAPTER THREE

Normal Pulmonary and Bronchial Vasculature

Knowledge of the structure of the normal lung vessels is a prerequisite for the study of the pulmonary vasculature in cases of pulmonary hypertension.

The lung, with its pulmonary and bronchial circulations, has a more complex vasculature than most other organs. There are structural differences not only between arteries and veins but also between pulmonary and bronchial vessels and, particularly in the pulmonary arterial tree, between vessels of larger and smaller caliber. Moreover, age is shaping the walls of the lung vessels, and thus the same type of vessel may be markedly different in an infant, a young adult, or an old individual.

DEVELOPMENT

The primitive truncus arteriosus is partitioned by a truncus septum, which eventually becomes continuous with the ventricular septum in such a way that the ostium of the aorta is in contact with the left, and the ostium of the pulmonary trunk with the right ventricle.

It has usually been accepted that the truncus septum grows distally and with torsion so that it is responsible not only for the formation of ascending aorta and pulmonary trunk but also for the spiral course of both vessels. This view has recently been challenged by Asami (1969) and Los (1976). Los believes that the truncus septum partitions only the origins of the large vessels and that ascending aorta and pulmonary trunk are derivatives of aortic arches. The fourth aortic arches were shown by him to grow downward in front of the sixth aortic arches, together with a septum aortico-pulmonale which becomes continuous with the truncus septum. In this way ascending aorta and pulmonary trunk are formed by the aortic arches. The torsion of these arteries results from an asymmetrical outgrowth of the aortic arches.

17

In any case, the sixth aortic arches will be continuous with the pulmonary trunk. A branch from either sixth aortic arch represents the right and left main pulmonary artery respectively. The dorsal part of the right sixth arch disappears along with the right dorsal aorta. The corresponding part of the left sixth aortic arch persists during fetal life as the ductus arteriosus. The branches of both sixth arches, representing the later main pulmonary arteries, grow into the lung buds and connect with the plexus of vessels within these buds (Congdon, 1922; Barry, 1951).

A single pulmonary vein grows from the dorsal wall of the left atrium immediately to the left of the septum primum. This vein and four of its branches expand to form the spatium pulmonale which initially is connected with the left atrium by a rather narrow opening. When at a later stage this opening widens, the spatium pulmonale becomes incorporated into the left atrium, constituting the larger part of it.

The four branches of the primitive pulmonary veins extend by a process of dichotomization in the direction of the lung buds. Here they form the proximal pulmonary veins either by making contact with the splanchnic venous plexus or by forming a plexus by itself (Los, 1969).

Little is known about the development of the bronchial arteries and veins. They probably represent splanchnic segmental vessels cranial to the coelomic cavity (Camarri and Marini, 1965; Hamilton et al., 1972).

COURSE

The pulmonary circulation conducts the blood from the right cardiac ventricle through the lungs to the left atrium. The pulmonary trunk arises from the infundibular portion of the right ventricle. Its orifice here is circular and provided with the pulmonary valve. Corresponding to the three cusps of this valve there is a slight dilatation of the initial portion of the trunk, its sinus.

The origin of the pulmonary trunk is situated in front of the aortic orifice, although slightly more cranial and to the left. The trunk runs obliquely upward to the left and dorsal over a distance of approximately 4.5 cm and divides, just under the aortic arch, in the right and left main pulmonary arteries.

The course of the left main pulmonary artery is more or less in line with that of the pulmonary trunk, that is, in cranio-dorsal direction and to the left. It runs ventral to the thoracic aorta and the left main bronchus and reaches the hilus of the left lung after arching over the angle formed by the main bronchus and the upper lobe bronchus.

The inside of the left pulmonary artery usually shows a small scar at the site of the original orifice of the ductus arteriosus, of which the remnant can be recognized in the ligamentum arteriosum between the left pulmonary artery and the aorta.

In contrast to the left pulmonary artery, the right main pulmonary artery makes a right angle with the pulmonary trunk. It runs horizontally to the right, dorsal to the aorta, and in front of the right main bronchus to the hilus of the right lung.

On entering the hilus of the lung, the main pulmonary arteries divide respectively into the lobar arteries and segmental arteries. There is such a great deal of variation in the number and course of these arteries and in the extent of the areas supplied by them (Frodl, 1951, Cory and Valentine, 1959), that there is hardly a "normal" pattern. Usually there are either one or two lobar arteries to each lobe but sometimes a single lobe is supplied by multiple arteries. The segmental arteries very often are not confined to one segment but supply adjacent areas of other segments.

The lobar and segmental arteries and their branches generally accompany the corresponding bronchi. This close association remains clearly recognizable until the respiratory bronchioles divide into the alveolar ducts. By that time the pulmonary arterioles gradually dissolve in the alveolar capillary network.

In addition, there are many, usually small, branches that do not follow the bronchial tree but are perpendicular to the main branches. These so-called supernumerary branches (Elliott and Reid, 1965) will be discussed later (p. 29).

In a postmortem arteriogram of the normal adult lung the caliber of the arteries tapers down gradually. The more peripheral branches provide a rather dense background filling (Figure 3-1).

From the alveolar and pleural capillary networks, the blood is drained by the

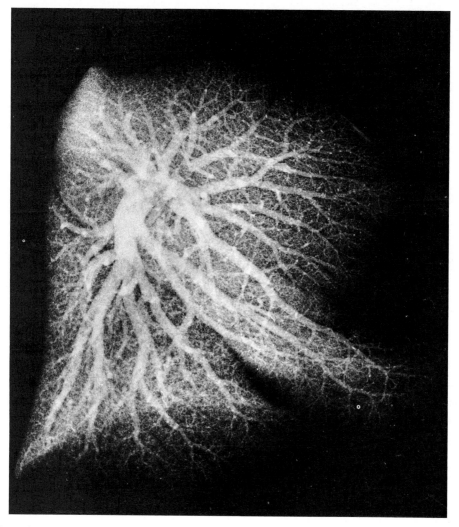

Figure 3-1.   Postmortem arteriogram of a normal lung in a 22-year-old man. The caliber of the pulmonary arteries tapers down gradually. There is a rather dense background filling.

pulmonary venules. These unite to form pulmonary veins that follow a course along the interlobular fibrous septa. While accepting successive tributary veins, the caliber increases, so that finally one lobar pulmonary vein drains each lobe.

Although in the course and pattern of the lobar veins, just as in that of the lobar arteries, there is much variation, usually two large pulmonary venous trunks emerge at the hilus of each lung. The superior pulmonary veins carry the blood from the upper lobes and, on the right side, from the middle lobe as well. The inferior pulmonary veins drain the lower lobes. These large pulmonary veins run a short course before entering the upper part of the left atrium. The orifices of the inferior veins lie somewhat more posteriorly and caudally to those of the superior veins. Neither in their course nor at their orifice do they possess valves.

The bronchial arteries may show a great variety in their number, their origin, and in their extrapulmonary course as well. Usually, there are two bronchial arteries on the left side and one on the right (Miller, 1947; Von Hayek, 1953). Exceptions to this rule, however, are numerous and two arteries (Tobin, 1952) or a single artery on each side (Lauweryns, 1962) occur commonly. Other variations in numbers have been demonstrated, for instance one left and four right bronchial arteries (Lauweryns, 1962).

The origin of the left bronchial artery or arteries, as a rule, is from the thoracic aorta. That of the right bronchial artery or arteries is more variable. The origin may be from the aorta or from one of the intercostal arteries but it may also arise from others such as the subclavian artery.

Clearly, the extrapulmonary course depends on the origin and thus varies greatly. On the left side, however, there is usually a straight course from the ventral side of the aorta to the left main bronchus. In most instances, the course of the right bronchial arteries is through the mediastinum, dorsal or ventral to the esophagus, to the right main bronchus.

The bronchial arteries then follow the bronchi. On their way to the hilus of the lungs, they provide branches supplying the mediastinum, esophagus, lymph nodes, and the walls of pulmonary arteries. In the hilus they form a richly anastomosing network from where several branches supply the mediastinal pleura. The true bronchial arteries accompany the bronchi and their divisions within the lung, supplying the walls of these bronchi. Their course is somewhat tortuous and often spiral. The larger bronchi usually contain two to three bronchial arteries, apart from very small branches, in their walls.

The drainage by way of the bronchial veins has been divided by Marchand et al. (1950) into a peripheral and a central system. Small radicles, beginning in the walls of terminal bronchioles, unite to form bronchial veins. These form plexuses around the bronchi. The bronchial veins, up to the level of approximately the third order bronchi, have wide anastomosing connections with the pulmonary veins and drain their blood via the latter vessels to the left atrium.

The central or pleurohilar veins drain the blood from the largest bronchi and from a part of the pleura. They form a plexus in the hilar area. From here the blood is conducted via various systemic veins to the right atrium.

STRUCTURE OF PULMONARY VASCULATURE

Pulmonary Trunk and Main Arteries

The pulmonary trunk is comparable in size to the aorta but its wall is thinner (Figure 3-2). On the average the thickness of the media is only approximately half or slightly over half that of the aorta (Figure 3-3).

Also the structure of the wall is different. The aorta is the characteristic example of an elastic artery with a regular and dense arrangement of parallel elastic laminae, alternating with scarce collagen fibers and smooth muscle cells in its media.

In pulmonary trunk and main pulmonary arteries, there is in principle a similar structural pattern but the elastic laminae are usually interrupted and fragmented. The individual fibers are irregular with alternating thick and slender portions (Heath et al., 1959). The spaces between the elastic fibers, which are much wider than in the aorta, contain acid mucopolysaccharides and a varying, but usually marked, amount of collagenous fibers (Figure 3-4).

This configuration of elastic tissue is a reflection of the relatively low pressure in the pulmonary circulation. When the pulmonary arterial pressure remains high after birth, as in some cases of congenital cardiac disease, there is a much denser pattern of elastic fibers in the media of the pulmonary trunk, so that this vessel resembles the aorta (Heath et al., 1959).

Although this is a general rule, it is good to realize that there is a great variation in the elastic pattern of the pulmonary trunk. In some individuals the elastic fibers in its wall are exceedingly scarce (Figure 3-5), but there are others, and such cases are not at all uncommon, in whom the elastic configuration of the pulmonary trunk closely resembles that of the aorta (Figure 3-6).

The intima in children and young adults is very thin and consists of a single layer of endothelial cells overlying the inner elastic membrane (Figure 3-7).

Vasa vasorum supplying the walls of the pulmonary trunk and main arteries are

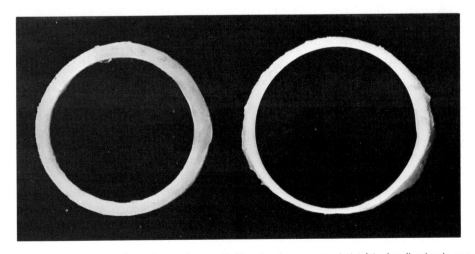

Figure 3-2.   Transverse slices of normal aorta (*left*) and pulmonary trunk (*right*) after fixation in normally expanded state, in a 58-year-old woman. The vessels have approximately the same caliber but the wall of the pulmonary trunk is thinner than that of the aorta (×1.7).

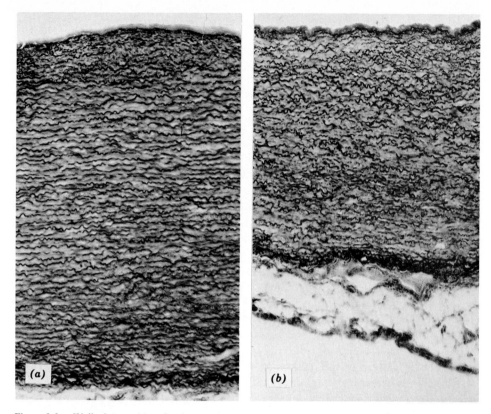

Figure 3-3.   Wall of aorta (*a*) and pulmonary trunk (*b*) from the same patient as Figure 3-2. The thickness of the wall of the pulmonary trunk is approximately 60 percent of that of the aorta (El.v.G., ×55).

derived from coronary, bronchial, and other systemic arteries (Parke, 1970). Their branches can be observed in the outer third of the media. They penetrate regularly down to the middle of the media (Tobin, 1960) and even further (Figure 3-8). The venous drainage takes place to some extent to the coronary sinus system but mainly to extracardiac veins (Parke, 1970).

Age Changes

With increasing age the capacity of the pulmonary trunk increases considerably (Meyer et al., 1957). In its wall, elastic tissue tends to diminish and to be replaced by collagen. Its content of calcium, although low as compared to that of the aorta, also increases (Gray et al., 1953) as does its content of total fat (Hevelke, 1965).

The most conspicuous age changes are observed in the intima. Some degree of intimal fibrosis is common in adults (Figure 3-9). It tends to increase with age. Patches of atheroma in the form of yellow streaks are common in individuals over the age of 40 years (Brenner, 1935). Often this is only obvious on close inspection, since these patches are generally small and little elevated so that they can be easily overlooked. Usually they are found near branching points, either at the bifurcation or at the sites of ramification of large branches (Figure 3-10).

In contrast to aortic atherosclerosis, pulmonary atherosclerosis of more than mild severity is rare, unless there is pulmonary hypertension or hypercholesterolemia.

Heath and his coworkers (1960) have stressed the importance of elevated pressure for its development. The histologic features of pulmonary arterial atherosclerotic plaques are essentially the same as of those in systemic arteries.

Obviously the structural composition of the arterial wall has an important bearing upon its mechanical properties. These have been studied either by using whole specimens of pulmonary trunk and main arteries (Meyer et al., 1957; Kolb and Hägele, 1968), or circumferential strips of the pulmonary trunk (Harris et al., 1965).

The extensibility of the pulmonary trunk is greater than that of the aorta. It decreases, however, with advancing age (Meyer et al., 1957; Harris et al., 1965), probably as a result of the change in structural composition with the increase of collagen. In these preparations the eventual role of the smooth muscle cells is neglected, although these may well influence the wall stiffness of the pulmonary artery (Patel et al., 1959).

Perinatal Period

In the fetus and newborn the pulmonary trunk and the aorta resemble each other both in size and in medial thickness (Figure 3-11). Also, the elastic configuration is identical and characterized by a regular and dense pattern of parallel elastic laminae (Figure 3-12).

Under normal circumstances, after birth there is a gradual change in the pulmonary artery from the "aortic type" of elastic configuration to an "adult type."

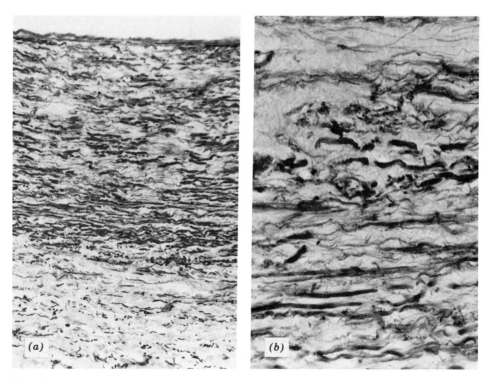

Figure 3-4. (a) Wall of normal pulmonary trunk in a 5-year-old boy. The elastic membranes are interrupted and fragmented (El.v.G., ×140). (b) Detail from same wall. The elastic fibers are plump, irregular, and widely separated by collagen (El.v.G., ×350).

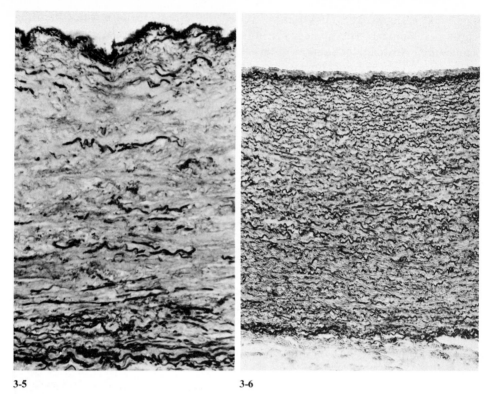

3-5   3-6

Figure 3-5. Wall of normal pulmonary trunk in a 60-year-old woman. Elastic fibers are exceedingly scarce (El.v.G., ×140).

Figure 3-6. Wall of normal pulmonary trunk in a 48-year-old woman. Dense configuration of elastic membranes, resembling that of the aorta (El.v.G., ×55).

This means that gradually the elastic laminae become swollen, disrupted, and fragmented. This process may become apparent at the age of 4 months and may be completed after 2 years (Heath et al., 1959).

Particularly after the age of one year, elastic tissue disappears rapidly from the pulmonary trunk along with a slight increase of collagen (Farrar et al., 1965). Also, the thickness of the wall of the pulmonary trunk in its relation to that of the aorta decreases during the first year of life to its normal ratio of roughly 60 percent.

"Glomus Pulmonale"

Chemoreceptors sensitive to alterations of the composition of the blood are known to occur along large systemic arteries in the form of carotid and aortic glomera. In 1960 a glomus was described by Krahl in the adventitia of the posterior wall of the pulmonary trunk. This glomus was supposed to be vascularized by a small branch from the pulmonary trunk, in which case it would function as a chemoreceptor to pulmonary arterial blood.

Since then it has been shown (Becker, 1966) that such a branch may be present occasionally in fetuses of rabbits and man but that it is always absent or obliterated after birth. The so-called glomus pulmonale is supplied by a branch from the left coronary artery and is thus to be regarded as one of the coronary glomera and not as a chemoreceptor for the pulmonary circulation.

Elastic Pulmonary Arteries

Within the lung the branches of the main arteries after successive ramification gradually decrease in caliber and in thickness of the wall. Their structure, however, remains of the elastic type down to a caliber of approximately one millimeter. The elastic laminae, in principle, remain regular and intact (Figure 3-13). The peculiar disordered configuration with extensive disruption of elastic fibers, characteristic of the pulmonary trunk and main arteries, is not present in the intrapulmonary elastic arteries.

The transition from elastic to muscular type of pulmonary artery (Figure 3-14) takes place at a caliber between 1000 and 500 μ. In this range the elastic arteries gradually lose their elastic tissue, whereby the elastic laminae within the media disappear more and more with the exception of internal and external elastic laminae.

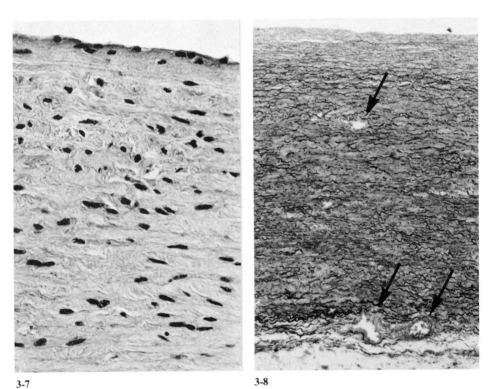

3-7   3-8

Figure 3-7. Wall of normal pulmonary trunk in a 5-year-old boy. The intima consists of a single layer of endothelial cells (H. and E., ×350).

Figure 3-8. Wall of normal pulmonary trunk in a 58-year-old woman. Vasa vasorum (arrows) in adventitia and penetrating over halfway into the media (El.v.G., ×55).

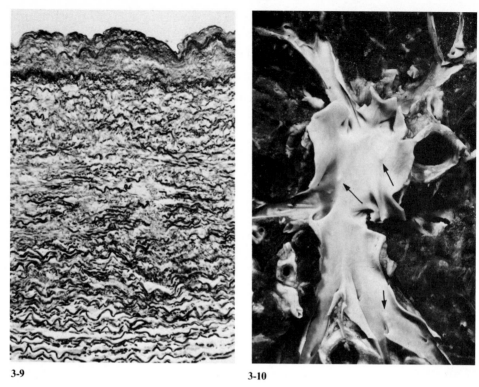

3-9   **3-10**

Figure 3-9. Wall of normal pulmonary trunk in a 61-year-old woman. There is a fairly thin layer of intimal fibrosis (El.v.G., ×140).

Figure 3-10. Normal main pulmonary arteries cut open from hilum, in a 46-year-old woman. Small, insignificant patches of atheroma (arrows) can be seen particularly at the sites of ramification.

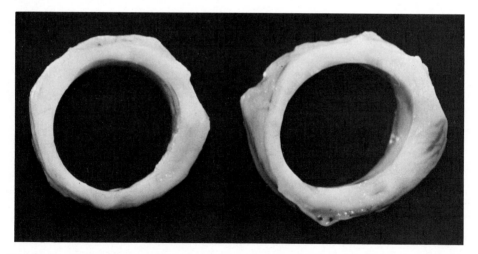

Figure 3-11. Transverse slices of normal aorta (*left*) and pulmonary trunk (*right*) in a newborn female infant. The vessels have approximately the same caliber and wall thickness (×7).

26

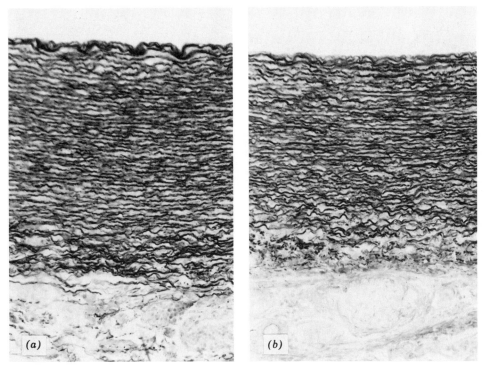

Figure 3-12. Wall of aorta (*a*) and pulmonary trunk (*b*) from the same infant as Figure 3-11. The wall of the pulmonary trunk has an identical elastic configuration as that of the aorta (El.v.G., ×140).

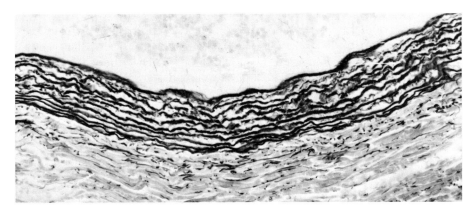

Figure 3-13. Normal elastic pulmonary artery in a 20-year-old man. Note the regular pattern of intact elastic laminae (El.v.G., ×230).

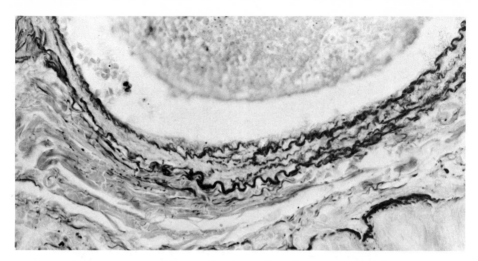

Figure 3-14. Pulmonary artery of the transitional type of a caliber of approximately 600 μ in a 5-year-old boy. In some areas incomplete elastic laminae are recognizable within the media (El.v.G., ×230).

Age Changes

In old age the structure of the elastic pulmonary arteries does not change significantly although there is occasional interruption of the laminae, while some intimal fibrosis of the patchy excentric type may occur. Atheromatous patches are confined to the lobar and segmental pulmonary arteries. In smaller elastic arteries they are not found in normal individuals.

Perinatal Period

The number of elastic pulmonary arteries in the fetal and neonatal lung is relatively low. Ferencz (1967) assumes that the number increases during further development.

The structure of these arteries is essentially the same as in the adult, but the transition to muscular pulmonary arteries takes place at a smaller caliber range. Pulmonary arteries with a regular configuration of elastic laminae may be observed in the newborn at an external vascular diameter of 150 μ or less.

A peculiar feature of the neonatal elastic pulmonary arteries, which has drawn little attention, is intimal proliferation. It forms a loose layer of intimal cells (Figure 3-15). This layer, rarely thicker than 20 μ, is continuous over long stretches and not confined to sites of ramification. It is observed in approximately 30 percent of newborn infants without cardiovascular disease. We have observed it even in premature stillborn infants. Its incidence decreases sharply after the age of 6 months. After the age of one year not even remnants of this proliferative process can be found. There is no clue as to its significance.

Muscular Pulmonary Arteries and Arterioles

Pulmonary arteries of an external diameter between 500 μ and approximately 70 μ are of the muscular type. At a caliber between 1000 and 500 μ, as we have seen, the wall shows a transition from elastic to muscular structure.

Muscular pulmonary arteries and arterioles form an important part of the pulmonary vasculature, since it has become clear that their tone plays a role in regulating resistance and pressure in the pulmonary circulation. Normally, when the pressure is low and the thickness of the muscular layer is thin, the effect of various stimuli, like certain drugs, is small and sometimes remains undetectable. This may account for the contradictory results of many workers in this field with regard to their vasoactivity (p. 3).

When under abnormal circumstances, as in pulmonary hypertension, the pressure is high and the pulmonary arterial media thick, the vasoconstrictive and vasodilatative effects of the agents can be distinctly demonstrated (p. 10).

In principle, the muscular pulmonary arteries follow the bronchi and bronchioli, ramifying in the same way. They diminish in caliber, however, more rapidly than the bronchi they accompany. At a peripheral level the diameter of the arterial branches is therefore much smaller, as compared to that of the adjacent bronchioles, than when they accompany larger bronchi (Miller, 1947).

In addition to these conventional branches, there are however numerous small arteries that do not follow the bronchial tree. These so-called supernumerary branches (Elliott and Reid, 1965) arise from elastic or large muscular pulmonary arteries perpendicularly or somewhat obliquely and supply adjacent lobules (Figure 3-16). Although often they do not show up on an angiogram, possibly due to their right angles of origin, Elliott and Reid (1965) state that they outnumber the conventional branches particularly in the periphery of the lung. Their structure is the same as that of the "ordinary" muscular pulmonary arteries. These branches have also been termed "abrupt" (Robertson, 1967) and "monopodial" (Cumming et al., 1969).

Therefore, since branching of the pulmonary arterial tree is not consistently dichotomous but rather asymmetrical, Singhal et al. (1973) proposed to number the orders of the branches from the periphery upward, rather than numbering orders or generations downward (Weibel, 1963). Assessed in this way, diameter and length of branches of successive orders taper down gradually to the periphery (Singhal et al., 1973).

The media of a muscular pulmonary artery consists of smooth muscle fibers with a circular of near-circular orientation (Figure 3-17). Between the individual muscle

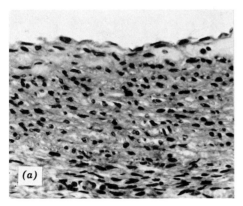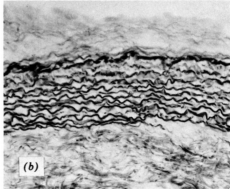

Figure 3-15. Elastic pulmonary artery in a male infant aged 7 days. There is a loose layer of intimal proliferation (*a*: H. and E., *b*: El.v.G., ×230).

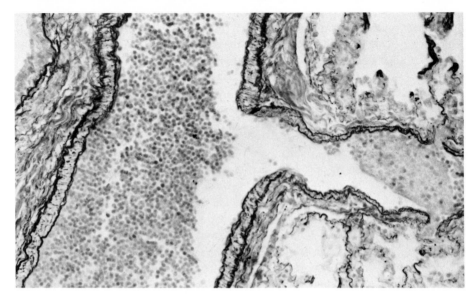

Figure 3-16. A supernumerary artery arising perpendicularly from a large muscular pulmonary artery and supplying adjacent lobules of lung tissue in a 4-year-old girl (El.v.G., ×230).

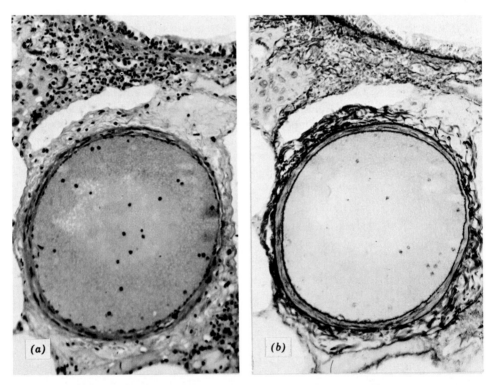

Figure 3-17. Normal muscular pulmonary artery with a thin media and wide lumen in an 18-year-old man (*a*: H. and E., *b*: El.v.G., ×140).

fibers there are only scarce collagen and reticulin fibers. These may be difficult to recognize in a histologic section but show up clearly in electron-microscopic preparations (Figure 3-18). The media is bounded by distinct external and internal elastic laminae. In systemic arteries the internal elastic lamina is present but the external is usually incomplete or absent.

As compared to systemic arteries of the muscular type, the pulmonary arteries have a thin wall, particularly a thin muscular media and a wide lumen (Figure 3-17). The differences in vascular resistance and pressure are thus reflected.

Generally the media-diameter ratio is fairly constant so that the medial thickness can be predicted when the diameter is known (Elliott and Reid, 1965). Even so it is often striking that in lungs of normal individuals, occasional muscular pulmonary arteries have thick walls, even up to 20 or 25 percent. The number of these thick-walled vessels is usually so small that the mean medial thickness is not significantly affected. These arteries give the impression of being constricted, also by the pronounced crenation of their internal elastic lamina (Figure 3-19). This suggests that the functional state of the lung vessels is not necessarily the same in all areas of the lung at a given time.

The question can be raised as to how far vasoconstriction, as functional change of the artery, is recognizable in histologic specimens after death of the individual or of the tissue. From experiments in which pulmonary arterial vasoconstriction has been induced in rats (Wagenvoort et al., 1974) and rabbits (Van Zandwijk et al., 1976), it is clear that contraction of arteries may remain demonstrable (Figure 3-20) even if fixation of the lung tissue was delayed for several hours.

The medial thickness usually is assessed morphometrically by expressing its value as a percentage of the external diameter. When this is done for a large number of arteries, the mean medial thickness of normal individuals generally appears to range from 3 to 7 percent of their external diameter, with the great majority between 4 and 6 percent. Values in excess of 7 percent are encountered uncommonly, and then it is questionable whether such values can be considered normal.

Granston (1958) applied this method to muscular pulmonary arteries of all calibers and described a relative medial thickness varying from 3 to 8 percent with an average of 4 percent. Heath and Best (1958) found the ratio to be 4.2 to 5.8 percent for arteries less than 100 μ in external diameter. In the larger arteries the variation was somewhat greater: 2.8 to 6.8 percent.

In our own studies (Wagenvoort and Wagenvoort, 1965) based on lungs of 63 normal individuals, we found a range from 3.5 to 8.2 percent with an average of 5.1 percent. This is somewhat higher than the result of an earlier series: 2.9 to 4.8 percent, average 4.3 percent (Wagenvoort, 1960), but here the pulmonary arteries were injected under controlled pressure, which obviously caused some dilatation. When high injection pressures are used, the results of morphometry sometimes may be affected significantly but not always predictably.

We did not find differences between males and females, nor between left and right lungs or between various parts of the same lung. We could not confirm the finding of Heath and Best (1958) that the pulmonary arteries in the lingula were more thick-walled than elsewhere. Simons and Reid (1969) as well found no differences between upper and lower lobes, even though in the lower parts of the lung the blood flow is considerably greater than in the upper lobes (West and Dollery, 1960).

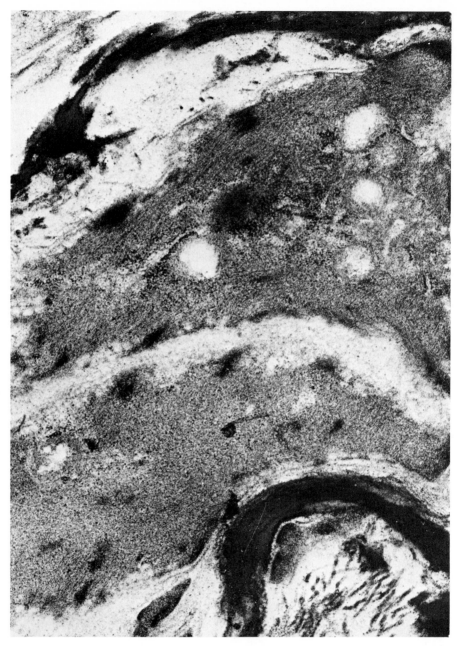

Figure 3-18. Electronmicrograph of media of normal muscular pulmonary artery in a 53-year-old man. The media is bounded by the crenated external (bottom) and internal (top) elastic laminae. Two smooth muscle cells, recognizable by fibrillar structure of cytoplasm and by multiple fusiform densities, are separated by a tissue space containing reticulin fibers. Some collagen fibers are present between the muscle and the internal elastic lamina and also in the adventitia (bottom) ($\times 37,000$).

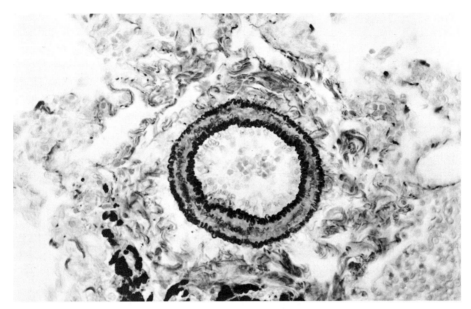

Figure 3-19. Normal muscular pulmonary artery with a thick media, probably in contracted state, from the same case as that of Figure 3-17. Such thick-walled arteries are normally very scarce (El.v.G., ×350).

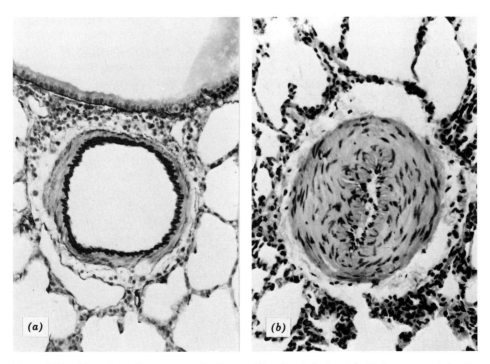

Figure 3-20. Muscular pulmonary arteries in a rabbit after inducing left-sided vasoconstriction by mechanical injury to the left main pulmonary artery. All arteries in the right lung (a) are normal, those in the left lung (b) are almost all severely constricted (a: El.v.G., b: H. and E., ×230).

When the caliber of the pulmonary arteries decreases to an external diameter in the range of 70 μ, they lose their muscular coat. This does not happen abruptly and that explains the difficulty of defining a pulmonary arteriole. The loss of the muscular coat is gradual in that there is a transition of an arterial segment with a single, although complete, layer of smooth muscle cells to a nonmuscular vessel (Figure 3-21). In between, there is a segment in which the muscle fibers have a spiral course in such a way that muscularized segments alternate with segments without a muscular media, but this sequence is usually not recognizable in a single histologic section. Thus the diameter at which the transition takes place has a great range.

Definitions based on absence of muscular coat (Wade and Ball, 1957), size, for instance below 100 μ (Brenner, 1935), or topography, that is, lying in alveolar walls and not accompanying bronchioles (O'Neal et al., 1957) are unsatisfactory. An artery with a discontinuous and incomplete media (Vandendorpe, 1936; Von Hayek, 1953) or, in other words, an artery with a complete media in its beginning and none in its remaining course (Edwards, 1957), indicates more correctly the transitional segment. Unless serial sections are available, the exact identification of such pulmonary arterioles remains difficult.

When a pulmonary arteriole has lost its smooth muscle tissue, its wall consists of a single elastic membrane as continuation of the external elastic lamina and a layer of endothelial cells. When pulmonary arterioles are no longer accompanied by bronchioles, they cannot be safely distinguished in histologic sections from pulmonary venules, unless they are traced in serial sections to recognizable vessels of larger caliber.

The intima of normal muscular pulmonary arteries and arterioles is composed of a single layer of endothelial cells. Electron microscopy reveals that these cells rest on a thin basement membrane (Figure 3-22). Sometimes collagen fibers are interspersed between the basement membrane and the internal elastic lamina.

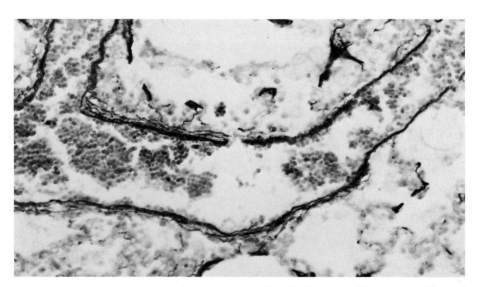

Figure 3-21. Normal pulmonary arteriole in a 4-year-old girl. Segments with a recognizable media alternate with nonmuscularized areas (El.v.G., ×230).

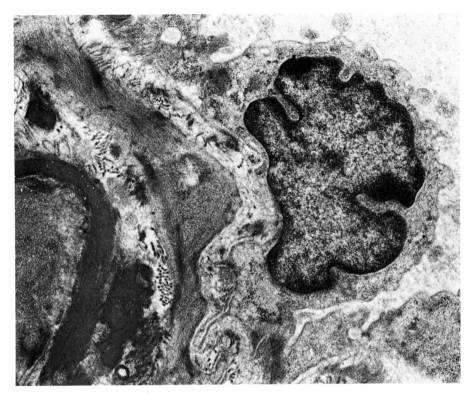

Figure 3-22.   Electronmicrograph of intima of normal muscular pulmonary artery in a 53-year-old man. The endothelium (with one nucleus) rests on a thin basement membrane. Between this membrane and the internal elastic lamina (left) there is deposition of collagen and reticulin fibers and one cell with the characteristics of a smooth muscle cell. This intimal thickening is an age change (×18,000).

The adventitia of the muscular pulmonary arteries, consisting of more or less dense collagen and elastic fibers, varies greatly in thickness. In larger arteries it may be twice or three times as thick as the media; in smaller branches its thickness may be less than half that of the media.

Vasa vasorum, formed by branches of the bronchial arteries, may supply the larger muscular pulmonary arteries, but they supply only the adventitia and do not penetrate into the media.

Age Changes

Age changes affect the media of muscular pulmonary arteries only to a limited extent. Apart from the first year of life (p. 38), the average medial thickness remains remarkably constant during life. In old individuals the medial thickness is often unequal throughout the circumference of an arterial cross-section (Wagenvoort and Wagenvoort, 1965), while the elastic laminae are often coarse and irregular (Figure 3-23).

Simons and Reid (1969) and Semmens (1970) found an increase in medial thickness after the age of 65, but it is very likely that their results were influenced by their

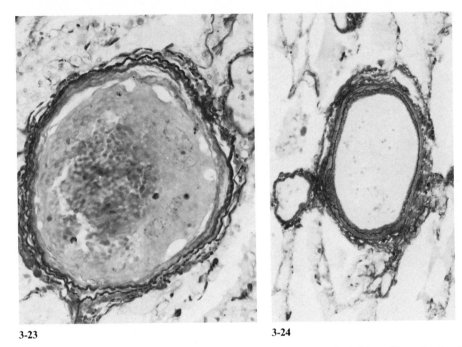

3-23   3-24

Figure 3-23.   Muscular pulmonary artery in a 60-year-old man. The media is thin and irregular. In addition there is minimal intimal fibrosis (El.v.G., ×230).

Figure 3-24.   Muscular pulmonary artery in a 20-year-old man. Minimal intimal fibrosis must be regarded as an age change (El.v.G., ×90).

technique. In both studies measurements were made after injection of the pulmonary arterial tree. The arterial branches of young individuals will yield more to the injection pressure with subsequent thinning of the media than will those of older individuals because arterial branches stiffen with age as a result of intimal fibrosis.

The effect of age on the intima is much more marked than on the media. Intimal fibrosis, as a rule, is absent in children and adolescents, although thin layers (Figure 3-24) or small patches are occasionally observed. The number of these patches increases gradually after the age of 20. When the intimal thickness is measured in a large number of arteries and expressed as a percentage of their internal diameter, the mean intimal thickness in the age group of 20 to 40 years is usually in the range of 2 to 6 percent. In older individuals this degree of intimal fibrosis rises sharply (Brenner, 1935) and may reach values of between 8 and 20 percent and occasionally over 25 percent, although there is considerable individual variation (Figure 3-25) (Wagenvoort and Wagenvoort, 1965).

This senile form of intimal fibrosis is patchy and irregularly distributed. The patches are usually cushion-like or crescent-shaped, and this appearance suggests that it is brought about by organization of thrombi—a view also held by Delarue et al. (1958). The incidence of intimal fibrosis is higher in the apex than in the lower parts of the lungs. We believe that this may be related to the low flow in the apex, which may influence the tendency to thrombosis in periods of lung infections or other diseases.

Pulmonary arterioles in old individuals often show a thick concentric layer of acellular fibrosis which may proceed to complete hyalinization of the wall (Figure 3-26).

Auerbach et al. (1963) described thickening of the pulmonary arterial and arteriolar walls with increasing age, without specifically indicating the contributions of media or intima to this increased thickness. They found even thicker walls in smokers than in nonsmokers. The occurrence of longitudinal muscle bundles in intimal thickening of normal muscular pulmonary arteries has been claimed, particularly in old individuals and in smokers (Naeye and Dellinger, 1971). Semmens (1970) did not find such longitudinal muscle in the intima, and we also could not confirm this.

These remarks apply to the arrangement of smooth muscle cells in the intima, recognizable under the light microscope. Electron-microscopic studies reveal that all or most of the cells in these age-related intimal fibrotic plaques have the characteristics of smooth muscle cells (Figure 3-22), although their arrangement is haphazard and their identification is not possible with light microscopy.

It is important to be aware of incidence and form of the age-related intimal fibrosis that occurs independent of elevated pulmonary arterial pressure when studying cases of pulmonary hypertension, in which intimal fibrosis may have an entirely different significance.

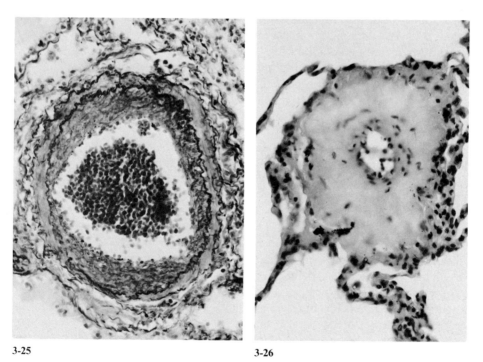

3-25   3-26

Figure 3-25. Muscular pulmonary artery in a 48-year-old man, with pronounced intimal fibrosis as an age change (El.v.G., ×230).

Figure 3-26. Pulmonary arteriole in a 75-year-old woman with complete hyalinization of its wall as an age change. Tracing the vessel in serial sections was necessary for identification as an arteriole (H. and E., ×230).

Perinatal Period

The perinatal age is a period of marked change in the pulmonary circulation (p. 6). This change affects all vessels of the lung but particularly the muscular pulmonary arteries and arterioles.

During fetal life there is a constant remodelling and increase of these vessels, a process which continues long after birth (Reid, 1967). At the time of birth the number of muscular pulmonary arteries and arterioles is small and so is their caliber. In the first few months of life their number increases rapidly along with the multiplication of alveoli (Davies and Reid, 1970).

This is also borne out in postmortem arteriograms. There is very little background filling in an arteriogram made of a fetal or neonatal lung (Figure 3-27), as compared to that in older children or adults (Figure 3-1). This indicates that the small arterioles are fewer in number and also so narrow that the contrast medium does not penetrate in the peripheral vasculature.

The branching pattern of the fetal pulmonary arteries has been described by Hislop and Reid (1972). They were able to demonstrate that supernumerary arteries (p. 29) were present before birth, as early as 12 weeks' gestation.

In early fetal life the media of the muscular pulmonary arteries has essentially the same structure as in the neonatal period and, as a matter of fact, in adult life, although this is not always easily apparent. There is a muscular media between two elastic laminae, but the latter are extremely thin and difficult to demonstrate in an elastic stain. Also, the muscle fibers are immature and pale. The size of individual muscle fibers remains constant during fetal life (Naeye, 1966).

During the entire gestational period, the lumen of the muscular pulmonary arteries is narrow, while their media is thick. The medial thickness expressed as a percentage of the external diameter remains constant. In fetuses of 20 weeks' gestational age (Figure 3-28) and in newborn infants (Figure 3-29), it is in the range of 15 to 25 percent (Wagenvoort et al., 1961).

The total amount of arterial muscle tissue, however, increases during fetal life. This has been demonstrated by calculating the surface area of medial muscle per square centimeter of lung parenchyma (Wagenvoort et al., 1961). Similar results were obtained by comparing the area of the media with that of the intima (Naeye, 1961). This increase in arterial muscle, which is not based on increasing medial thickness, is clearly an expression of growth and multiplication of arterial branches. Also in fetal lambs it has been shown that there is an increase in the number of resistance vessels while the medial thickness remains constant (Levin et al., 1976).

Civin and Edwards (1951) demonstrated the transition from the thick-walled, narrow prenatal pulmonary arteries to the thin-walled, wide arteries, occurring in postnatal life. This was confirmed by many subsequent studies (Dammann and Ferencz, 1956; Rosen et al., 1957; Granston, 1958; Lucas et al., 1961).

Since this process is a reflection of the sudden hemodynamic change in pulmonary circulation at birth, one might expect an abrupt transition from the fetal to the postnatal type of pulmonary arteries. To a certain extent this is what happens. However, in the first 2 or 3 days after birth, the relative medial thickness is usually in the same range as in a stillborn infant. Possibly the reason for this is the tendency to almost complete collapse of neonatal lungs upon opening the thoracic cavity. In

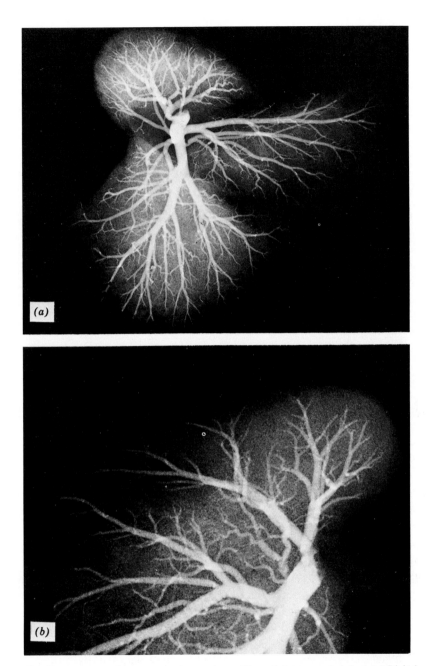

Figure 3-27. Postmortem pulmonary arteriogram in a stillborn full-term male infant. (*a*) Right lung. (*b*) Detail of left lung at higher magnification to show lack of background filling.

somewhat older infants collapse of the lungs is less pronounced, and this may influence the width and thereby the wall thickness of the pulmonary arteries.

From the second or third day of life there is a marked widening of the lumen and concomitant thinning of the media of the arteries, particularly during the first 2 or 3 postnatal weeks (Figure 3-30). Thereafter, the medial thickness decreases more gradually to reach, after one or one and a half years, a ratio that is the same as in the adult (Wagenvoort et al., 1961).

The rapid thinning of the media in the first weeks is very likely related to the marked and sudden dilatation of the pulmonary vascular bed after birth. In this respect it is of interest that during the first 4 weeks of life the smallest arterioles, with their distinct impact upon resistance, tend to dilate before the larger arteries.

The gradual decrease of medial thickness in the following year may be due to medial atrophy since the arterial tone, presumably associated with the lowering of pulmonary arterial resistance and pressure, may be reduced. An effect of further arterial dilatation cannot be excluded.

Other authors (Civin and Edwards, 1951; Herzenberg and Eskelund, 1961) gave ages between 6 and 8 months as the moment at which the process of postnatal thinning of the pulmonary arterial media is completed. These differences are clearly related to the very slow and gradual drop in the media-diameter ratio after the first months of life.

The intima of the fetal pulmonary arteries and arterioles consists largely of endothelial cells. In the contracted state of the vessels, these cells bulge into the lumen so that they contribute to a large extent to its narrowing. In this way some arterioles are completely obstructed.

Longitudinal muscle bundles within the intima of pulmonary arterioles (Figure 3-31) are regularly observed in fetuses and newborn infants (Von Hayek, 1949). They tend to contribute to occlusion of these vessels but their mode of function is unknown. We did not find them in infants older than 10 days (Wagenvoort, 1962).

Capillaries

From the pulmonary arterioles thin-walled amuscular branches arise at approximately right angles. These terminal arterioles or precapillaries in turn give rise to the alveolar capillaries (Figure 3-32) which form a dense network in the alveolar walls (Miller, 1947). This network is built up roughly by hexagonal meshes, formed by short capillary segments of 10 to 15 μ long (Weibel, 1963). Weibel and Gomez (1962) found an average alveolar capillary diameter of 8.3 μ with individual variations, presumably related to the degree of filling of the pulmonary vasculature.

The capillary networks of adjacent alveoli communicate so that the pulmonary arterial blood perfuses more than one alveolus on its way from arteriole to venule (Knisely, 1960; Staub, 1963; Reeves et al., 1965). The distance between these two points has been assessed as 600 to 800 μ in the dog and 550 to 650 μ in the cat (Staub and Schultz, 1968).

No differences could be demonstrated between the alveolar capillary networks in upper and lower lobes (Reid and Heard, 1962).

The walls of alveolar capillaries are composed of endothelial cells overlying a basement membrane (Figure 3-33). This is revealed by electron-microscopic studies

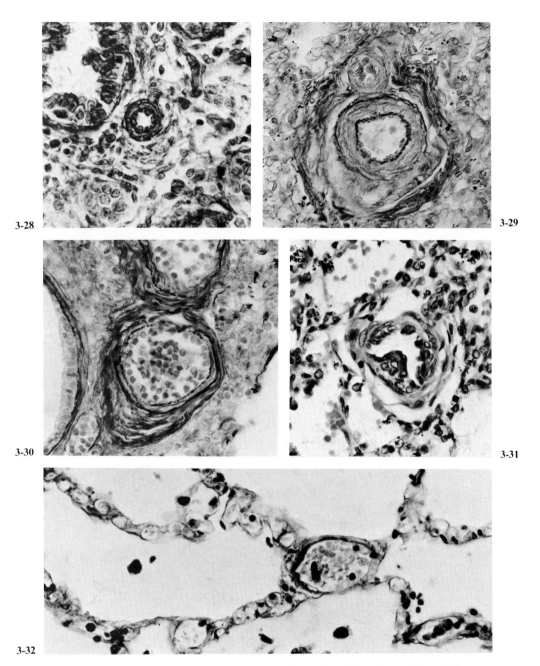

Figure 3-28. Thick-walled muscular pulmonary artery in a male stillborn fetus of 21 weeks' gestation (El.v.G., ×350).

Figure 3-29. Thick-walled muscular pulmonary artery in a stillborn full-term male infant (El.v.G., ×350).

Figure 3-30. Muscular pulmonary artery in a 3-week-old female. Many arteries exhibit considerable thinning of their media (El.v.G., ×350).

Figure 3-31. Muscular pulmonary artery in a stillborn full-term male infant. A bundle of longitudinal smooth muscle bundles narrows the lumen (H. and E., ×350).

Figure 3-32. Alveolar walls with alveolar capillaries and one precapillary in a 19-year-old man (H. and E., ×350).

41

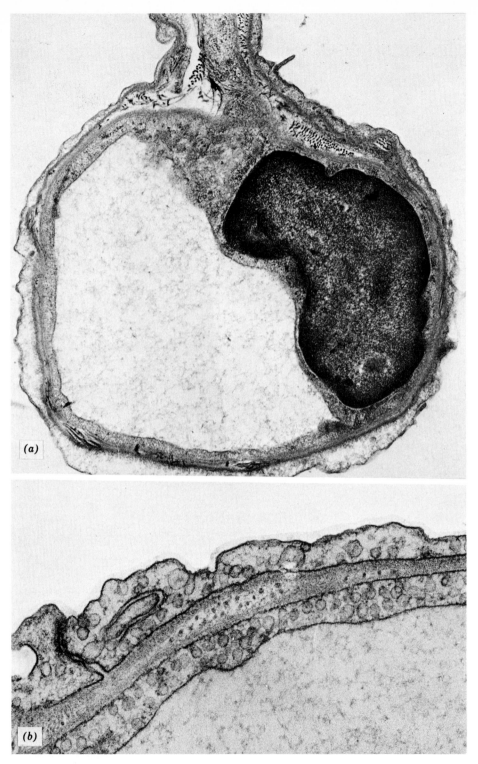

Figure 3-33. Electronmicrograph of alveolar capillary in a 55-year-old man. (*a*) The body of an endothelial cell contains a nucleus. (*b*) The free wall of the capillary consists of five layers from lumen to alveolar space: a layer of endothelium with an intercellular junction, the endothelial basement membrane, a thin interstitial space with reticulin and occasional collagen fibers, the epithelial basement membrane and a layer of alveolar epithelium (*a*: ×15,000, *b*: ×40,000).

(Schulz, 1959; Low, 1961). On the other side of the alveolar wall there is a continuous layer of epithelium that is extremely thin outside the areas of the nuclei. The epithelium also rests on a thin basement membrane. Between the two basement membranes there is usually a thin, although variable, layer containing occasional reticulin fibers. In some areas this layer is so attenuated that the basement membranes fuse. The whole thickness of the air-blood barrier has been estimated to be in the order of 1.6 to 1.8 μ (Weibel, 1970).

The occurrence of pericytes on human alveolar capillaries was established by Schulz (1956) and recently more extensively studied in lungs of men and various animals by Weibel (1974). They are rarer and have fewer branches than on systemic capillaries.

Pulmonary Venules and Veins

The blood from the alveolar capillary networks is collected in the venous system. The capillaries gather in the collecting venules, which then merge at acute angles to form pulmonary venules (Reeves et al., 1965). The wall of these venules consists of endothelium overlying a broad basement membrane. On the other side of this membrane occasional smooth muscle cells may be present. With increasing caliber of the venules the number of these smooth muscle cells increases and an elastic membrane develops between muscle and endothelium. When these muscle cells are absent or scarce, the structure of the pulmonary venules is so similar to that of the nonmuscular portion of the arterioles that these vessels cannot be distinguished confidently in a histologic section (Figure 3-21). Localization of venules is not helpful since both pulmonary arterioles and venules lie in alveolar walls, unrelated to bronchi or interlobular fibrous septa. For identification, branches must be traced in serial sections to larger vessels.

Gradually the pulmonary venules join and form pulmonary veins (Figure 3-34). At

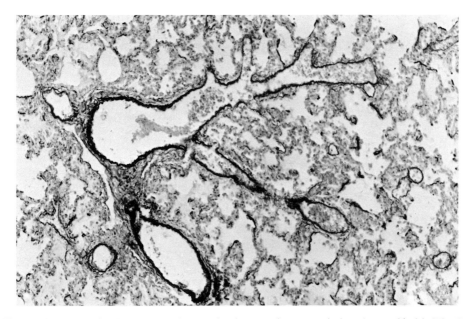

Figure 3-34. Normal pulmonary venules merging into a pulmonary vein in a 4-year-old girl. (El.v.G., ×90).

a caliber of 60 to 100 μ these veins enter the interlobular fibrous septa, as far as possible from the pulmonary arteries. Their localization may now distinguish them from the arteries but differences in wall structure between the two types of vessels also become apparent.

The venous wall, while being thinner than that of an artery of equal size, is composed of irregularly arranged elastic membranes, generally with a distinct internal elastic lamina (Figure 3-35). Smooth muscle fibers, usually in small irregular bundles, are lying scattered between the elastic fibers (Wagenvoort, 1970). Moreover, there is a varying amount of collagen in the media. The intima consists of an endothelial sheet overlying the internal elastic lamina. Valves are absent. There is no sharp demarcation of the media and the adventitia, which consists of dense bundles of collagen interspersed with elastic fibers.

This structural pattern, in principle, is retained in the larger pulmonary venous trunks. From the hilar region onward the extrapulmonary part of the veins contains an outer layer of cardiac muscle as an extension of the left atrial wall. The extent of cardiac muscle, which may sometimes be observed within the lung, varies greatly (Nathan and Eliakim, 1966).

Occasionally small cell proliferation in the adventitia of pulmonary veins within the lung have been found and have been interpreted as hyperplastic nodules of chemoreceptor cells (Edwards and Heath, 1972) or as chemodectomas (Korn et al., 1960), suggesting that they developed from cells sensitive to oxygen or carbon dioxide. These minute tumors are rare and their ultrastructural characteristics do not resemble those of chemoreceptive paraganglia (Kuhn and Askin, 1975). The cells from which they should have been developed have not been clearly identified.

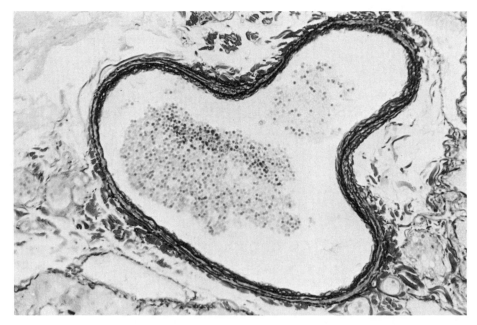

Figure 3-35.   Normal pulmonary vein in a 28-year-old man. There is a haphazard arrangement of elastic fibers within the media (El.v.G., $\times 140$).

Age Changes

In the older age groups there is an increasing tendency to fragmentation of elastic laminae in the venous media. The resulting loss of elasticity is reflected by the irregular shape of the vessels in cross section. Intimal fibrosis, often of an acellular hyaline type, is very common in venules and veins, although this rarely leads to severe narrowing of the lumen (Figure 3-36).

Perinatal Period

In the newborn, the pulmonary veins are even more thin-walled than in adults (Wagenvoort, 1970), particularly as contrasted to the thick-walled arterioles. There is, however, no essential difference in the structure of its wall as compared to that of the adult pulmonary veins.

Bronchial Vessels

As compared to the pulmonary vessels, the bronchial arteries and veins are of limited importance in most forms of pulmonary hypertension. Even so, their recognition in histologic sections is necessary, and a brief discussion of their normal structure therefore is justified.

The bronchial arteries accompany the bronchi, supplying both the bronchial adventitia outside the cartilage and the bronchial mucosa. When the bronchi lose their cartilage, recognizable bronchial arteries soon disappear after having broken up into a capillary network.

As with other systemic arteries, bronchial arteries have a fairly thick muscular media with a well-defined internal elastic lamina. An external elastic lamina is either absent or thin and often fragmented (Figure 3-37).

The intima is usually thin with a single layer of endothelial cells. However, crescent-shaped bundles or circular layers of smooth muscle fibers in a reduplication of the internal elastic lamina may result in thickening of the intima (Figure 3-38). These bundles may even completely occlude the lumen (Figure 3-39). Their significance is still under discussion. A function in the sense of blocking mechanisms has been assumed by Von Hayek (1940). Weibel (1958) believed that the bundles developed as a reaction to the stretching of the bronchus, but Wagenaar (1975) demonstrated that this is unlikely and interpreted them as reparative changes developing with age.

Both pulmonary and bronchial arteries accompany bronchi, but the latter are always small in comparison to the large bronchi they serve as nutrient vessels. They also may be found in the adventitia of large elastic pulmonary arteries. The bronchial arteries usually lie adjacent to bronchial veins and nerve bundles.

The capillary networks in the walls of bronchi and bronchioli are situated both inside and outside the bronchial muscle coat (Miller, 1947) and communicate freely with those of adjacent alveolar walls (Reid and Heard, 1962).

From these capillaries, the bronchial venules arise which themselves form plexuses around bronchi. While small channels may be present in the walls of terminal bronchioles, in the larger bronchi there is usually one plexus in the bronchial mucosa

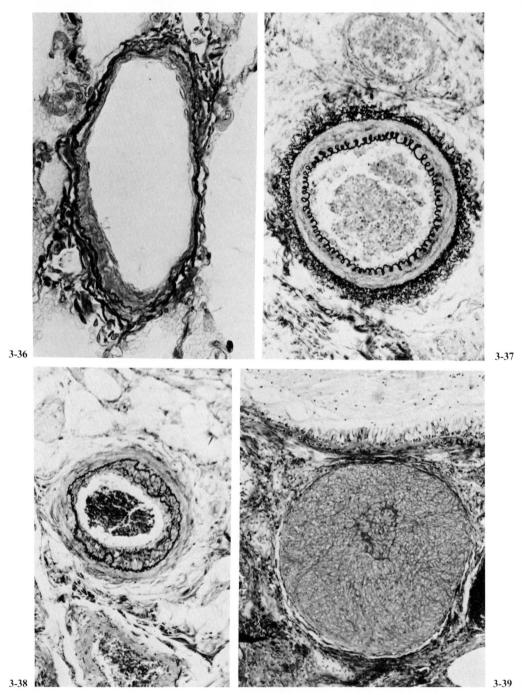

Figure 3-36. Pulmonary vein with some intimal fibrosis as an age change from the same case as that of Figure 3-35 (El.v.G., ×350).

Figure 3-37. Normal bronchial artery in a 22-year-old man. There is a distinct internal elastic lamina and a condensation of elastic fibers in the adventitia (El.v.G., ×140).

Figure 3-38. Bronchial artery in a 73-year-old man. The intima is thickened by a crescent-shaped layer of longitudinal smooth muscle cells (El.v.G., ×140).

Figure 3-39. Bronchial artery totally obstructed by longitudinal smooth muscle cells in a 49-year-old woman. Remnants of the media are recognizable in the lower left corner (El.v.G., ×90).

46

connected with another in the bronchial adventitia. Not only at this level but also in the further course of the bronchial veins, which arise from these plexuses, there are extensive communications with pulmonary veins (Figure 3-40) that can easily be detected when serial sections are used or when the pulmonary veins are injected. All the blood, derived from this bronchial venous system, reaches the left atrium.

In addition there are veins, arising from the vascular networks in the pleura and from the hilar region, which eventually drain into the right atrium, at the right side by way of the azygos vein and at the left side by way of the hemiazygos or left innominate veins.

The structure of these bronchial and pleuro-hilar veins does not differ essentially from that of the pulmonary veins. Their walls, however, are generally thinner, even at similar caliber than the pulmonary venous walls. In contrast to the pulmonary veins, the bronchial veins contain delicate bicuspid valves. These valves are relatively more frequent in infants and children than in adults. Since these valves may protrude into the lumen of pulmonary veins at the site of anastomoses, sometimes the erroneous impression is gained that the latter are provided with valves (Figure 3-41).

Anastomoses

Vessels connecting various types of blood vessels in the lung at other than capillary level do occur although there is often disagreement as to their significance. It is generally agreed that under normal conditions there are no anastomoses between pulmonary arteries nor between pulmonary veins.

The existence of pulmonary arteriovenous anastomoses always has been con-

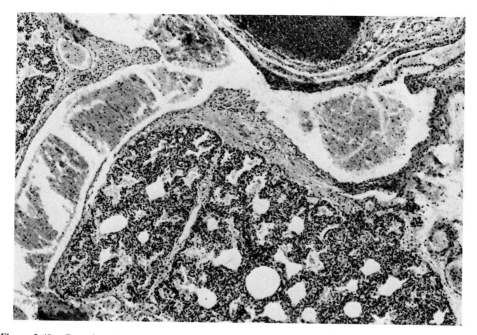

Figure 3-40. Bronchopulmonary venous anastomosis in a 4-year-old boy. A bronchial vein provided with a valve (upper right corner) connects with a large pulmonary vein (H. and E., ×50).

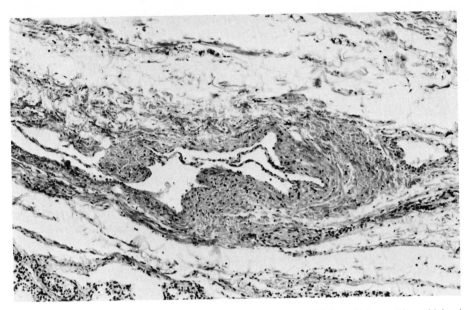

Figure 3-41. Bronchopulmonary venous anastomosis in a 2-year-old boy. Valves of bronchial veins extend into the pulmonary venous lumen and may be misinterpreted as pulmonary venous valves (H. and E., ×90).

troversial. The injection of glass spherules or plastic beads into the pulmonary artery with subsequent collection from the pulmonary veins has been taken by some authors as proof of the existence of these anastomoses (Prinzmetal et al., 1948; Niden and Aviado, 1956). The risks of these methods have been discussed earlier (Wagenvoort et al., 1964). Liebow (1962) found no evidence of these anastomoses in corrosion casts.

Morphologic demonstration of pulmonary arteriovenous anastomoses by using serial sections appears to be exceedingly difficult. Von Hayek (1942) has claimed their presence but others (Verloop, 1948; Weibel, 1959; Wagenvoort and Wagenvoort, 1967; Robertson, 1973) were unable to find them, while Florange (1960) observed them very rarely. Since in these studies muscular pulmonary arteries and arterioles generally were traced down to a level where they lose their muscular coat, the existence of occasional connections between nonmuscular pre- and postcapillary vessels cannot be excluded, although positive morphologic evidence for this supposition is lacking.

With regard to the anastomoses between bronchial and pulmonary arteries, there is general agreement that they do occur in normal lungs (Figure 3-42) but their frequency is disputed. Some authors (Von Hayek, 1940, 1953; Verloop, 1948) believe that they are common, while others (Weibel, 1959; Wagenvoort et al., 1964) maintain that they are fairly rare and usually of small caliber in the absence of cardiac or pulmonary disease. There is no doubt that their number can increase considerably under pathologic conditions. Probably in infants they are relatively more common than in adults (Wagenvoort and Wagenvoort, 1967).

In the perinatal period, bronchopulmonary and pulmobronchial arteries can be easily found in histologic serial sections. Bronchopulmonary arteries are branches of bronchial arteries supplying the alveolar capillaries (Figure 3-43). They may be derived from bronchial arteries accompanying bronchi, as well as from pleural arteries. Pulmobronchial arteries are branches from pulmonary arteries which supply the interstitium of the lung and the walls of bronchi. Under normal conditions both types of vessels tend to decrease in number or to disappear completely within the first years of life (Wagenvoort and Wagenvoort, 1966, 1967; Robertson, 1967, 1973).

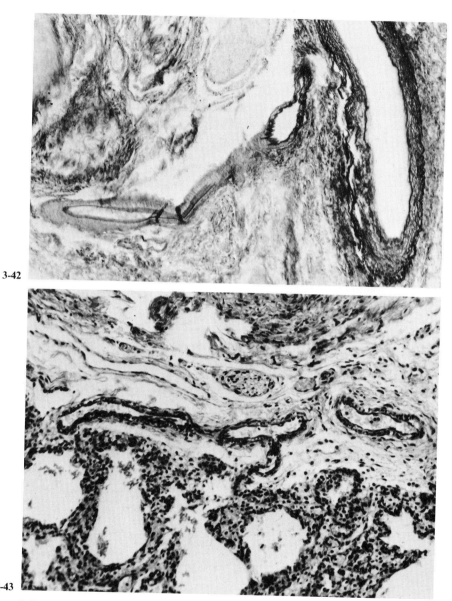

Figure 3-42. Bronchopulmonary arterial anastomosis in a stillborn male infant of 34 weeks' gestation. The anastomosis connects a bronchial (left) with a pulmonary artery (right) (El.v.G., ×50).

Figure 3-43. Bronchopulmonary artery in a stillborn female infant of 32 weeks' gestation. A bronchial artery provides small branches supplying the lung tissue (H. and E., ×140).

Anastomoses between the branches of bronchial arteries and veins have been found by Weibel (1959) and also, but rarely, by Wagenvoort and Wagenvoort (1967) and Robertson (1973). Anastomoses between pulmonary and bronchial veins are very frequent as has been discussed on p. 20.

In pathologic conditions and notably in several forms of pulmonary hypertension, the significance of many of these anastomotic vessels may become much greater. Not only will they often increase in number and size (Liebow et al., 1948, 1949) but also types of anastomoses that normally do not occur may be found in the diseased lungs.

Pulmonary Lymphatics

There are extensive networks of lymphatics in the lungs that can be divided into pleural or superficial networks and interstitial or deep networks. Lymphatics are not present in alveolar walls but can be found in the pleura (Figure 3-44) as well as in the connective tissue septa of the lungs, even in very delicate ones, around pulmonary arteries and veins, and in the walls of bronchi, both in mucosa and adventitia. Usually there are one to three larger lymphatics accompanying the blood vessels, while smaller branches form networks around arteries and veins (Miller, 1947). The superficial and deep networks anastomose in the region of the hilum and drain to the hilar and tracheobronchial lymph nodes.

The lymph capillaries consist of endothelial cells overlying a basement membrane. With increasing caliber, more and more collagen and elastic fibers strengthen the walls of the lymphatics, while irregularly arranged smooth muscle cells (Figure 3-45) often are present in the larger ones. The cytoplasm of the endothelium contains thin as well as thick filaments suggesting an active regulation of intercellular junctions and therefore of its permeability (Lauweryns et al., 1976). Valves are common in lymphatics; they are usually bicuspid and extremely thin (Figure 3-46).

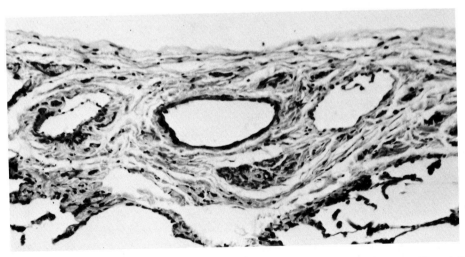

Figure 3-44. Pleural lymphatics on either side of a small vein in a 48-year-old woman (H. and E., ×140).

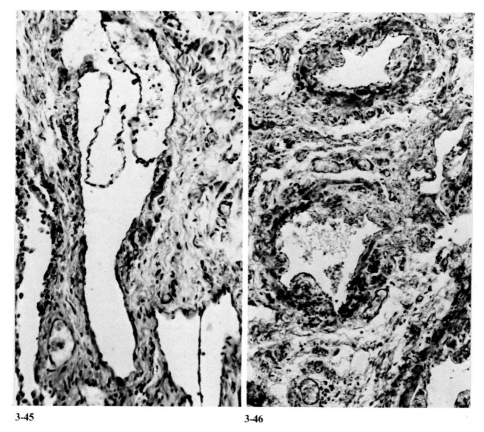

3-45   3-46

Figure 3-45.   Parabronchial lymphatics with an irregular layer of smooth muscle cells in their walls in a 64-year-old man (H. and E., ×90).
Figure 3-46.   Lymphatics in a connective tissue septum in the lungs of a 31-year-old woman. They contain delicate bicuspid valves (H. and E., ×140).

Pulmonary lymphatics are often collapsed in normal lungs so that they are seemingly limited in number. Injection, for instance by Indian ink, may reveal their true numbers and extension. This also becomes apparent when they are dilated as in chronic congestion.

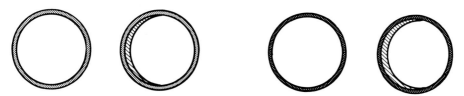

Normal pulmonary vessels: Arteries (*left*) and veins (*right*) with thin media and wide lumen, without or with some intimal fibrosis as an age change.

REFERENCES

Asami, I.: Beitrag zur Entwicklung des Kammerseptums im menschlichen Herzens mit besonderer Berücksichtigung der sogenannten Bulbusdrehung. *Z. Anat. u. Entwickl. Gesch.* **128:** 1, 1969.

Auerbach, O., Stout, A. E., Hammond, E. C., and Garfinkel, L.: Smoking habits and age in relation to pulmonary changes. Rupture of alveolar septums, fibrosis and thickening of walls of small arteries and arterioles. *New Engl. J. Med.* **269,** 1045, 1963.

Barry, A.: The aortic arch derivatives in the human adult. *Anat. Rec.* **111:** 221, 1951.

Becker, A. E.: The glomera in the region of the heart and great vessels. A microscopic-anatomic study. *Path. Europ.* **1:** 410, 1966.

Brenner, O.: Pathology of the vessels of the pulmonary circulation. *Arch. Intern. Med.* **56:** 211, 1935.

Camarri, E., and Marini, G.: La circulation bronchique à l'état normal et pathologique. Edition Doin, Paris, 1965.

Civin, W. H., and Edwards, J. E.: The postnatal structural changes in the intrapulmonary arteries and arterioles. *Arch. Path.* **51:** 192, 1951.

Congdon, E. D.: Transformation of the aortic arch system during development of the human embryo. *Contr. Embryol. Carneg. Instit.* **14:** 47, 1922.

Cory, R. A. S., and Valentine, E. J.: Varying patterns of the lobar branches of the pulmonary artery. *Thorax* **14:** 267, 1959.

Cumming, G., Henderson, R., Horsfield, K., and Singhal, S. S.: The functional morphology of the pulmonary circulation. In A. P. Fishman and H. H. Hecht (eds.), *The Pulmonary Circulation and Interstitial Space.* University of Chicago Press, Chicago and London, 1969.

Dammann, J. F., and Ferencz, C.: The significance of the pulmonary vascular bed in congenital heart disease. I. Normal lungs. II. Malformations of the heart in which there is pulmonary stenosis. *Am. Heart J.* **52:** 7, 1956.

Davies, G., and Reid, L.: Growth of the alveoli and pulmonary arteries in childhood. *Thorax* **25:** 669, 1970.

Delarue, J., Chomette, G., Auriol, M., and Abalanet, R.: Modifications vasculaires observées dans le poumon du vieillard. *Arch. Anat. Path.* **6:** 295, 1958.

Edwards, C., and Heath, D.: Pulmonary venous chemoreceptor tissue. *Brit. J. Dis. Chest* **66:** 96, 1972.

Edwards, J. E.: Functional pathology of the pulmonary vascular tree in congenital cardiac disease. *Circulation* **15:** 164, 1957.

Elliott, F. M., and Reid, L.: Some new facts about the pulmonary artery and its branching pattern. *Clin. Radiol.* **16:** 193, 1965.

Farrar, J. F., Blomfield, J., and Reye, R. D. K.: The structure and composition of the maturing pulmonary circulation. *J. Path. Bact.* **90:** 83, 1965.

Ferencz, C., Libi-Sylora, M., and Greco, J.: Age-related characteristics of the human pulmonary arterial tree. *Circulation* **34:** suppl. II, 107, 1967.

Florange, W.: Anatomie und Pathologie der Arteria bronchialis. *Ergebn. Allg. Path.* **39:** 152, 1960.

Frodl, F. K. O.: De bloedvaten van de long. *Ned. Tijdschr. v. Geneesk.* **95:** 2752, 1951.

Granston, A. S.: Morphologic alterations of the pulmonary arteries in congenital heart disease. *Proc. Inst. Med.* Chicago **22:** 116, 1958.

Gray, S. H., Handler, F. P., Blache, J. O., Zuckner, J., and Blumenthal, H. T.: Aging processes of aorta and pulmonary artery in negro and white races (Comparative study of various segments). *Arch. Path.* **56:** 238, 1953.

Hamilton, W. J., Boyd, W. D., and Mossman, H. W.: *Human Embryology,* ed. 4. W. Heffer and Sons Ltd., Baltimore and Cambridge, 1972.

Harris, P., Heath, D., and Apostolopoulos, A.: Extensibility of the human pulmonary trunk. *Brit. Heart J.* **27:** 651, 1965.

Heath, D., and Best, P. V.: The tunica media of the arteries of the lung in pulmonary hypertension. *J. Path. Bact.* **76:** 165, 1958.

Heath, D., Wood, E. H., DuShane, J. W., and Edwards, J. E.: The structure of the pulmonary trunk at different ages in cases of pulmonary hypertension and pulmonary stenosis. *J. Path. Bact.* **77**: 443, 1959.

Heath, D., Wood, E. H., DuShane, J. W., and Edwards, J. E.: The relation of age and blood pressure to atheroma in the pulmonary arteries and thoracic aorta in congenital heart disease. *Lab. Invest.* **9**: 259, 1960.

Herzenberg, H., and Eskelund, V.: The morphological development of pulmonary arteries during the first years of life. *Acta Paediat.* **50**: 263, 1961.

Hevelke, G.: Alterswandlungen der menschlichen Lungenschlagader dargestellt am Phospholipidgehalt. *Münsch. Med. Wschr.* **107**: 2309, 1965.

Hislop, A., and Reid, L.: Intra-pulmonary arterial development during fetal life-branching pattern and structure. *J. Anat.* **113**: 35, 1972.

Knisely, W. H.: In vivo architecture of blood vessels supplying and draining alveoli. *Amer. Rev. Resp. Dis.* **81**: 735, 1960.

Kolb, P., and Hägele, U.: Die Volumen-Druck-Beziehung des extrapulmonalen Abschnittes der menschlichen Lungenschlagader und ihre Zuordnung zu Lebensalter Körperlänge und Herzgewicht. *Z. Kreislaufforsch.* **57**: 641, 1968.

Korn, D., Bensch, K., Liebow, A. A., and Castleman, B.: Multiple minute pulmonary tumors resembling chemodectomas *Amer. J. Path.* **37**: 641, 1960.

Krahl, V. E.: The glomus pulmonale. A preliminary report. *Bull. Sch. Med. Maryland* **45**: 36, 1960.

Kuhn, C., and Askin, F. B.: The fine structure of so-called minute chemodectomas. *Human Path* **6**: 681, 1975.

Lauweryns, J.: De longvaten. Architectoniek en rol bij de longontplooiing. *Presses Acad. Europ.*, Brussel, 1962.

Lauweryns, J. M., Baert, J., and De Loecker, W.: Fine filaments in lymphatic endothelial cells. *J. Cell Biol.* **68**: 163, 1976.

Levin, D. L., Rudolph, A. M., Heymann, M. A., and Phibbs, R. H.: Morphological development of the pulmonary vascular bed in fetal lambs. *Circulation* **53**: 144, 1976.

Liebow, A. A.: Recent advances in pulmonary anatomy. In *Ciba Foundation Symposium on Pulmonary Structure and Function*. Churchill, London, 1962.

Liebow, A. A., Hales, M. R., and Lindskog, G. E.: Enlargement of the bronchial arteries and their anastomoses with the pulmonary arteries in chronic pulmonary disease. *Amer. J. Path.* **24**: 691, 1948.

Liebow, A. A., Hales, M. R., and Lindskog, G. E.: Enlargement of bronchial arteries and their anastomoses with pulmonary arteries in bronchiectasis. *Amer. J. Path.* **25**: 211, 1949.

Los, J. A.: Embryology. In H. Watson, *Paediatric Cardiology*. Lloyd Luc Ltd., London, 1969.

Los, J. A.: Een eenvoudig ruimtelijk schema voor het classificeren van stoornissen in het septeringsproces van het menselijke hart naar morfogenetische criteria. *Nederl. Tijdschr. v. Geneesk.* **120**: 100, 1976.

Low, F. N.: The extracellular portion of the human blood-air barrier and its relation to tissue space. *Anat. Rec.* **139**: 105, 1961.

Lucas, R. V., St. Geme, J. W., Anderson, R. C., Adams, P., and Ferguson, D. J.: Maturation of the pulmonary vascular bed: A physiologic and anatomic correlation in infants and children. *Amer. J. Dis. Child.* **101**: 467, 1961.

Marchand, P., Gilroy, J. C., and Wilson, V. H.: An anatomical study of the bronchial vascular system and its variations in disease. *Thorax* **5**: 207, 1950.

Meyer, W. W., Richter, H., Schollmeyer, P., and Simon, E.: Das Fassungsvermögen und die Volumendehnbarkeit des aortalen Windkessels und der Pulmonalis in Abhängigkeit von Alter, Arteriosklerose und Hochdruck. *Verh. Deutsch. Ges. Kreislaufforsch.* **23**: 346, 1957.

Miller, W. S.: *The Lung*, ed. 2, Charles C Thomas, Springfield, Ill. 1947.

Naeye, R. L.: Arterial changes during the perinatal period. *Arch. Path.* **71**: 121, 1961.

Naeye, R. L.: Development of systemic and pulmonary arteries from birth through early childhood. *Biol. Neonat.* (Basel) **10**: 7, 1966.

Naeye, R. L., and Dellinger, W. S.: Pulmonary arterial changes with age and smoking. *Arch. Path.* **92:** 284, 1971.

Nathan, H., and Eliakim, M.: The junction between the left atrium and the pulmonary veins. *Circulation* **34:** 412, 1966.

Niden, A. H., and Aviado, D. M.: Effects of pulmonary embolism on the pulmonary circulation with special reference to arteriovenous shunts in the lung. *Circulation Res.* **4:** 67, 1956.

O'Neal, R. M., Ahlvin, R. C., Bauer, W. C., and Thomas, W. A.: Development of fetal pulmonary arterioles. *Arch. Path.* **63:** 309, 1957.

Parke, W. W.: The vasa vasorum of the ascending aorta and pulmonary trunk and their coronary-extracardiac relationship. *Amer. Heart J.* **80:** 802, 1970.

Patel, D. J., Schilder, D. P., Mallos, A. J., and Casper, G. T.: Mechanical properties of the pulmonary artery. *Circulation* **20:** 748, 1959.

Prinzmetal, M., Ornitz, E. M., Simkin, R., and Bergman, H. C.: Arterio-venous anastomoses in liver, spleen and lungs. *Amer. J. Physiol.* **152:** 48, 1948.

Reeves, J. T., Leathers, J. E., and Quigley, M. B.: Microradiography of pulmonary arterioles, capillaries and venules of the rabbit. *Anat. Rec.* **151:** 531, 1965.

Reid, A., and Heard, B. E.: Preliminary studies of human pulmonary capillaries by india ink injection. *Med. Thorac.* **19:** 215, 1962.

Reid, L.: The embryology of the lung. In A. V. S. de Reuck, and R. Porter, (eds.), *Ciba Foundation Symposium: Development of the Lung.* Churchill, London, 1967.

Robertson, B.: The normal intrapulmonary arterial pattern in infancy and early childhood. A microangiographic and histological study. *Acta Path. Microbiol. Scand.* **71:** 481, 1967.

Robertson, B.: *Micro-angiography of the Lung in Infancy and Childhood.* Proprius, Stockholm, 1973.

Rosen, L., Bowden, D. H., and Uchida, I.: Structural changes in pulmonary arteries in the first year of life. *Arch. Path.* **63:** 316, 1957.

Schulz, H.: Elektronenoptische Untersuchungen der normalen Lunge und der Lunge bei Mitralstenose. *Virchows Arch.* **328:** 582, 1956.

Schulz, H.: *Die Submikroskopische Anatomie und Pathologie der Lunge.* Springer, Heidelberg, 1959.

Semmens, M: The pulmonary artery in the normal aged lung. *Brit. J. Dis. Chest* **64:** 65, 1970.

Simons, P., and Reid, L.: Muscularity of pulmonary artery branches in the upper and lower lobes of the normal young and aged lung. *Brit. J. Dis. Chest* **63:** 38, 1969.

Singhal, S., Henderson, R., Horsfield, K., Harding, K., and Cumming, G.: Morphometry of the human pulmonary arterial tree. *Circulation Res.* **33:** 190, 1973.

Staub, N. C.: The interdependence of pulmonary structure and function. *Anesthesiol.* **24:** 831, 1963.

Staub, N. C., and Schultz, E.: Pulmonary capillary length in dog, cat and rabbit. *Resp. Physiol.* **5:** 371, 1968.

Tobin, C. E.: The bronchial arteries and their connections with other vessels in the human lung. *Surg. Gynec. Obstet.* **95:** 741, 1952.

Tobin, C. E.: Some observations concerning the pulmonic vasa vasorum. *Surg. Gynec. Obstet.* **111:** 297, 1960.

Vandendorpe, F.: Structure de l'artériole pulmonaire chez l'homme. *Ann. Anat. Path.* **13:** 652, 1936.

Van Zandwijk, N., Wagenvoort, C. A., and Groen, A. S.: Unpublished data, 1976.

Verloop, M. C.: The arteriae bronchiales and their anastomosing with the arteria pulmonalis in the human lung: a micro-anatomical study. *Acta Anat.* **5:** 171, 1948.

Von Hayek, H.: Über verschluszfähige Arterien in der menschlichen Lunge. *Anat. Anz.* **89:** 219, 1940.

Von Hayek, H.: Über Kurzschlüsse und Nebenschlüsse des Lungenkreislaufes. *Anat. Anz.* **93:** 155, 1942.

Von Hayek, H.: Epitheloide Sperrarterien in der Neugeborenenlunge und Histamin-Wirkung. Zur postfetalen Kreislaufumstellung. *Zschr. Anat. Entwickl. Gesch.* **114:** 9, 1949.

Von Hayek, H.: *Die Menschliche Lunge.* Springer Verlag, Berlin, 1953.

Wade, G., and Ball, J.: Unexplained pulmonary hypertension. *Quart. Med. J.* **26:** 83, 1957.

Wagenaar, S. S.: Histologie en histopathologie van bronchiale arterien. Een morphometrische en experi-mentele studie. Thesis. Amsterdam, 1975.

Wagenvoort, C. A.: Vasoconstriction and medial hypertrophy in pulmonary hypertension. *Circulation* **22:** 535, 1960.

Wagenvoort, C. A.: The pulmonary arteries in infants with ventricular septal defect. *Med. Thorac.* **19:** 354, 1962.

Wagenvoort, C. A.: Morphologic changes in intrapulmonary veins. *Human Path.* **1:** 205, 1970.

Wagenvoort, C. A., Neufeld, H. N., and Edwards, J. E.: The structure of the pulmonary arterial tree in fetal and early postnatal life. *Lab. Invest.* **10:** 751, 1961.

Wagenvoort, C. A., Heath, D., and Edwards, J. E.: *The Pathology of the Pulmonary Vasculature.* Charles C Thomas, Springfield, Ill., 1964.

Wagenvoort, C. A., and Wagenvoort, N.: Age changes in muscular pulmonary arteries. *Arch. Path.* **79:** 524, 1965.

Wagenvoort, C. A., and Wagenvoort, N.: The pulmonary vascular bed in the normal fetus and newborn. In D. E. Cassels, *The Heart and Circulation in the Newborn and Infant.* Grune and Stratton, New York, London, 1966.

Wagenvoort, C. A., and Wagenvoort, N.: Arterial anastomoses, bronchopulmonary arteries, and pulmobronchial arteries in perinatal lungs. *Lab. Invest.* **16:** 13, 1967.

Wagenvoort, C. A., Wagenvoort, N., and Dijk, H. J.: Effect of fulvine on pulmonary arteries and veins of the rat. *Thorax* **29:** 522, 1974.

Weibel, E.: Die entstehung der Längsmuskulatur in der Ästen der A. bronchialis. *Z. Zellforsch.* **47:** 440, 1958.

Weibel, E.: Die Blutgefässanastomosen in der menschlichen Lunge. *Z. Zellforsch.* **50:** 653, 1959.

Weibel, E. R.: *Morphometry of the Human Lung.* Academic Press, New York, 1963.

Weibel, E. R.: Morphometric estimation of pulmonary diffusion capacity. I. Model and Method. *Resp. Physiol.* **11:** 54, 1970.

Weibel, E. R.: On pericytes, particularly their existence on lung capillaries. *Microvascular Research* **8:** 218, 1974.

Weibel, E. R., and Gomez, D. M.: Architecture of the human lung. *Science* **137:** 577, 1962.

West, J. B., and Dollery, C. T.: Distribution of blood flow and ventilation-perfusion ratio in the lung, measured with radio-active CO_2. *J. Appl. Physiol.* **15:** 405, 1960.

CHAPTER FOUR

Pulmonary Hypertension
in Cardiac Left to Right Shunts

Congenital cardiac malformations with a large left to right shunt between systemic and pulmonary circulations often are associated with pulmonary arterial hypertension. In fact, most of the earlier reports of vascular disease in the lungs dealt with patients with congenital cardiac defects. The pulmonary arterial alterations are commonly severe and, by reducing the vascular bed available to the pulmonary circulation, may lead to a progressively increased vascular resistance in the lung and to a reversal of the shunt.

The most widespread and pronounced lesions in the lung vessels usually are observed in cases of post-tricuspid shunts (Harris and Heath, 1962), such as large ventricular septal defect, truncus arteriosus persistens, single ventricle, patent ductus arteriosus, and aorta-pulmonary septal defect. Particularly when there are complicated malformations such as a common atrioventricular canal or a transposition of the large arteries associated with a ventricular septal defect, the pulmonary vascular lesions tend to be very severe. In isolated patent ductus arteriosus severe vascular disease is less common.

In all these instances of large post-tricuspid congenital cardiac shunts, pulmonary hypertension is present from birth and the alterations in the lung vessels appear early in life.

In contrast, in pretricuspid shunts like atrial septal defect or anomalous pulmonary venous drainage to the left atrium, the pulmonary arterial pressure initially is not or only mildly elevated. The flow through the pulmonary circulation may be very large in these instances but the vasculature of the lung has a capacity for adaptation to this increased flow so that severe pulmonary hypertension does not develop until in later adult life and even then uncommonly. Consequently, marked pulmonary vascular disease is also uncommon in these cases.

In principle, pulmonary hypertension may result from an acquired left to right shunt for instance following perforation of a ventricular septum due to myocardial infarction or after rupture of an aortic aneurysm into the pulmonary artery. The life-threatening nature of these situations, however, will rarely permit the development of marked pulmonary vascular disease.

Generally, if pulmonary hypertension is present in cases of congenital cardiac defects, the pulmonary vascular changes conform to the same pattern, whether the shunt is pretricuspid or post-tricuspid and irrespective of the type of cardiac anomaly (Edwards, 1957; Wagenvoort et al., 1964). This pattern will be discussed in this chapter.

PULMONARY TRUNK, MAIN ARTERIES, AND ELASTIC PULMONARY ARTERIES

In prenatal life the hemodynamic situations in the large conducting arteries of systemic and pulmonary circulation respectively are comparable. Consequently there are no differences in caliber or in thickness or structure of the vascular wall between aorta and pulmonary trunk in fetal life. In both vessels there are long, regular elastic laminae running parallel to each other.

After birth, when under normal circumstances the pressure in the pulmonary artery becomes much lower than in the aorta, there is a gradual change. While the flow through both vessels remains equal, there is no appreciable difference in caliber between the two vessels with age. But the ratio in thickness of the wall of pulmonary trunk and aorta respectively decreases gradually until, as we have seen (p. 24), the thickness of the wall of the pulmonary trunk is only slightly more than half that of the aorta. While the elastic configuration of the aorta remains in principle the same, that of the pulmonary artery changes gradually. Its elastic laminae become irregular, disrupted, and sparse.

If pulmonary hypertension is present from birth, as in the cardiac abnormalities under discussion, the diameter of the pulmonary trunk tends to become greater than that of the aorta and the relative thickness of its wall tends to remain unchanged so that it equals that of the aorta (Figure 4-1). Moreover, the elastic configuration of these vessels keep their uniform, intact, and regular elastic laminae (Figure 4-2). This "aortic configuration" of the pulmonary trunk, as it was labeled by Heath et al. (1959), is a fairly constant feature in pulmonary hypertension, although there are exceptions. In our experience in some cases of marked elevation of the pulmonary arterial pressure present from birth, the aortic configuration is either not very distinct or absent (Figure 4-3). Conversely, in normal adults there is a considerable variation in the elastic pattern of the pulmonary trunk (p. 21).

The media of the elastic intrapulmonary arteries in pulmonary hypertension is thicker than normal but otherwise, as a rule, has the same structure as in normal individuals.

Atherosclerosis

Under normal circumstances, pulmonary atherosclerosis in a very mild form is common, particularly in older individuals (Brenner, 1935). Grossly it can be recognized when the vessels are cut open as small yellow streaks or patches, sometimes in

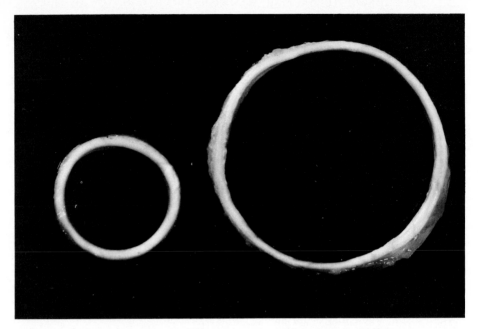

Figure 4-1. Transverse slices of aorta (*left*) and pulmonary trunk (*right*) after fixation in expanded state, in a 31-year-old man with a ventricular septal defect of the endocardial cushion type and pulmonary hypertension. The pulmonary trunk is extremely dilated, while its wall thickness is in the same range as that of the aorta (×1.7).

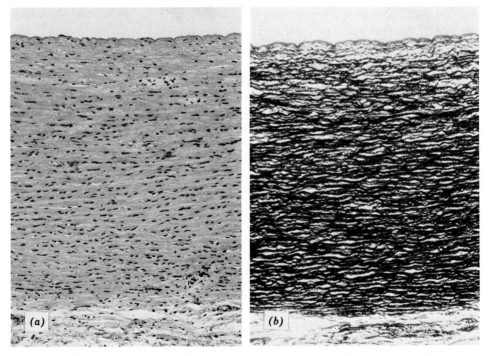

Figure 4-2. Wall of pulmonary trunk in a 4-year-old boy with a ventricular septal defect. There is an "aortic" configuration of the media with regular and continuous elastic laminae. (*a*: H. and E., *b*: El.v.G., ×90).

pulmonary trunk and main pulmonary arteries but often—and then sometimes missed at autopsy—in the large intrapulmonary branches notably at their sites of ramification.

In pulmonary hypertension, atheroma is much more pronounced (Figure 4-4) and is common even in children. It is related to the degree of elevation of pressure, but it is nonspecific in that it occurs in any form of pulmonary hypertension (Heath et al., 1960). The plaques of lipid-containing foam cells, often embedded in fibrous tissue, are not limited to the largest pulmonary arteries but may occur in elastic arteries as small as 500 to 300 μ (Figure 4-5), constituting the smallest caliber arteries in the body in which distinct atheromatous changes do occur.

As in systemic arteries, the media at the site of the atheromatous plaque often shows thinning. Marked calcification of the plaques does occur (Timpanelli and Steinberg, 1961) but is uncommon and ulceration is rare.

Aneurysms

Aneurysms of the large pulmonary arteries are sometimes observed in the absence of pulmonary hypertension but more often when the pressure in the pulmonary arteries is elevated, irrespective of the cause for the pulmonary hypertension. Saccular

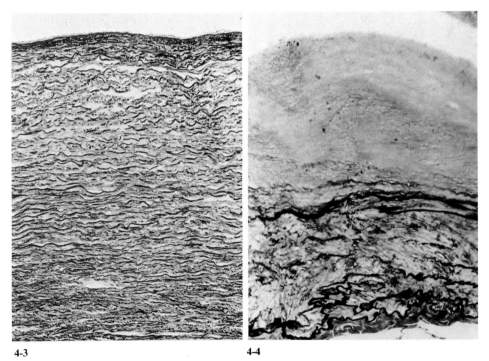

4-3   4-4

Figure 4-3. Wall of pulmonary trunk in a 17-year-old man with a patent ductus arteriosus. In this case there is no distinct "aortic" configuration, since the elastic membranes are interrupted and fragmented (El.v.G., × 90).

Figure 4-4. Wall of left main pulmonary artery with marked atherosclerosis in a 45-year-old woman with a large atrial septal defect and pulmonary hypertension (El.v.G., ×140).

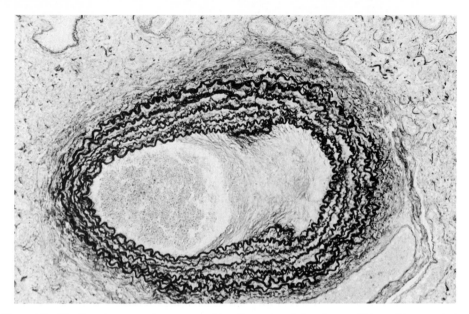

Figure 4-5.   Elastic pulmonary artery narrowed by atherosclerosis in a 5-year-old boy with a ventricular septal defect (El.v.G., ×90).

aneurysms have been described in patients with ventricular septal defect (Davis et al., 1963; Loire et al., 1970), in atrial septal defect (Kajchuk, 1973), and particularly in patent ductus arteriosus (Hartwell and Tilden, 1943; Deterling and Clagett, 1947; Krückemeijer, 1953; Foord and Lewis, 1959; Shull et al., 1970). The aneurysms may be located in the pulmonary trunk (Figure 4-6) or in intrapulmonary elastic arteries

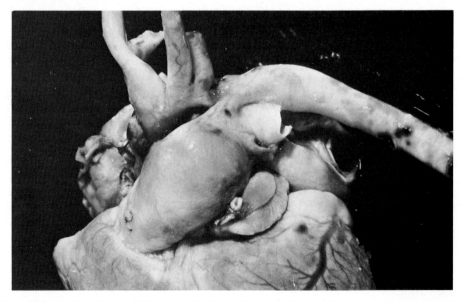

Figure 4-6.   Basis of heart with large arteries in an 18-month-old boy with a common atrioventricular canal. There is a saccular aneurysm of the pulmonary trunk.

(Figure 4-7) but are usually observed in the main pulmonary arteries. In several cases, they are associated with bacterial endocarditis and are clearly mycotic in origin. Sometimes the aneurysm developed after surgical closure of the patent ductus (Kerwin and Jaffe, 1959; Williams et al., 1971). In some instances a congenital weakness of the wall of elastic pulmonary arteries may be basic to their origin (Plokker et al., 1975).

Dissecting aneurysms of the pulmonary trunk or its branches also are observed particularly in patients with patent ductus arteriosus (Ravines, 1960; Kapanci, 1965a; d'Arbela, 1970). Rupture of the pulmonary artery is rare (Ohela and Teir, 1954).

Compression of Airways

Dilatation of main pulmonary arteries in patients with pulmonary hypertension may compress adjacent bronchi particularly of the right lung. This may contribute to accumulation of exudate in the bronchial tree. When the pressure returns to normal after corrective surgery of the cardiac anomaly, the deformity of these bronchi may persist for some time (Edwards, 1967; Stanger et al., 1969). Also, displacement of

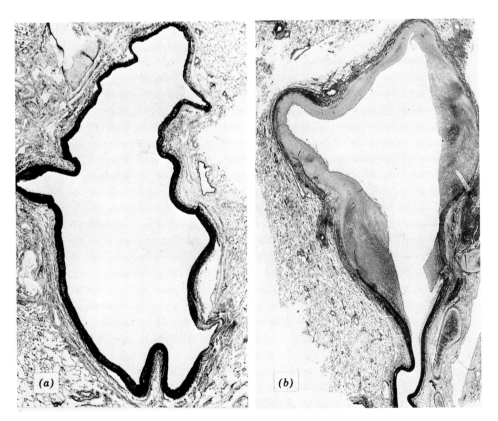

(a)   (b)

Figure 4-7. Aneurysms of elastic pulmonary arteries within the lung of a 26-year-old woman with a ventricular septal defect. In one artery (a) the intima is normal, in the other (b) the wall is thickened as a result of organized thrombosis (El.v.G., ×8).

the aortic arch by the left pulmonary artery may result in an accentuated indentation into the left side of the trachea on a chest roentgenogram (Edwards and Burchell, 1960). Hoarseness may result from impingement on the left recurrent laryngeal nerve at the site of this indentation.

MUSCULAR PULMONARY ARTERIES AND ARTERIOLES

The muscular pulmonary arteries, particularly those of small caliber, form the most reactive part of the vasculature of the lung. These vessels have the greatest influence on pulmonary vascular resistance and are also the vessels most extensively affected in pulmonary arterial hypertension.

In postmortem angiograms (Figure 4-8), but also in histologic sections, these arteries often appear coiled (Figure 4-9). All layers of their wall may be affected in pulmonary hypertension. As a result of obliterative intimal lesions, many arteries in the postmortem arteriogram appear to be cut off so that a "pruning" effect is produced (Figure 4-8).

Medial Hypertrophy

Among the various arterial alterations, medial hypertrophy stands out for two reasons: it is the first and the most common lesion in pulmonary hypertension.

The term "medial hypertrophy" will be used throughout this book, although an increase in the number of smooth muscle cells, or medial hyperplasia, is for the greater part responsible for the thickening of the media (Figure 4-10). There is no doubt, however, that the individual muscle fibers also are increased in size, constituting true hypertrophy, thus contributing to the medial thickness. Moreover, the term "medial hypertrophy" is generally accepted in medical literature.

Medial hypertrophy is a common lesion as it is widespread throughout the lung; it is present in almost all patients with pulmonary arterial hypertension. In spite of occasional assertions to the contrary, it is doubtful if this lesion is ever absent in patients with a significant elevation of the pulmonary arterial pressure. If the vessels are adequately studied, using morphometric methods, it will appear that the average media is thickened, even though in more severe cases, secondary thinning by dilatation or by atrophy resulting from marked intimal fibrosis (p. 67) may influence the average thickness. There are, however, some forms of pulmonary hypertension in which medial hypertrophy is limited to, or at least predominant in, the smallest pulmonary arteries (p. 237).

Since thickening of the media is so common in any form of elevated pulmonary arterial pressure, it can hardly be used in differentiating various types of pulmonary hypertension.

That medial hypertrophy is the first vascular change in cases of pulmonary arterial hypertension is evident from experimental work. In dogs when a shunt is created between systemic and pulmonary circulations, medial hypertrophy of pulmonary arteries may develop within 2 weeks, long before any other vascular changes become apparent (Ferguson et al., 1955; Geer et al., 1965). It is the only lesion generally to be observed in infants with pulmonary hypertension. Other

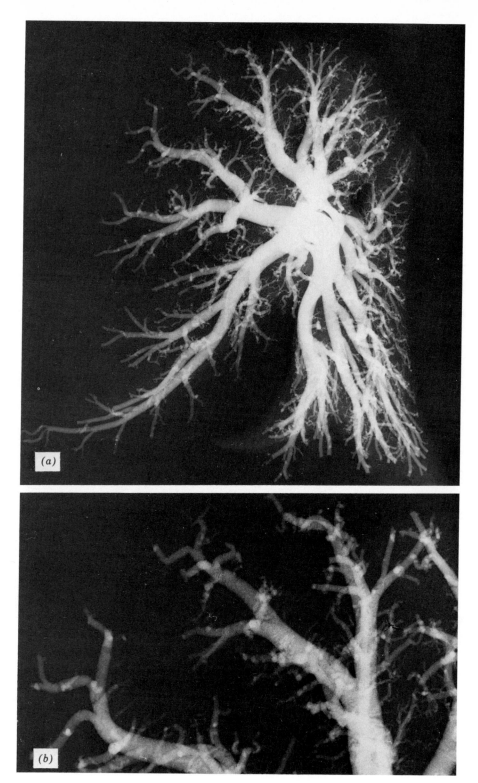

Figure 4-8. Postmortem pulmonary arteriogram (*a*) in a 3-year-old girl with a ventricular septal defect and pulmonary hypertension. There is little background filling, the vasculature has a "pruned tree" appearance and there are many coiled arteries (*b*).

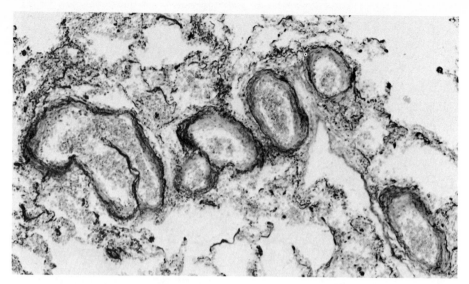

Figure 4-9. Coiled muscular pulmonary artery in a 23-year-old woman with a ventricular septal defect (El.v.G., ×90).

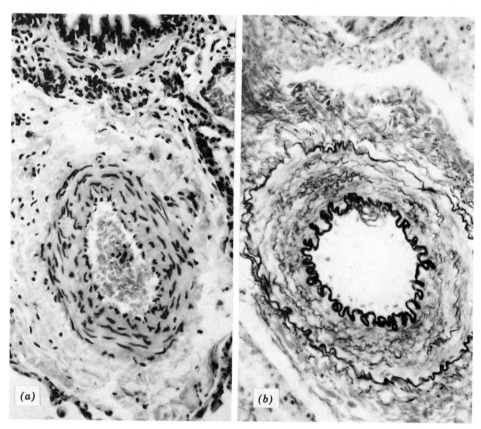

Figure 4-10. Medial hypertrophy of muscular pulmonary arteries in a 3-year-old girl with complete transposition of the large vessels and a ventricular septal defect (*a*) and in an 11-month-old boy with a common atrioventricular canal (*b*) (*a*: H. and E., *b*: El.v.G., ×225).

vascular alterations like intimal fibrosis are uncommon below the age of one or 2 years and rare in the first months of life. In contrast, medial hypertrophy may be present practically from birth in infants with congenital cardiac defects and may be very severe in the first months of life (Wagenvoort, 1962).

The term "persistency" or "carry-over of the fetal type of vessel" has been used (Edwards, 1957) to indicate that the fetal muscular pulmonary arteries which, as we have seen (p. 38), have a thick media, fail to exhibit the fairly abrupt thinning in the early postnatal period, as they do in normal infants. This sometimes has been interpreted as if medial hypertrophy in these cases is a congenital vascular mal-formation. However, during fetal life and at the time of birth, infants with a ventricular septal defect have the same medial thickness of pulmonary arteries as normal fetuses and infants. There is even evidence that after birth there is an initial thinning of the media (Wagenvoort et al., 1961), no doubt due to the markedly increased pulmonary flow and vascular dilatation on mechanical expansion of the lungs. Then, however, the abnormal postnatal hemodynamic situation existing in these infants takes effect and within one to 3 weeks medial hypertrophy develops. The normal downward trend in thickness of the media is interrupted and within one or 2 months the media may be much thicker than at the time of birth (Figure 4-11). In view of this development it is clear that medial hypertrophy is a postnatal adaptation and not a congenital disorder.

The increase of medial smooth muscle finds its expression not only in thickening of the muscular layer but also in an extension of media in a peripheral direction. While normally a continuous muscular coat is absent in arterioles of a caliber below 70 μ, in pulmonary hypertension new muscle fibers develop in these small vessels so that a distinct media may be present in arterioles of 30 μ or even 20 μ in diameter (Figure 4-12). This extension over the length of the arterial pathway may contribute considerably to the effectiveness of medial hypertrophy in determining vascular resistance.

As we have discussed in Chapter One, pulmonary arteries and arterioles have a vascular tone, supplied by the smooth muscle fibers of their media. This tone may vary and, although normally of little effect as a result of the thin muscular layer in the arteries, these vessels may actively dilate and constrict. Prolonged vasoconstriction leads to medial hypertrophy. This is a fair assumption since everywhere in the body increased activity of muscle fibers produces hypertrophy of muscle.

Obviously the increased amount of vascular smooth muscle may produce a more effective vasoconstriction. This explains why the effect of drugs, acting as constrictors or dilators, is much more apparent in patients with pulmonary hypertension and marked medial hypertrophy than in normal individuals (Harris and Heath, 1962).

Vasoconstriction may cause problems for the pathologist assessing the degree of medial hypertrophy. When an artery is constricted, the thickness of its wall increases and its lumen narrows. It is often assumed that after death the effect of constriction subsides but this is generally not true. We know, also from experiments in which vasoconstriction has been produced, that the thick-walled constricted artery as a rule remains in that state, even in histologic sections (p. 31). This means that a thick media may result from either vasoconstriction or from medial hypertrophy or from a combination of both (Short, 1962). The problem may be solved by assessing the amount of medial muscle tissue in relation to the amount of lung tissue in which it occurs in the histologic sections (Wagenvoort, 1960), but this

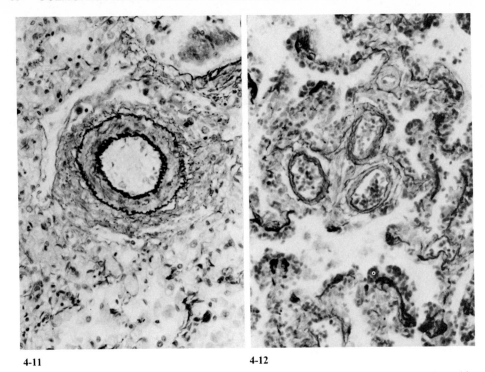

4-11   4-12

Figure 4-11.   Muscular pulmonary artery with marked medial hypertrophy in a 2-month-old boy with a ventricular septal defect (El.v.G., ×225).

Figure 4-12.   Pulmonary arterioles with muscularization in a 4-year-old boy with a ventricular septal defect. There is a distinct muscular media in arterioles of a diameter from 20 to 30 μ (El.v.G., ×225).

method is laborious and time consuming. Fortunately, such studies have shown that the contribution of vasoconstriction to the thickening of the media is limited as compared to that of hypertrophy. In man, if the average pulmonary arterial media is distinctly thickened, then there is medial hypertrophy even if vasoconstriction contributes to the thickening. This relationship does not apply to some animals. In the rabbit a pronounced increase of medial thickness may be brought about by constriction alone (Van Zandwijk et al., 1976).

It also must be realized that the lung vessels as seen in histologic sections are collapsed and therefore do not reflect their state during life. The internal elastic lamina is almost always crenated, but the degree of crenation increases when there is vasoconstriction. Attempts to overcome this difficulty by infusing the vessels with formalin or other fluids are hazardous, even when "physiologic pressures" are used. When the vascular tone is lost after death, the muscle fibers do not resist an intravascular pressure the same way living muscle fibers do, and the arteries may be blown up in an irregular way by relatively low pressures.

A better method is to instill formalin or another fixative into the trachea while the lungs are in situ. When the lungs are distended in this way, collapse of the lung vessels is prevented. The pulmonary arteries in cross-section generally have a circular and smooth circumference. The presence of vasoconstriction, however, remains recognizable by crenation of the elastic laminae, as is demonstrated in experiments (p. 238).

Levin et al. (1976) advocated arterial injection with a fixative under physiologic pressures. They worked with fetal lambs that were injected immediately after death. In this situation the results may be reliable, but we cannot agree with them that a similar method should be used in human material for reasons just explained. If one wants to study bronchi and bronchioli, the pulmonary vessels should be injected; if on the other hand, one wants to study the lung vessels, these should not be manipulated, but instillation of bronchi with the fixative is useful.

Often it is not possible to use the instillation technique in human lungs from autopsy and never in lung biopsies. In our experience a reliable and reproducible assessment of the medial thickness is to apply morphometry to vessels in collapsed, formalin-fixed lung tissue, and to compare them with those from similarly treated control lungs. If pulmonary hypertension is present, the mean medial thickness will be over 7 percent of the external diameter. In older children and adults it is often in the range of 10 to 15 percent. In infants much higher mean values (20 to 25 percent) may be obtained, with mean values for individual arterioles up to 30 or 35 percent.

Marked intimal fibrosis may lead to secondary atrophy of the media (Figure 4-13), while this layer may also become thinner when dilatation lesions develop. Since these severe alterations are virtually absent in infants and younger children, this in part may explain that their arterial media is thicker than in adults, but even so, there is little doubt that in infants the pulmonary arteries have a greater capacity for developing medial hypertrophy than in adults.

Sometimes in infants with congenital shunts between systemic and pulmonary circulations, who succumb shortly after birth, the muscular pulmonary arteries are dilated and relatively thin-walled. These infants apparently die from pulmonary edema (Dammann and Ferencz, 1956; Heath et al., 1958). It is likely that in these instances the pulmonary arteries gave way to the elevated pressure before the arterial smooth muscle was adequately adapted to it.

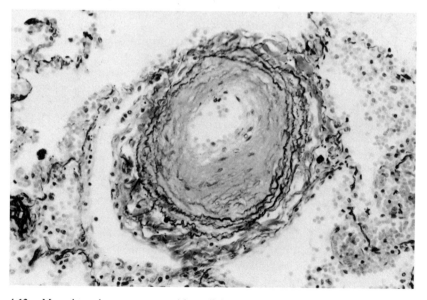

Figure 4-13. Muscular pulmonary artery with medial atrophy due to severe intimal thickening in a 23-year-old woman with a ventricular septal defect (El.v.G., ×225).

Intimal Proliferation and Fibrosis

If pulmonary hypertension develops in patients with congenital cardiac disease with a shunt, intimal thickening is a common although not a very early occurring lesion. Infants and young children with these cardiac anomalies rarely show vascular alterations other than medial hypertrophy. Small thrombi occasionally are observed although in our experience not as often as reported by Naeye (1966). After the age of 2 the chance that the intima is affected, increases.

Advanced intimal fibrosis has great consequences for the pulmonary circulation. By narrowing or obstructing muscular pulmonary arteries and arterioles, the vascular resistance rises further. This resistance was already raised in the stage of vasoconstriction and medial hypertrophy but then the vessels may potentially dilate and the resistance may fall, notably when the cardiac anomaly is repaired. Edwards (1957) introduced the term "high resistance-high reserve" for this type of vascular bed. In the presence of extensive obliterative intimal lesions there is a "high resistance-low reserve" vascular bed. Closure of the defect will not substantially reduce the vascular resistance, and the pressure may remain the same or may increase since there is no longer a safety valve provided by the defect. Postoperative right cardiac failure may result in death of the patient.

Cellular Intimal Proliferation

The process of thickening of the intima begins with proliferation of cells. It is a fairly common lesion, present in the lungs of many patients with congenital cardiac shunts. Usually other arteries or other segments of the same artery show intimal fibrosis.

The earliest stages in the development of this lesion are not often observed. However, they may be seen in occasional pulmonary arteries in the presence of congenital cardiac shunts. These changes are more widespread in cases of subacute pulmonary hypertension. If in patients with tetralogy of Fallot, who underwent a complete surgical repair, the patch used for closure of the ventricular septal defect becomes partially detached, the pulmonary vasculature is exposed for the first time to high pressures, the pulmonic stenosis now having been removed. A similar situation may occur when too large a surgical anastomosis is created between systemic and pulmonary circulations and gives rise to pulmonary hypertension.

In these instances, if the patient dies shortly after operation and lung tissue is available for study, it may appear that numerous muscular pulmonary arteries and arterioles show the very early lesions of cellular intimal proliferation (Wagenvoort et al., 1964). From such uncommon cases we know that this growth of intimal cells may begin within 2 weeks and may have formed a fairly thick layer within 2 months after the sudden elevation of pulmonary arterial pressure occurred.

It is interesting to realize that intimal lesions may develop in a very short time when pulmonary hypertension develops very suddenly, whereas the lesions develop rarely within the first years of life if pulmonary hypertension is congenital. The obvious explanation is that the thick media of the pulmonary arteries in the perinatal period, subsequently strengthened by medial hypertrophy, can adequately cope with the elevated pressure for a long time, while in the cases of sudden postoperative pulmonary hypertension these vessels are thin and unprepared.

It appears regularly that the proliferating cells of the intima are arranged perpendicularly to the internal elastic lamina (Figure 4-14) and sometimes can be demonstrated to penetrate this lamina. This suggests that these cells are not, or not only, derived from the endothelial layer but may be formed by medial cells. This would be consistent with the observation by others that in systemic arteries multipotent cells from the media are involved in the development of intimal thickening (Backwinkel et al., 1973; Webster et al., 1974).

It also is borne out by our own observations that in electron-micrographs the cells in the areas of intimal fibrosis have all the characteristics of smooth muscle cells, although they usually are arranged haphazardly. It is likely that in all forms of intimal fibrosis, thus also in age changes and in chronic pulmonary venous hypertension, the constituents of the intimal thickening are smooth muscle cells rather than fibroblasts or endothelial cells. Thrombosis with subsequent organization does not seem to play a part in the process.

In the course of time the loose reticulated layer of intimal cells becomes thicker and also more compact (Figure 4-15). From the beginning the whole circumference of the pulmonary artery, as seen in cross section in a histologic slide, is involved and cellular proliferation tends to be concentric. Eventually, mucoid changes by accumulation of mucopolysaccharides within the layer, may be added to the picture, although this is not always prominent.

Intimal Fibrosis

Gradually collagen fibers are deposited in the cellular intimal layer, which becomes more and more fibrosed (Figure 4-16). Elastic fibers may follow, although with greater variation. Elastosis of the intima may be either completely absent or very marked.

Intimal fibrosis is thus the stage following that of active cellular proliferation. Both show widespread distribution within the pulmonary arterial tree, often extending over a long distance along the vessels, and usually concentric arrangement in the arterial cross section. Apart from the content of collagen and elastic fibers, intimal fibrosis differs from cellular proliferation by its laminar, onionskin-like configuration (Figure 4-17). This concentric laminar intimal fibrosis is a highly characteristic feature of this form of pulmonary hypertension.

In other forms of pulmonary hypertension intimal fibrosis may present itself in occasional arteries as a concentric layer. Sometimes we see this in embolic pulmonary hypertension and more often in mitral stenosis, although in most arteries it is excentric. In these conditions, however, the laminar, onionskin arrangement generally is missing.

If there is elastosis of the intima, an elastic stain sometimes may give the impression of a concentric laminar configuration which may be mistaken for this type of intimal fibrosis but in pulmonary hypertension due to cardiac shunts, the onionskin layering usually can be observed in a hematoxylin stain (Figure 4-18).

In the late stages of the disease complete obstruction of pulmonary arteries and arterioles is common. When the patient is in this stage of high resistance-low reserve vascular bed with rigid and occluded pulmonary arteries, repair of the underlying cardiac malformation will be of little avail and is even likely to hasten death.

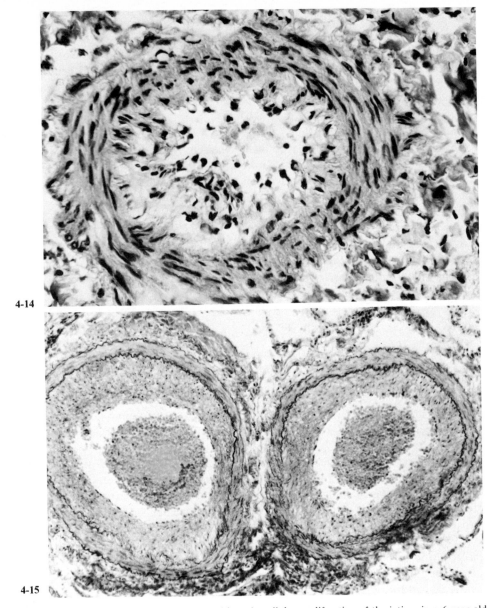

4-14

4-15

Figure 4-14. Muscular pulmonary artery with early cellular proliferation of the intima in a 6-year-old girl with a ventricular septal defect. Intimal cells tend to be arranged perpendicularly to the media (H. and E., ×350).

Figure 4-15. Two branches of a muscular pulmonary artery, narrowed by pronounced cellular intimal proliferation in a 5-year-old girl with a ventricular septal defect (El.v.G., ×140).

Therefore, such cases generally will not be subjected to surgery. This explains the usually great difference between the findings in autopsy material from such cases and those in lung biopsies taken at operation. In the latter, the intimal changes tend to be comparatively mild.

If such lung biopsies are regularly taken at operation and studied, there appears to be a correlation between the degree of intimal fibrosis and the pressure existing in

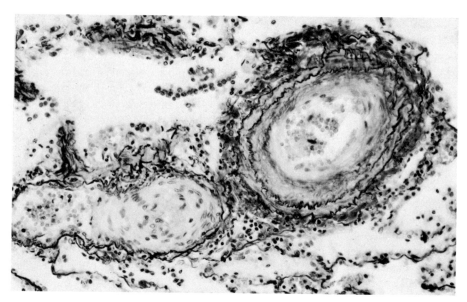

Figure 4-16. Muscular pulmonary artery with early fibrosis of the intima in a 5-year-old girl with a ventricular septal defect. A branch (left) is occluded by cellular intimal proliferation (El.v.G., ×225).

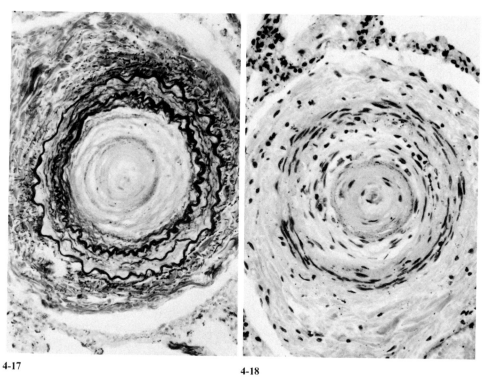

4-17

4-18

Figure 4-17. Muscular pulmonary artery with concentric laminar intimal fibrosis in a 3-year-old boy with common atrioventricular canal (El.v.G., ×225).

Figure 4-18. Muscular pulmonary artery from the same case as Figure 4-17. Concentric laminar intimal fibrosis is also distinct in a hematoxylin stain (H. and E., ×225).

the pulmonary circulation (Wagenvoort et al., 1967). No such correlation could be found with the degree of pulmonary flow, at least if those cases are omitted in which pulmonary vascular disease was so advanced that the flow was secondarily reduced.

This lack of correlation between intimal fibrosis and pulmonary flow was particularly striking in patients with atrial septal defect in whom, even in the presence of very large flow, the pulmonary arteries were often almost or even entirely free of intimal fibrosis as long as there was no marked elevation of pressures.

In this respect our experience is at variance with that of Heath and Edwards (1958), who maintain that in atrial septal defect intimal fibrosis is common in the smaller arterioles, particularly in older patients, and that is the result of the increased flow.

There is no doubt that with increasing age, patients with a large atrial septal defect tend to develop an elevated pulmonary arterial pressure, although even then severe pulmonary hypertension is uncommon. In the absence of pulmonary hypertension, however, we found that even in most adult patients with atrial septal defect, intimal fibrosis was not significantly increased as compared to that which is seen regularly as an age change.

Fibrinoid Necrosis and Arteritis

If in patients with congenital cardiac shunts pulmonary hypertension becomes severe, in addition to medial hypertrophy and intimal fibrosis, areas of arterial necrosis may become apparent (Figure 4-19). This necrosis never occurs over long distances but usually is confined to fairly small areas of the arterial wall. Either the whole circumference or part of it is affected, and sometimes the process is limited to a small spot corresponding to a few smooth muscle fibers.

Often the segment with fibrinoid necrosis is located in a small artery shortly after its ramification from a larger branch (Figure 4-20). In some instances there is marked intimal fibrosis of the parent artery and around the orifice of the branch with narrowing of the lumen.

In the areas of necrosis there is loss of muscle fiber nuclei, and fibrin is deposited in the wall of the artery. In an hematoxylin stain this material stands out by its bright eosinophilic color. The media initially is swollen at the site of fibrinoid necrosis; this is particularly apparent when part of the circumference is affected (Figure 4-21). The wall in this area is thicker than at the opposite side. In the lumen a fibrin clot usually is formed (Figure 4-22), at least when the greater part of the cross-sectional circumference is affected.

The fibrinoid necrosis in these instances may well be comparable to that described in the systemic circulation (Byrom, 1954; Lober and Lillehei, 1954; Singleton et al., 1959).

Often the internal or external elastic laminae or both, become interrupted in the necrotic area. Either by retraction of the elastic membranes or by their destruction, they may be missing over a large portion of the vascular circumference.

An inflammatory reaction to this vascular necrosis may occur. In some cases it is completely absent; in others it may be pronounced, and then it consists usually of polymorphonuclear leucocytes (Figure 4-23). These not only lie within the wall, thus contributing to the swelling of the media, but may extend both into the fibrin clot

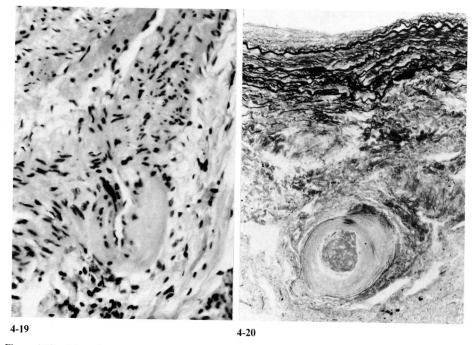

4-19   4-20

Figure 4-19. Muscular pulmonary artery with fibrinoid necrosis in a 3-year-old girl with complete transposition of the large vessels and a ventricular septal defect (H. and E., ×225).

Figure 4-20. Muscular pulmonary artery with fibrinoid necrosis in a 3-year-old boy with common atrioventricular canal. The necrosis usually is situated in a branch not far from its parent artery (top) (El.v.G., ×90).

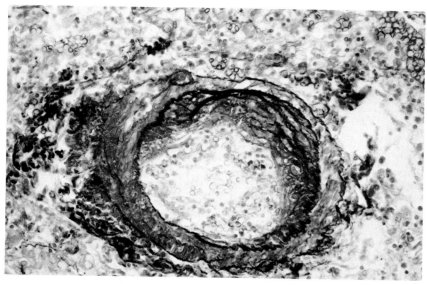

Figure 4-21. Muscular pulmonary artery with fibrinoid necrosis in a part of its circumference in a 13-year-old girl with a patent ductus arteriosus. The media in the affected area (left) is swollen (El.v.G., ×225).

73

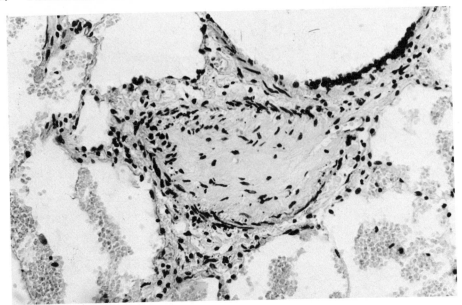

Figure 4-22.   Muscular pulmonary artery with fibrinoid necrosis in a 20-year-old woman with a ventricular septal defect. The lumen is occluded by a fibrin clot (H. and E., ×225).

within the lumen and into the adventitia. Often the cellular exudate spreads further than the vascular wall, extending into the alveolar spaces. In the course of time lymphocytes and plasma cells may replace the polymorphonuclear leucocytes.

If the patient survives, the older stages of pulmonary arteritis may be recognized, although the inflammatory exudate tends to disappear completely. The arterial wall,

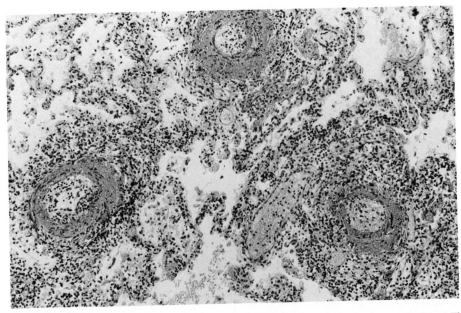

Figure 4-23.   Necrotizing pulmonary arteritis in a 13-year-old girl with a patent ductus arteriosus. The inflammatory exudate extends far into the surrounding lung tissue (H. and E., ×90).

however, has become very thin and fibrous, with the media completely absent in some areas. In those instances the wall consists of an elastic membrane overlying the adventitia and lined by an intima which may be thickened. The part played by fibrinoid necrosis and arteritis in the formation of plexiform lesions is discussed later (p. 78).

Fibrinoid necrosis with or without arteritis is not a pathognomonic feature, since it may occur in other forms of pulmonary hypertension. It is, however, so much more common in pulmonary hypertension due to cardiac shunts and in primary pulmonary hypertension (p. 130) than in other conditions, that it may help in establishing a morphologic diagnosis.

In some patients the lungs contain only very few pulmonary arteries with fibrinoid necrosis and arteritis, in others numerous vessels are affected, particularly the small pulmonary arteries and arterioles. Arteries with an external diameter in excess of 150 μ rarely are involved.

The mechanism basic to fibrinoid necrosis of pulmonary arteries is not known, but it is likely that severe pulmonary hypertension and particularly intense spastic contraction of the medial smooth muscle tissue produces the areas of necrosis. Subsequently fibrin may seep into the wall from the lumen (Wagenvoort, 1959). The following arguments favor such a hypothesis. Fibrinoid necrosis is observed in cases of severe pulmonary hypertension and particularly in such cases in which marked vasoconstriction seems likely, as in congenital cardiac shunts and primary pulmonary hypertension (Wood, 1959). The process begins in the media and often immediately after a ramification from a larger artery, thus in an area in which the wall is likely to be submitted to relatively greater stress. As we have seen, in some instances the orifice of the branch, immediately proximal to the area with fibrinoid necrosis, is narrowed by intimal fibrosis. This suggests that a jet lesion sometimes may also elicit necrosis of the media. Similar changes may be observed in systemic arteries exposed to prolonged hypertension or to sudden increase of pressure as after excision of a coarctation of the aorta. The inflammatory cellular exudate in all likelihood is reactive to the necrosis of the muscle fibers. Experimental work also suggests a relation between vasoconstriction and medial necrosis (p. 104). How far damage to the endothelium is essential to the process of fibrinoid necrosis, and if so, whether such damage is concomitant with, secondary to, or even preceding the medial necrosis remains to be solved.

The picture of hypertensive pulmonary arteritis may resemble that of polyarteritis nodosa and probably has been confused with this condition at times. According to Spencer (1957) in polyarteritis nodosa the inflammatory reaction is more widespread, but as we have shown, this is not always a safe mark of distinction. In patients with a ventricular septal defect or primary pulmonary hypertension exhibiting pulmonary arteritis, there are to our knowledge never lesions of polyarteritis nodosa in systemic arteries, while conversely in patients with polyarteritis nodosa, as a rule the pulmonary arteries are not, or hardly, affected (Sweeney and Baggenstoss, 1949).

Plexiform Lesions

In addition to fibrinoid necrosis and arteritis, there are other vascular alterations occurring only in the more severe cases of vasoconstrictive pulmonary hypertension.

One of these is the so-called plexiform lesion. Plexiform lesions are rather complex and also highly characteristic changes. Although they are not easily overlooked in histologic sections, particularly not when stained with hematoxylin, they may be missed when an insufficient number of blocks of lung tissue is studied. Cases of congenital heart disease with pulmonary hypertension exhibiting these alterations in the pulmonary arteries are not at all rare, but the incidence of these changes in a given case varies greatly. Often they are so frequent that one section contains many examples but sometimes 10 histologic sections or more have to be studied before one plexiform lesion can be found.

Plexiform lesions are situated in muscular pulmonary arteries with an external diameter usually in the range of 100 to 200 μ and usually shortly after its ramification from a larger vessel.

Their description varies with their stage of development. In its most characteristic form there is a local dilatation of a small segment of the arterial branch often with destruction of a part of its wall (Figure 4-24). Remnants of fibrinoid necrosis and an inflammatory exudate are often present in this area but this also depends on the phase of development of the lesion. The widened lumen in the area contains a plexus of small slits or channels separated by strands of proliferating intimal cells with dark nuclei. The channels open up at the distal end of the lesion into a markedly dilated and thin-walled but patent portion of the artery.

The parent artery, from which the branch containing the plexiform lesion has arisen, always has a hypertrophic media. It also may show concentric laminar intimal fibrosis, with narrowing of the orifice, but this is by no means a constant feature. Sometimes part of the plexus of channels and cellular strands extend retrograd into the parent artery (Figure 4-25). In such instances dependent on the plane of sec-

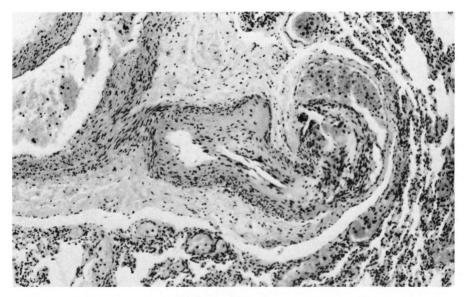

Figure 4-24. Plexiform lesion in a branch of a pulmonary artery in a 3-year-old boy with a common atrioventricular canal. Distal to the plexus there is a dilated thin-walled segment of the branch (H. and E., ×90).

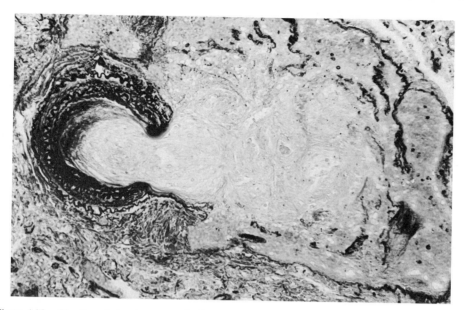

Figure 4-25. Plexiform lesion in a muscular branch of an elastic pulmonary artery (left) in a 5-year-old boy with a ventricular septal defect. The plexiform lesion extends retrograd into the parent artery (El.v.G., ×140).

tion, it may seem that a large artery with intact wall contains a plexiform lesion, while it is essentially part of an alteration in one of its branches.

The pathogenesis of the plexiform lesions has given rise to much speculation and confusion. As the segment with the plexus connects a distinct muscular pulmonary artery with the dilated, very thin-walled distal portion of the vessel, which may be taken for a vein, the lesions often have been interpreted as pulmonary arteriovenous anastomoses (Kucsko, 1949, 1953; Spencer, 1950; Rutishauser and Blanc, 1950; Unschold, 1952; Gordon et al., 1954; Jewett and Ober, 1956; Hufner and McNicol, 1958; McCormack, 1959).

When the plexiform lesions are studied in serial sections, it can be demonstrated that in principle there are no anastomosing channels but that the distal part of the vessel can be traced to small arterioles and alveolar capillaries (Brewer, 1955; Wagenvoort, 1959; Naeye and Vennart, 1960). Occasional tiny connections with a branch of a bronchial artery or of a pulmonary vein (Brewer, 1955; Heath, 1957, Brewer and Heath, 1959) have been described but these are obviously not essential.

The plexiform structures also have been taken for multiple angiomas (Plaut, 1940) and for congenital malformations of the vessels (Zur Linden, 1924; Rutishauser and Feuardent, 1952; Moschcowitz et al., 1961; Stanisic, 1967).

Our arguments for an acquired nature of these lesions in part have been pointed out before (Wagenvoort et al., 1964). The statement of Moschcowitz and associates (1961) that plexiform lesions do not occur in acquired heart disease with pulmonary hypertension, such as mitral stenosis, but only in congenital heart disease, cannot be accepted as an argument for a congenital nature of these structures. Plexiform lesions occur *only* in congenital heart disease when pulmonary hypertension is present. They occur never in patients with pulmonic stenosis or tetralogy of Fallot, except for those uncommon cases in which too large a surgical shunt, created between systemic and pulmonary circulations, caused pulmonary hypertension (Ross et al., 1958; Wagenvoort et al., 1960).

The production of plexiform lesions in animals with experimental pulmonary hypertension due to a shunt between systemic and pulmonary circulations (see below) provides additional proof that the lesions are acquired.

Moreover, as mentioned, various stages can be recognized in the development of the plexiform lesions even within the same lung. Such a gradual development not only is consistent with an acquired rather than with a congenital origin but also permits a better understanding of their pathogenesis. Although plexiform lesions are very rare in young infants they have been observed at ages between 3 weeks and 4 months (Hruban and Humphreys, 1960; Wagenvoort, 1962; Kanjuh et al., 1964; Kapanci, 1965b). In these instances very early stages always are seen.

As we have stated before (Wagenvoort, 1959, 1973), we believe that plexiform lesions gradually develop in areas affected by necrotizing arteritis for the following reasons. Both vascular alterations occur only in the more severe cases of pulmonary hypertension and both are found in the same class of muscular pulmonary arteries and arterioles with a preference for an area shortly after a ramification from a larger vessel. Generally, in a plexiform lesion the wall of the aneurysm-like segment containing the plexus, shows signs of destruction which are suggestive of previous necrotizing arteritis and in many instances active fibrinoid necrosis is present in this segment. The lumina of the channels in the plexus very often contain remnants of a clot consisting of fibrin and platelets. Polymorphonuclear or more often mononuclear inflammatory cells also are seen regularly in or around the lesions. Though this has been denied by some authors (Moschcowitz et al., 1961), it may suffice to point out that many others, who were under the impression that plexiform lesions represented arteriovenous anastomoses, used the term "anastomositis" to stress the rather common finding of an inflammatory reaction (Kucsko, 1949; Chiari, 1950; Unschold, 1952).

From the various stages that may be recognized in the development of the plexiform lesions and particularly from the rather uncommon early stages, the following course of events can be deduced. Fibrinoid necrosis of a small segment of a pulmonary arterial branch leads to destruction of a part of the media with subsequent aneurysm-like dilatation and the formation of a fibrin clot in the lumen often with admixture of platelets. By organization of this clot by strands of intimal cells (Figures 4-26, 4-27, 4-28, 4-29, 4-30) the plexus is formed. Small capillary-like channels within the plexus (Figure 4-31) provide some sort of continuity of the lumen. The distal part of the artery undergoes marked poststenotic dilatation. In the course of time the inflammatory component subsides, the fibrin disappears, the strands of intimal cells become somewhat more fibrosed, and the channels inbetween wider (Figures 4-32 and 4-33).

Additional proof for such a pathogenesis of the plexiform lesion has been provided by experiments. In dogs with a surgical creation of a shunt between systemic and pulmonary circulations, fibrinoid necrosis and arteritis preceded the development of plexiform lesions (Downing et al., 1963; Harley et al., 1968; Saldana et al., 1968).

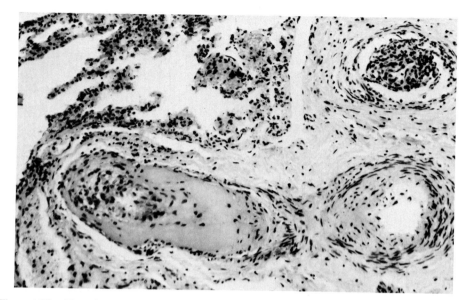

Figure 4-26. Muscular pulmonary arteries in a 3-year-old boy with a common atrioventricular canal. The parent artery (lower right) is narrowed by intimal fibrosis. One branch (left) shows necrotizing arteritis with early organization of the fibrin clot. Another branch (upper right) contains an early plexiform lesion (H. and E., ×140).

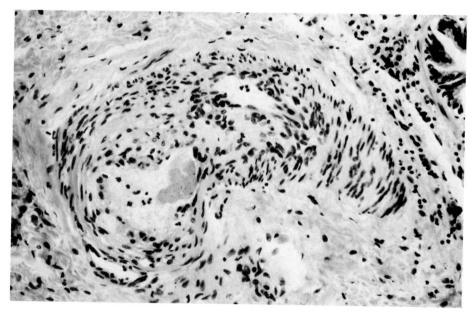

Figure 4-27. Muscular pulmonary artery from the same case as Figure 4-26 with some areas of fibrinoid necrosis and with early organization of a fibrin clot. Remnants of fibrin and platelets are recognizable in the lumen (H. and E., ×225).

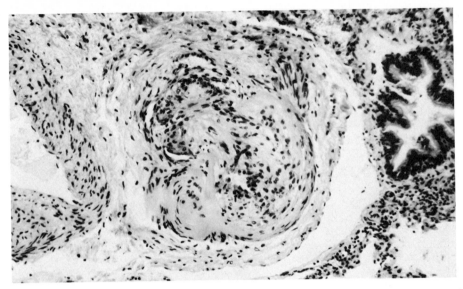

Figure 4-28. Muscular pulmonary artery with early plexiform lesion from the same case as Figure 4-26. There is fibrinoid necrosis of the media and active proliferation of intimal cells (H. and E., ×140).

Dilatation Lesions

Heath and Edwards (1958) introduced the term "dilatation lesions" to indicate all arterial alterations in which dilatation, resulting from sustained pulmonary arterial hypertension, plays a part. Therefore, this term included the plexiform lesions. Since the plexiform lesion is so characteristic and easily recognizable in histologic sections

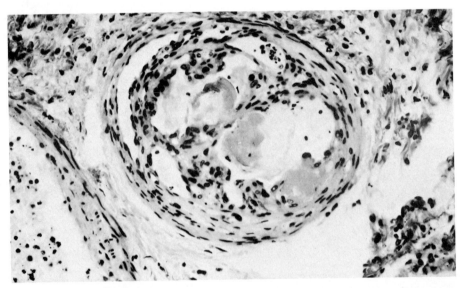

Figure 4-29. Muscular pulmonary artery with early plexiform lesion from the same case as Figure 4-26. Strands of intimal cells are proliferating within a clot composed of fibrin and platelets (H. and E., ×225).

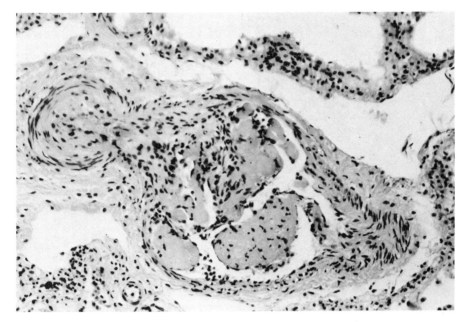

Figure 4-30. Muscular pulmonary artery with early plexiform lesion in an 11-month-old male infant with a common atrioventricular canal. There is organization and recanalization of a fibrin clot (H. and E., ×140).

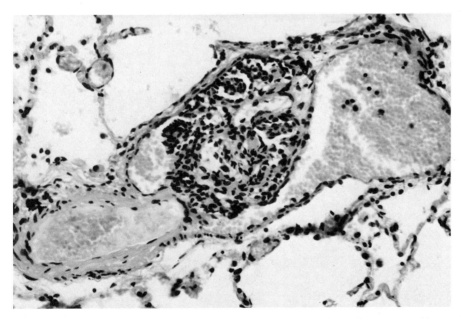

Figure 4-31. Muscular pulmonary artery with characteristic plexiform lesion in a 20-year-old woman with a ventricular septal defect. A fully developed plexus of channels is flanked by a parent artery (left) showing fibrinoid necrosis and by a dilated thin-walled distal segment (right) of the artery (H. and E., ×225).

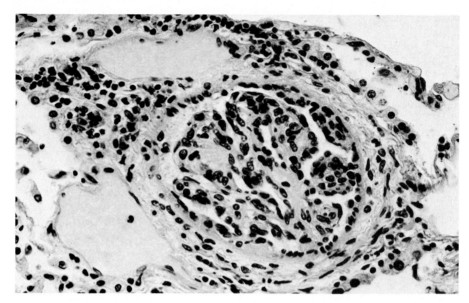

Figure 4-32. Muscular pulmonary artery with plexiform lesion in a 45-year-old woman with a large atrial septal defect and pulmonary hypertension. The lesion is more advanced with collagen deposition in the strands between the channels (H. and E., ×350).

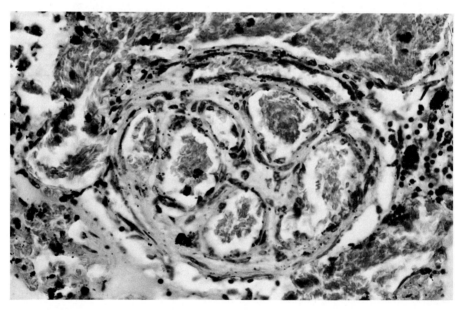

Figure 4-33. Muscular pulmonary artery with an old stage of plexiform lesion in a 22-year-old woman with patent ductus arteriosus. Without the use of serial sections, this lesion cannot be distinguished from an old organized and recanalized thromboembolus (H. and E., ×350).

and since dilatation is not its most striking feature, we prefer to limit the use of the term "dilatation lesions" to those alterations in which dilatation is the predominant, if not the only, feature.

In longstanding vasoconstrictive pulmonary hypertension, dilatation, often over a considerable length of the vessels, will lead to thinning of the arterial wall. This may decrease the average thickness of the arterial media considerably (p. 62). Such an artery may mimic a normal pulmonary artery. Even virtually all the media may disappear so that "vein-like branches of hypertrophied muscular pulmonary arteries" (Heath and Edwards, 1958) are formed (Figure 4-34). An abrupt transition of a thick media to a very thin media may be observed. These vessels often are tortuous and may form clusters of dilated vessels. The fairly uncommon "angiomatoid lesion" is essentially a dilatation lesion in which widening of the channels and particularly dilatation and tortuosity of the surrounding distal branches, produces a fairly large, angioma-like mass (Figure 4-35).

Dilatation lesions, generally, are common in severe pulmonary hypertension, particularly in adult patients. Very often they are found in lungs, containing plexiform lesions but they may occur in the absence of these alterations. Fibrinoid necrosis, in all probability is not responsible for their development. The parent artery, or the initial portion of the branch in which dilatation lesions occur, is often severely narrowed by intimal fibrosis (Figure 4-36). It is therefore likely that also dilatation lesions are an expression of a poststenotic dilatation.

ALVEOLAR CAPILLARIES

Apart from congestion, sometimes observed in cases of pulmonary hypertension due to cardiac left to right shunts, the alveolar capillaries are generally unremarkable

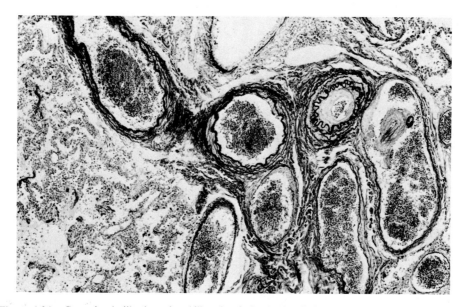

Figure 4-34. Several vein-like branches (dilatation lesions) of coiled muscular pulmonary artery in a 5-year-old girl with ventricular septal defect (El.v.G., ×90).

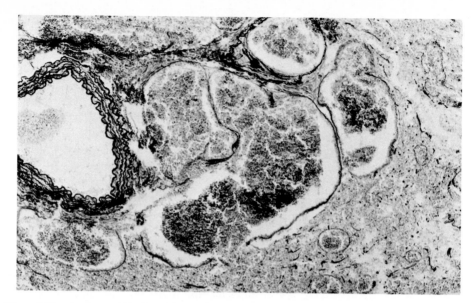

Figure 4-35. Angiomatoid lesion (dilatation lesion) in a muscular branch of an elastic pulmonary artery (left) in a 4-year-old boy with ventricular septal defect (El.v.G., ×90).

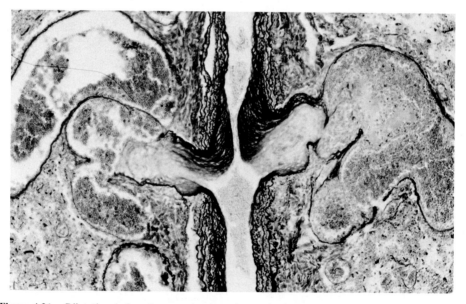

Figure 4-36. Dilatation lesions in muscular branches at both sides of an elastic pulmonary artery (center) from the same case as Figure 4-35. There is fibrous stenosis at the origin of both branches (El.v.G., ×90).

when observed with the light microscope. Electron-microscopic studies revealed some thickening of the alveolar-capillary membrane, particularly of the endothelial layer while the basement membrane is not or only in some cases thicker than normal (Turunen and Stjernvall, 1959; Coalson et al., 1967).

PULMONARY VEINS AND VENULES

The pulmonary veins and venules as a rule are unaffected in these patients. In complicated cases there may be thickening of the venous media and intima but this is infrequent.

HEMOSIDEROSIS

Iron pigment, derived from desintegrated erythrocytes after diapedesis or bursting of a small vessel, is accumulated in siderophages or is deposited in the interstitial connective tissue of lung or pleura. Although there is generally some degree of hemosiderosis in pulmonary hypertension due to congenital heart disease, it is certainly not a specific or characteristic alteration. Other parenchymal lesions in the lungs are even less common in these instances. A granulomatous reaction around cholesterol-laden macrophages is sometimes observed (Glancy et al., 1968) but we agree with Littler et al. (1969) that this may be found in a wide variety of conditions.

PLEXOGENIC PULMONARY ARTERIOPATHY

The pattern of pulmonary vascular lesions, just described, as it is observed in patients with cardiac left to right shunts, is characteristic but not pathognomonic for these cases since the same type of vascular disease is observed in the lungs of patients with primary pulmonary hypertension, for example. To indicate this morphologic pattern the term "plexogenic pulmonary arteriopathy" has been proposed by the W.H.O. Committee on Primary Pulmonary Hypertension (1975).

This term implies that the most typical alteration, the plexiform lesion, is an end-result in the development, even though it is not necessarily present in all cases. In its fully developed stage, plexogenic pulmonary arteriopathy is characterized by medial hypertrophy, concentric-laminar intimal fibrosis, necrotizing arteritis, dilatation lesions, and plexiform lesions. When the pattern is incomplete, and particularly when the vascular disease did not advance beyond the stage of medial hypertrophy, it may be impossible to make an accurate diagnosis.

We will come back to the morphologic pattern of plexogenic pulmonary arteriopathy in subsequent chapters and especially in relation to primary pulmonary hypertension (p. 127).

PROGNOSIS IN RELATION TO VASCULAR LESIONS

The various lesions described in the pulmonary arteries in patients with congenital heart disease with a shunt have prognostic significance. It is clear, however, that the natural history of these conditions shows a wide spectrum of clinical and hemodynamic patterns. There are many patients in whom the pulmonary arterial pressure remains stationary or even falls after the first or second year of life without surgical intervention and apparently without spontaneous closure of a ventricular septal defect. For that reason some authors believe that fear of progressive pulmonary vascular disease has no place in deciding on conservative versus surgical approach (Nadas et al., 1960; Lynfield et al., 1961; Hoffman and Rudolph, 1965).

On the other hand, a gradual progression of hypertensive pulmonary vascular disease has been observed in 5 to 20 percent of the cases (Weidman and DuShane, 1974a), and this progression is sometimes so rapid that its development may elude the clinicians in spite of close follow-up (Anderson et al., 1967). For these reasons and in view of the fact that the risk of the more severe changes increases after the age of 2, an early repair of the cardiac anomaly seems advisable, particularly when the defect is large (Friedli et al., 1974; Vogel et al., 1974; Weidman and DuShane, 1974b).

Surgical closure of a ventricular septal defect or of a patent ductus arteriosus does not always forestall progression of pulmonary hypertension and vascular pathology, particularly when the patients are over the age of 2 at the time of operation (Weidman and DuShane, 1974a). Progression of pulmonary hypertension also has been noted following spontaneous closure of a ventricular septal defect. (Shemtov et al., 1973).

An infant, described by Bessinger et al. (1975), developed severe hypertensive pulmonary vascular disease including plexiform lesions, in spite of ligation of a patent ductus arteriosus at the age of four months. It died 3 years later. These researchers raised the possibility that the vascular disease had a primary cause rather than being the result of the patent ductus.

In pulmonary hypertension when the increased pressure is of short duration, as in infants, or of moderate elevation, medial hypertrophy is usually the only lesion. The thickening of the media may subside after reparation of the cardiac disorder (see also Chapter Fifteen) and the pulmonary circulation may be restored to normal.

When medial hypertrophy is followed by cellular intimal proliferation and intimal fibrosis, the prognosis after operation depends on the severity of these changes. Mild intimal lesions have little influence but with increasing obstruction of the vascular bed the changes for survival after corrective operation, diminish rapidly.

In the full-blown form of plexogenic pulmonary arteriopathy the prognosis is severe. When a fixed right to left shunt is established, at present there is nothing that can be done for the patient (Heath et al., 1958; Edwards, 1967). This stresses the importance of prevention by early surgical procedures.

GRADING

Heath and Edwards (1958) introduced a grading system on the basis of this progressive development. In grade 1 there is only medial hypertrophy; in grades 2 and 3 cellular intimal proliferation and intimal fibrosis, respectively, are added to the picture. In grade 4, in addition to progressive fibrotic obliteration, plexiform lesions appear, followed by the other dilatation lesions (grade 5) and necrotizing arteritis (grade 6). Minor alterations to this grading system have been proposed later (Harris and Heath, 1962).

This grading system has definitely stimulated the interest of pathologists in hypertensive pulmonary vascular disease. In using it, it should be realized that it was devised for pulmonary hypertension in cases of congenital heart disease with a shunt, and that it is not applicable to other forms of pulmonary hypertension, with the exception of primary pulmonary hypertension. While the first three grades clearly reflect a succession in the development of the lesions, this is unlikely for the grades 4 through 6. As we have discussed, we believe that necrotizing arteritis precedes the formation of plexiform lesions, even though the active stages of arterial necrosis and inflammation need not to be present, when plexiform lesions occur. Any of the alterations—necrotizing arteritis, plexiform lesions, or dilatation lesions—may be observed alone in the absence of the others, or in combination with the others. All are indicative of severe pulmonary hypertension. In our experience, when present in a lung biopsy taken at operation, none of these lesions carried a more severe prognosis than the others.

Even if, for these reasons, grades 4 through 6 from the classification of Heath and Edwards should be combined into a single grade, it must not be overlooked that, although the qualitative aspects of the vascular changes expressed in the grading system are certainly important, the quantitative aspects are even more so. Mild intimal fibrosis of pulmonary arteries is of little consequence when a cardiac defect is closed, but severe obliterative changes form a contraindication to surgery. Moreover, some patients have been reported who had plexiform lesions in their lung biopsies but who subsequently were in good health many years after closure of their ventricular septal defects although this is not the regular course of events (Anderson et al., 1967; Wagenvoort and Wagenvoort, 1974). In our opinion grading of vascular lesions cannot replace an adequate description in which qualitative and quantitative aspects are combined (Wagenvoort, 1973). This does not significantly add to the work load of the pathologist. Exact morphometric assessment of the lesions, which would be very laborious, as a rule is not necessary.

VARIOUS FORMS OF CARDIAC SHUNTS AND PULMONARY VASCULAR DISEASE

If pulmonary hypertension develops in patients with a congenital cardiac shunt, the result will be plexogenic pulmonary arteriopathy, irrespective of the type of congenital malformation. In other words, the pulmonary vascular lesions are in principle the same, whatever malformation gave rise to the shunt. The chances that severe pulmonary hypertension and pronounced vascular alterations develop are, however, widely different.

In pretricuspid shunts severe hypertensive pulmonary vascular disease is uncommon. This applies to atrial septal defects that produce pronounced pulmonary vascular alterations only in a relatively small percentage and then particularly in older individuals. In anomalous pulmonary venous drainage severe pulmonary hypertension and prominent changes in the lung vessels are even more rare.

Post-tricuspid shunts are more prone to give rise to severe pulmonary hypertension and this is particularly true in cases of large ventricular septal defects. In patients with such a malformation, the chances that the severe stages of plexogenic pulmonary arteriopathy eventually will develop, are very great. The same is true for any form of left to right shunt in which there is little or no pressure gradient over the communication between systemic and pulmonary circulations. Usually, in persistent truncus arteriosus pulmonary vascular disease is severe unless there is an associated stenosis of the pulmonary arteries. In patients with patent ductus arteriosus much depends on the width and the length of the ductus. Severe hypertensive pulmonary vascular disease affects a minority of these patients and is only common in those in whom the ductus is short and wide.

Common atrioventricular canal often is associated with severe pulmonary hypertension and plexiform lesions are sometimes present in young infants.

Complete transposition of the great vessels deserves special mention with regard to the development of hypertensive pulmonary vascular disease. Pulmonary hypertension is to be expected when the condition is associated with a ventricular septal defect or with a patent ductus arteriosus, as is often the case. It appears, however, that in these instances pulmonary arterial lesions tend to become more severe and to develop at a much younger age than in children who have a ventricular septal defect or patent ductus arteriosus without transposition (Ferguson et al., 1960; Ferencz, 1966; Shaker and Kidd, 1968; Wagenvoort et al., 1968).

When there is an intact ventricular septum and a closed ductus arteriosus, the

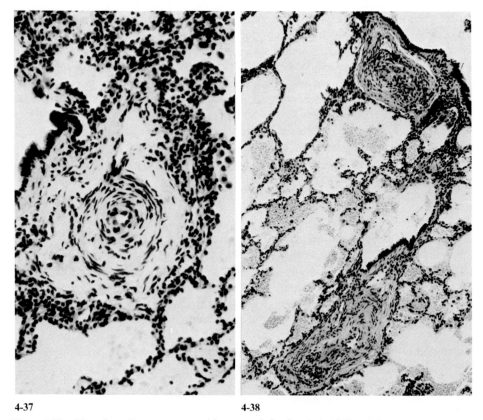

4-37   4-38

Figure 4-37. Muscular pulmonary artery with concentric laminar intimal fibrosis in a one-year-old male infant with complete transposition of the great vessels and intact ventricular septum (H. and E., ×225).
Figure 4-38. Two muscular pulmonary arteries with plexiform lesions from the same case as Figure 4-37 (H. and E., ×90).

pulmonary arterial pressure is usually normal or only mildly elevated. The pulmonary arteries, as a rule, are wide with a media that is normal or more or less atrophic (Wagenvoort et al., 1968). There are, however, occasional patients with transposition and intact ventricular septum who develop severe pulmonary hypertension and pronounced plexogenic pulmonary vascular disease (Figures 4-37 and 4-38) even at a very early age (Viles et al., 1969; Lakier et al., 1975; Clarkson et al., 1976). Even after a surgical correction severe pulmonary hypertension may develop (Rosengart et al., 1975).

Why transposition of the great vessels tends to be associated with pulmonary arterial lesions of such particular severity and such early onset in the presence of a shunt at ventricular level, and sometimes even in the absence of a defect, is unknown. It is, however, important that the clinicians are aware of it, since these patients may well be in need of earlier surgical management than others with pulmonary hypertension but without transposition (Newfeld et al., 1974).

Eisenmenger's Syndrome

The term "Eisenmenger's syndrome" is applied to cases of severe pulmonary hypertensive vascular disease due to congenital heart disease with a shunting defect and reversal of the shunt.

The defect may be at any level so that, in principle, a large variety of congenital cardiac malformations may give rise to the syndrome (Young and Mark, 1971).

It is clear that in these patients obstructive vascular alterations are usually present. Often these include arterial necrosis, plexiform lesions, and dilatation lesions but this is not necessarily so. Pulmonary plexogenic arteriopathy in these cases may go no further than severe intimal fibrosis. In children, reversal of the shunt has been observed when there was only medial hypertrophy (Wagenvoort and Wagenvoort, 1974). In such cases a corrective operation may be successful (Brammell et al., 1971), but generally patients with an Eisenmenger syndrome are considered inoperable even though, with conservative treatment, their life-span may be longer than is often expected (Young and Mark, 1971).

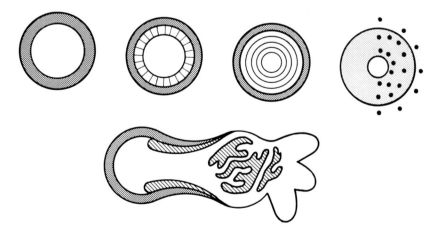

Plexogenic pulmonary arteriopathy: Arteries with medial hypertrophy, cellular intimal proliferation, concentric-laminar intimal fibrosis, fibrinoid necrosis without or with arteritis, plexiform lesions.

REFERENCES

Anderson, R. A., Levy, A. M., Naeye, R. L., and Tabakin, B. S.: Rapidly progressing pulmonary vascular obstructive disease. Association with ventricular septal defects during early childhood. *Amer. J. Cardiol.* **19:** 854, 1967.

Backwinkel, K. P., Themann, H., Schmitt, G., and Hauss, W. H.: Elektronenmikroskopische Untersuchungen über das Verhalten glatter Muskelzellen in der Arterienwand unter verschiedenen experimentellen Bedingungen. *Virch. Arch.* **359:** 171, 1973.

Bessinger, F. B., Blieden, L. C., and Edwards, J. E.: Hypertensive pulmonary vascular disease associated with patent ductus arteriosus: primary or secondary? *Circulation* **52:** 157, 1975.

Brammell, H. L., Vogel, J. H. K., Pryor, R., and Blount, S. G.: The Eisenmenger syndrome. A clinical and physiologic reappraisal. *Amer. J. Cardiol.* **28:** 679, 1971.

Brenner, O.: Pathology of the vessels of the pulmonary circulation. *Arch. Intern. Med.* **56:** 211, 1935.

Brewer, D. B.: Fibrous occlusion and anastomosis of the pulmonary vessels in a case of pulmonary hypertension associated with patent ductus arteriosus. *J. Path. Bact.* **70:** 299, 1955.

Brewer, D. B., and Heath, D.: Pulmonary vascular changes in Eisenmenger's complex. *J. Path. Bact.* **77:** 141, 1959.

Byrom, F. B.: The pathogenesis of hypertensive encephalopathy and its relation to the malignant phase of hypertension. Experimental evidence from the hypertensive rat. *Lancet* **ii:** 201, 1954.

Chiari, H.: Cor pulmonale. *Bull. Schweiz. Akad. Med. Wiss.* **6:** 432, 1950.

Clarkson, P. M., Neutze, J. M., Wardill, J. C., and Barratt-Boyes, B. G.: The pulmonary vascular bed in patients with complete transposition of the great arteries. *Circulation* **53:** 539, 1976.

Coalson, J. J., Jacques, W. E., Campbell, G. S., and Thompson, W. M.: Ultrastructure of the alveolar-capillary membrane in congenital and acquired heart disease. *Arch. Path.* **83:** 377, 1967.

Dammann, J. F., and Ferencz, C.: The significance of the pulmonary vascular bed in congenital heart disease. III. Defects between the ventricles or great vessels in which both increased pressure and blood flow may act upon the lungs and in which there is a common ejectable force. *Amer. Heart J.* **52:** 210, 1956.

D'Arbela, P. G., Mugerwa, J. W., Patel, A. K., and Somers, K.: Aneurysms of pulmonary artery with persistent ductus arteriosus and pulmonary infundibular stenosis. Fatal dissection and rupture in pregnancy. *Brit. Heart J.* **32:** 124, 1970.

Davis, B. T., Davison, P. H., and Heath, D.: Clinical pathologic conference. *Amer. Heart J.* **65:** 267, 1963.

Deterling, R. A., and Clagett, O. T.: Aneurysm of the pulmonary artery: Review of the literature and report of a case. *Amer. Heart J.* **34:** 471, 1947.

Downing, S. E., Pursel, S. E., Vidome, R. A., Brandt, H. M., and Liebow, A. A.: Studies on pulmonary hypertension with special reference to pressure-flow relationships in chronically distended and undistended lobes. *Med. Thorac.* **19:** 76, 1962.

Edwards, J. E.: Functional pathology of the pulmonary vascular tree in congenital cardiac disease. *Circulation* **15:** 164, 1957.

Edwards, J. E.: Ventricular septal defect. Unresolved problems. *Amer. J. Cardiol.* **19:** 832, 1967.

Edwards, J. E., and Burchell, H. B.: Effects of pulmonary hypertension on the tracheobronchial tree. *Dis. Chest.* **38:** 272, 1960.

Ferencz, C.: Transposition of the great vessels. Pathophysiologic considerations based upon a study of the lungs. *Circulation* **33:** 232, 1966.

Ferguson, D. J., Berkas, E. M., and Varco, R. L.: Process of healing in experimental pulmonary arteriosclerosis. *Proc. Soc. Exper. Biol.* **89:** 492, 1955.

Ferguson, D. J., Adams, P., and Watson, D.: Pulmonary arteriosclerosis in transposition of the great vessels. *Amer. J. Dis. Child.* **99:** 653, 1960.

Foord, A. G., and Lewis, R. D.: Primary dissecting aneurysms of peripheral and pulmonary arteries. Dissecting hemorrhage of media. *Arch. Path.* **68:** 553, 1959.

Friedli, B., Langford Kidd, B. S., Mustard, W. T., and Keith, J. D.: Ventricular septal defect with increased pulmonary vascular resistance. Late results of surgical closure. *Amer. J. Cardiol.* **33:** 403, 1974.

Geer, J. C., Glass, B. A., and Albert, H. M.: The morphogenesis and reversibility of experimental hyperkinetic pulmonary vascular lesions in the dog. *Exper. Molec. Path.* **4**: 399, 1965.

Glancy, D. L., Frazier, P. D., and Roberts, W. C.: Pulmonary parenchymal cholesterol-ester granulomas in patients with pulmonary hypertension. *Amer. J. Med.* **45**: 198, 1968.

Gordon, A. J., Donoso, E., Kuhn, C. L. A., Ravitch, M. M., and Himmelstein, A.: Patent ductus arteriosus with reversal of flow, *New Engl. J. Med.* **251**: 923, 1954.

Harley, R. A., Friedman, P. J., Saldana, M., Liebow, A. A., and Carrington, C. B.: Sequential development of lesions in experimental extreme pulmonary hypertension. *Amer. J. Path.* **52**: 52a, 1968.

Harris, P., and Heath, D.: *The Human Pulmonary Circulation. Its Form and Function in Health and Disease.* E. & S. Livingstone Ltd., Edinburgh and London, 1962.

Hartwell, A. S., and Tilden, I. L.: Aneurysm of the pulmonary artery. Report of a case in which the aneurysm apparently developed under observation. *Amer. Heart J.* **26**: 692, 1943.

Heath, D.: Cor triloculare biatriatum. *Circulation* **15**: 701, 1957.

Heath, D., and Edwards, J. E.: The pathology of hypertensive pulmonary vascular disease. A description of six grades of structural changes in the pulmonary arteries with special reference to congenital cardiac septal defects. *Circulation* **18**: 533, 1958.

Heath, D., Swan, H. J. C., DuShane, J. W., and Edwards, J. E.: The relation of medial thickness of small muscular pulmonary arteries to immediate postnatal survival in patients with ventricular septal defect or patent ductus arteriosus. *Thorax* **13**: 267, 1958.

Heath, D., Wood, E. H., DuShane, J. W., and Edwards, J. E.: The structure of the pulmonary trunk at different ages and in cases of pulmonary hypertension and pulmonary stenosis. *J. Path. Bact.* **77**: 441, 1959.

Heath, D., Wood, E. H., DuShane, J. W., and Edwards, J. E.: The relation of age and blood pressure to atheroma in the pulmonary arteries and thoracic aorta in congenital heart disease. *Lab. Invest.* **9**: 259, 1960.

Hoffman, J. I. E., and Rudolph, A. M.: The natural history of ventricular septal defect in infancy. *Amer. J. Cardiol.* **16**: 634, 1965.

Hruban, Z., and Humphreys, E. M.: Congenital anomalies associated with pulmonary hypertension in an infant. *Arch. Path.* **70**: 766, 1960.

Hufner, R. F., and McNicol, C. A.: The pathologic physiology of microscopic pulmonary vascular shunts. *Arch. Path.* **65**: 554, 1958.

Jewett, J. F., and Ober, W. B.: Primary pulmonary hypertension as a cause of maternal death. *Amer. J. Obstet. Gynec.* **71**: 1335, 1956.

Kajchuk, R., Gonzales-Lavin, L., and Replogle, R. L.: Pulmonary artery aneurysm associated with atrial septal defect and absent pulmonary valve. *J. Thorac. Cardiovasc. Surg.* **65**: 699, 1973.

Kanjuh, V. I., Sellers, R. D., and Edwards, J. E.: Pulmonary vascular plexiform lesion. *Arch. Path.* **78**: 513, 1964.

Kapanci, Y.: Médionécrose et ánévrysmes disséquants des artères intra-pulmonaires. Description d'un cas chez le nourrisson et étude morphogénétique de la médionécrose type Gsell-Erdheim. *Frankf. Z. Path.* **74**: 425, 1965a.

Kapanci, Y.: Hypertensive pulmonary vascular disease. Endothelial hyperplasia and its relations to intravascular fibrin precipitation. *Amer. J. Path.* **48**: 665, 1965b.

Kerwin, A. J., and Jaffe, F. A.: Postoperative aneurysm of the ductus arteriosus with fatal rupture of a mycotic aneurysm of a branch of the pulmonary artery. *Amer. J. Cardiol.* **10**: 397, 1959.

Krückemeyer, K.: Über das Vorkommen seltener Aneurysmen der Aorta und ihrer grossen Äste. *Zbl. Allg. Path., Path. Anat.* **90**: 363, 1953.

Kucsko, L.: Über eigentümliche Gefäszveränderungen in der Lunge (Anastomositis). *Wien. klin. Wschr.* **61**: 659, 1949.

Kucsko, L.: Über arterio-venöse Verbindungen in der menschlichen Lunge und ihre funktionelle Bedeutung. *Frankf. Z. Path.* **64**: 54, 1953.

Lakier, J. B., Stanger, P., Heymann, M. A., Hoffman, J. I. E., and Rudolph, A. M.: Early onset of pulmonary vascular obstruction in patients with aortopulmonary transposition and intact ventricular septum. *Circulation* **51**: 875, 1975.

Levin, D. L., Rudolph, A. M., Heyman, M. A., and Phibbs, R. H.: Morphological development of the pulmonary vascular bed in fetal lambs. *Circulation* **53:** 144, 1976.

Littler, W. A., Kay, J. M., Hasleton, P. S., and Heath, D.: Busulphan lung. *Thorax* **24:** 639, 1969.

Lober, P. H., and Lillehei, C. W.: Necrotizing panarteritis following repair of coarctation of aorta. *Surgery* **35:** 950, 1954.

Loire, R., Plauchu, G., and Tabib, A.: Anévrysme de l'artère pulmonaire. A propos de deux observations anatomo-cliniques. *Lyon Méd.* **223:** 1187, 1970.

Lynfield, J., Gasul, B. M., Arcilla, R., and Luan, L. L.: The natural history of ventricular septal defects in infancy and childhood. *Amer. J. Med.* **30:** 357, 1961.

McCormack, L. J.: Glomoid hyperplasia of the pulmonary vasculature; a phenomenon in severe pulmonary hypertension. *Amer. J. Path.* **35:** 668, 1959.

Moschcowitz, E., Rubin, E., and Strauss, L.: Hypertension of the pulmonary circulation due to congenital glomoid obstruction of the pulmonary arteries. *Amer. J. Path.* **39:** 75, 1961.

Nadas, A. S., Rudolph, A. M., and Gross, R. E.: Pulmonary arterial hypertension in congenital heart disease. *Circulation* **22:** 1041, 1960.

Naeye, R. L.: The pulmonary arterial bed in ventricular septal defect. Anatomic features in childhood. *Circulation* **34:** 962, 1966.

Naeye, R. L., and Vennart, G. P.: The structure and significance of pulmonary plexiform structures. *Amer. J. Path.* **36:** 593, 1960.

Newfeld, E. A., Paul, M. H., Muster, A. J., and Idriss, F. S.: Pulmonary vascular disease in complete transposition of the great arteries: A study of 200 patients. *Amer. J. Cardiol.* **34:** 75, 1974.

Ohela, K., and Teir, H.: Rupture of the pulmonary artery. Report of three cases. *Ann. Med. Intern. Fenn.* **43:** 39, 1954.

Plaut, A.: Hemangioendothelioma of the lung. Report of two cases. *Arch. Path.* **29:** 517, 1940.

Plokker, H. W. M., Wagenaar, S. S., Bruschke, A. V. G., and Wagenvoort, C. A.: Aneurysm of a pulmonary artery branch: an uncommon cause of a coin lesion. *Chest* **68:** 258, 1975.

Ravines, H. T.: Dissecting hematomas of intrapulmonary arteries in a case of pulmonary hypertension associated with patent ductus arteriosus. *J. Thorac. Cardiovasc. Surg.* **39:** 760, 1960.

Rosengart, R., Fishbein, M., and Emmanouilides, G. C.: Progressive pulmonary vascular disease after surgical correction (Mustard procedure) of transposition of great arteries with intact ventricular septum. *Amer. J. Cardiol.* **35:** 107, 1975.

Ross, R. S., Taussig, H. B., and Evans, M. H.: Late hemodynamic complications of anastomotic surgery for treatment of the tetralogy of Fallot. *Circulation* **18:** 553, 1958.

Rutishauser, E., and Blanc, W.: Anastomoses artério-veineuses glomiques du poumon avec syndrome d'insuffisance droite et cyanose. *Schweiz. Z. Allg. Path. Bakt.* **13:** 61, 1950.

Rutishauser, E., and Feuardent, R.: Schnittrekonstruktion glomusartiger Bildungen (Anastomositis) der Lunge. *Schweiz. Z. Allg. Path. Bakt.* **15:** 641, 1952.

Saldana, M. E., Harley, R. A., Liebow, A. A., and Carrington, C. B.: Experimental extreme pulmonary hypertension and vascular disease in relation to polycythemia. *Amer. J. Path.* **52:** 935, 1968.

Shaher, R., and Kidd, L.: Effect of ventricular septal defect and patent ductus arteriosus on left ventricular pressure in complete transposition of the great vessels. *Circulation* **37:** 232, 1968.

Shemtov, A., Fine, L. G., Rotem, Y., and Neufeld, H. N.: Occlusive pulmonary vascular disease in a child with a spontaneously closed ventricular septal defect. *Israel J. Med. Sc.* **9:** 469, 1973.

Short, D. S.: The problem of medial hypertrophy in pulmonary hypertension. *Med. Thorac.* **19:** 225, 1962.

Shull, W. K., Kapadia, S. B., and Zuberbuhler, J. R.: Aneurysm of the main pulmonary artery. Association with patent ductus arteriosus and ostium secundum defect. *Amer. J. Dis. Child.* **119:** 507, 1970.

Singleton, A. D., McGinnis, L. M. S., and Eason, H. R.: Arteritis following correction of coarctation of the aorta. *Surgery* **45:** 665, 1959.

Spencer, H.: Primary pulmonary hypertension and related vascular changes in the lungs. *J. Path. Bact.* **62:** 75, 1950.

Spencer, H.: Primary lesions in polyarteritis nodosa. *Brit. J. Tuberc.* **51:** 123, 1957.

Stanger, P., Lucas, R. V., and Edwards, J. E.: Anatomic factors causing respiratory distress in acyanotic congenital cardiac disease: special reference to bronchial obstruction. *Pediatrics* **43:** 760, 1969.

Stanisic, M.: Zur morphologischen Klassifikation der primären pulmonalen Arteriopathien mit pulmonaler Hypertonie. *Zbl. Allg. Path., Path. Anat.* **110:** 367, 1967.

Sweeney, A. R., and Baggenstoss, A. H.: Pulmonary lesions of periarteritis nodosa. *Proc. Staff Meet. Mayo Clin.* **24:** 35, 1949.

Timpanelli, A. E., and Steinberg, I.: Calcification of the pulmonary artery in patent ductus arteriosus with reversal of blood flow. *Amer. J. Med.* **30:** 405, 1961.

Turunen, M., and Stjernvall, L.: Submicroscopic structure of the pulmonary capillaries in patent ductus arteriosus. *Acta Chir. Scand.* **117:** 131, 1959.

Unschold, G.: Über einen Fall von Endarteritis pulmonalis unter dem Bild eines offenen Ductus Botalli bei einen 7½ jährigen Kind. *Arch. Klin. Chir.* **271:** 17, 1952.

Van Zandwijk, N., Wagenvoort, C. A., and Groen, A. S.: Unpublished data, 1976.

Viles, P. H., Ongley, P. A., and Titus, J. L.: The spectrum of pulmonary vascular disease in transposition of the great arteries. *Circulation* **40:** 31, 1969.

Vogel, J. H. K., Grover, R. F., Jamieson, G., and Blount, S. G.: Long-term physiologic observations in patients with ventricular septal defect and increased pulmonary vascular resistance. *Adv. Cardiol.* **11:** 108, 1974.

Wagenvoort, C. A.: The morphology of certain vascular lesions in pulmonary hypertension. *J. Path. Bact.* **78:** 503, 1959.

Wagenvoort, C. A.: Vasoconstriction and medial hypertrophy in pulmonary hypertension. *Circulation* **22:** 535, 1960.

Wagenvoort, C. A.: The pulmonary arteries in infants with ventricular septal defect. *Med. Thorac.* **19:** 162, 1962.

Wagenvoort, C. A.: Hypertensive pulmonary vascular disease complicating congenital heart disease: A review. *Cardiovasc. Clinics* **5:** 43, 1973.

Wagenvoort, C. A., DuShane, J. W., and Edwards, J. E.: Cardiac clinics. 151. Hypertensive pulmonary arterial lesions as a late result of anastomosis of systemic and pulmonary circulations. *Proc. Staff Meet. Mayo Clin.* **35:** 186, 1960.

Wagenvoort, C. A., Neufeld, H. N., DuShane, J. W., and Edwards, J. E.: The pulmonary arterial tree in ventricular septal defect. A quantitative study of anatomic features in fetuses, infants and children. *Circulation* **23:** 740, 1961.

Wagenvoort, C. A., Heath, D., and Edwards, J. E.: *The Pathology of the Pulmonary Vasculature.* Charles C Thomas, Springfield, Ill., 1964.

Wagenvoort, C. A., Nauta, J., Van der Schaar, P. J., Weeda, H. W. H., and Wagenvoort, N.: Effect of flow and pressure on pulmonary vessels. *Circulation* **35:** 1028, 1967.

Wagenvoort, C. A., Nauta, J., Van der Schaar, P. J., Weeda, H. W. H., and Wagenvoort, N.: The pulmonary vasculature in complete transposition of the great vessels judged from lung biopsies. *Circulation* **38:** 746, 1968.

Wagenvoort, C. A., and Wagenvoort, N.: Pathology of the Eisenmenger syndrome and primary pulmonary hypertension. *Adv. Cardiol.* **11:** 123, 1974.

Webster, W. S., Bishop, S. P., and Geer, J. C.: Experimental aortic intimal thickening. I. Morphology and source of intimal cells. *Amer. J. Path.* **76:** 245, 1974.

Weidman, W. H., and DuShane, J. W.: Course of pulmonary hypertension following surgical closure of ventricular septal defect. *Adv. Cardiol.* **11:** 131, 1974a.

Weidman, H. W., and DuShane, J. W.: Selection of patients for surgical correction of ventricular septal defect, congenital aortic valve stenosis, and pulmonary valve stenosis. *Adv. Cardiol.* **11:** 74, 1974b.

Williams, T. E., Schiller, M., Craenen, J., Hosier, J. M., and Sirak, H. D.: Pulmonary artery aneurysm. Successful excision and replacement of the main pulmonary artery. *J. Thorac. Cardiovasc. Surg.* **62:** 63, 1971.

Wood, P.: Pulmonary hypertension. *Modern Conc. Cardiovasc. Dis.* **28**: 513, 1959.

World Health Organization: Primary pulmonary hypertension. Report of Committee. 1975.

Young, D., and Mark, H.: Fate of the patient with the Eisenmenger syndrome. *Amer. J. Cardiol.* **28**: 658, 1971.

Zur Linden, W.: Isolierte Pulmonalsklerose im jungsten Kindesalter. *Virch. Arch. Path. Anat.* **252**: 228, 1924.

CHAPTER FIVE

Hepatic Injury
and Pulmonary Hypertension

In recent years there has been a growing number of reports indicating an association between severe hepatic injury, particularly cirrhosis of the liver, and pulmonary hypertension. A discussion of this rare combination therefore, is, necessary, although it is hampered by the paucity of case reports, the uncertainty of the mechanisms by which the pulmonary arterial pressure may be produced, and the contradictory results of the morphologic studies of the pulmonary vasculature.

PORTAL AND PULMONARY HYPERTENSION

Mantz and Craige (1951) were the first to describe coexistent portal and pulmonary hypertension in a patient with a stenotic portal vein and thrombosis of portacaval anastomotic vessels. The same case was included in a later report on thromboembolic pulmonary hypertension by Owen et al. (1953). Naeye (1960) reported on six patients with the combination of portal and pulmonary hypertension. In five of these there was advanced cirrhosis of the liver; in two cases this was associated with thrombosis of the portal vein. In the sixth patient there was portal vein thrombosis without cirrhosis. Thromboembolism was suggested as being responsible for the elevated pulmonary arterial pressure in most cases.

Since that time the association of cirrhosis of the liver and pulmonary hypertension has been reported in one patient by Kerbel (1962), in one by Cohen and Mendelow (1965), in two by Jöbsis (1966), in one by Segel et al. (1968), and in six by Senior et al. (1968). Three patients described by Levine et al. (1973) included one previously reported by Naeye (1960). In the patient described by Lal and Fletcher (1968) there was associated portal vein thrombosis.

This list may well be incomplete but even so it is clear that only very few patients who have portal hypertension, with or without severe hepatic injury, develop pulmonary hypertension. The question could be even raised whether the association is real or coincidence. The gradually increasing numbers of reports, however, suggest a genuine relationship between the two conditions. Moreover, it has become clear that in patients with hepatic cirrhosis there generally may be alterations in respiratory pattern and in both pulmonary and systemic circulations (Murray et al., 1958; Heinemann, 1960; Bayley et al., 1964).

Although it seems likely that in these patients the increase in pulmonary arterial pressure results from the hepatic injury, either directly or indirectly, the actual mechanism is enigmatic.

An increased circulating blood volume and cardiac output often is observed in patients with cirrhosis of the liver, and this has been implicated as causing a moderate elevation of the pulmonary arterial pressure (Murray et al., 1958; Bayley et al., 1964). On the other hand, even a markedly increased circulating blood volume in patients with liver cirrhosis may leave the pressure in the pulmonary artery unaffected (Massumi et al., 1965), and it is difficult to visualize how it could be responsible for severe pulmonary hypertension.

The common development of a porta-systemic collateral circulation, usually by way of esophageal or gastric varices, sometimes by a direct portacaval shunt, which may be either spontaneous or surgically created, has always figured greatly in the hypotheses concerning the relation between portal and pulmonary hypertension.

In the presence of portal vein thrombosis, thromboemboli may reach the pulmonary circulation by these pathways. Pulmonary hypertension could then be embolic in origin, as suggested by several authors (Mantz and Craige, 1951; Owen et al., 1953; Naeye, 1960).

Obviously, thrombosis of the portal vein and of portacaval shunts may be a source of pulmonary thromboembolism, and it is certainly possible that in some patients with portal hypertension, the elevation of the pulmonary arterial pressure must be explained in this way. This is particularly likely in patients suffering from recurrent pyogenic cholangitis. In some of these patients embolic pulmonary hypertension as a consequence of thrombosis of small hepatic veins has been described (Lai et al., 1968).

On the other hand, Senior and coworkers (1968), although accepting thromboembolism as a possible cause, have listed some points that throw doubt upon the embolic origin of the raised pressure in patients with portal hypertension. Thrombi were found in none of their patients in whom surgical decompression of the portal vein was performed. There was no recurrence of esophageal bleeding after the procedure, suggesting that the shunts were patent. Autopsy in two of their patients failed to show thrombosis of the portal vein or gross thromboemboli in the lung vessels. The absence of pulmonary thromboemboli also was stressed by others (Segel et al., 1968; Levine et al., 1973).

Another argument against the hypothesis that pulmonary hypertension in patients with hepatic or portal vein disease is based generally on chronic thromboembolism may be found in the morphologic picture of the pulmonary vascular disease in most of these instances. This is not immediately apparent from the various publications. In several of these, the vascular alterations have only been described summarily. Plexogenic pulmonary arteriopathy with concentric laminar intimal fibrosis, fibrinoid necrosis of pulmonary arterioles, and plexiform lesions was demonstrated in some patients (Segel et al., 1968; Levine et al., 1973). In other patients, the vascular lesions were interpreted as thromboembolic, although necrotizing arteritis and plexiform lesions either were described (Naeye, 1960; Cohen and Mendelow, 1965) or probably present in view of description and illustration (Mantz and Craige, 1951).

We had an opportunity to study material from two patients who had been reported previously, although briefly, by Jöbsis (1966). Both patients had cirrhosis of the liver (Figure 5-1). In neither of them could we find any evidence of recent or old

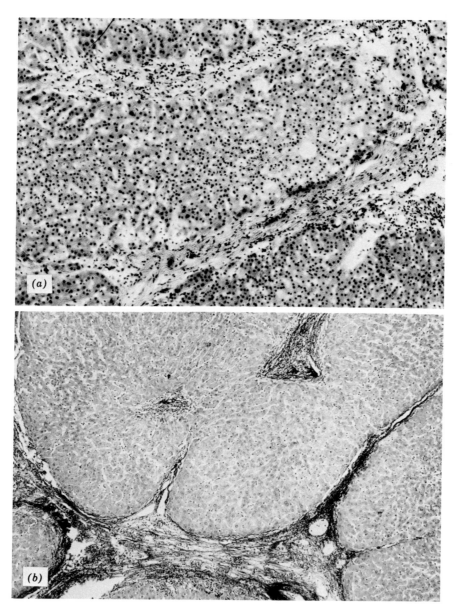

Figure 5-1. (*a*) Cirrhosis of the liver in a 19-year-old woman (patient 1) who had portal hypertension and died of pulmonary hypertension. (*b*) Cirrhosis of the liver in a 43-year-old man (patient 2) who had portal hypertension and died of pulmonary hypertension (*a*: H. and E., ×90; *b*: El.v.G., ×55).

thromboembolic lesions (Chapter Nine) but pulmonary vascular morphology was characterized by concentric-laminar intimal fibrosis (Figure 5-2), necrotizing arteritis (Figure 5-3) and plexiform lesions (Figures 5-4 and 5-5).

Since plexogenic pulmonary arteriopathy is characteristic for vasoconstrictive pulmonary hypertension as in congenital cardiac disease with a shunt (Chapter Four) or in primary pulmonary hypertension (Chapter Seven) and not for thromboembolic pulmonary hypertension (Chapter Eight), it is unlikely that emboli play a predominant part in producing the elevated pulmonary arterial pressure in patients with hepatic disease.

An entirely different mechanism may be based on humoral agents inducing vasoconstriction of pulmonary arteries. If intestinal metabolites, which normally are inactivated in the liver, bypass this organ and gain direct access from the portal to the pulmonary circulation, their effect could be a raised pulmonary resistance (Heinemann, 1960; Segel et al., 1968). Although no such intestinal metabolic agent has been identified as yet, the principle of such a mechanism seems very likely (Fishman, 1974). It also would be in line with the observation that not only different forms of hepatic cirrhosis, such as "juvenile," "Laennec," and "postnecrotic," but also portal vein obstruction without hepatic damage might cause pulmonary hypertension. It even seems likely that plexogenic pulmonary arteriopathy, associated with severe hepatic injury caused by Gaucher's disease (Roberts and Frederickson, 1967) or by Niemann-Pick's disease, as we have observed personally, may be explained in this way.

The concept of a humoral influence on the pulmonary circulation in these cases at present seems the most likely explanation although it is unproven. However, it may be significant that, when Crotalaria is administered to animals (Chapter Six), hepatic injury always preceeds pulmonary hypertension (Wagenvoort et al., 1974).

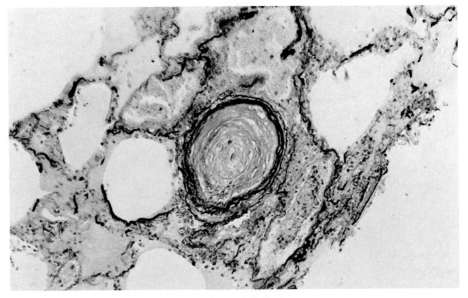

Figure 5-2.   Obliterating concentric laminar intimal fibrosis of a muscular pulmonary artery in patient 1 (El.v.G., ×140).

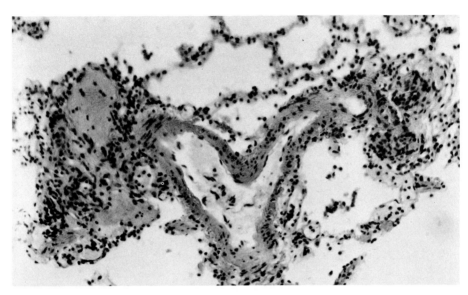

Figure 5-3. Muscular pulmonary artery with two branches in patient 2. The left branch shows fibrinoid necrosis and arteritis, the right branch contains an early stage of a plexiform lesion (H. and E., ×140).

The fact that so few patients with portal hypertension develop pulmonary hypertension is disturbing, unless individual susceptibility in the sense of hyper-reactivity of lung vessels (Grover et al., 1963) is accepted.

There is no convincing sex preference for the combination of portal and pulmonary hypertension. Of the 21 patients we collected from the literature, there were 12 males and 9 females. Their average age was 40 years, ranging from 10 to 76 years.

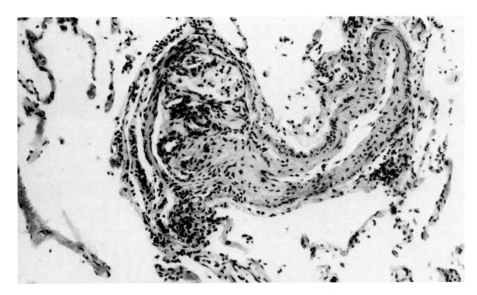

Figure 5-4. Muscular pulmonary artery with a plexiform lesion in patient 2 (H. and E., ×140).

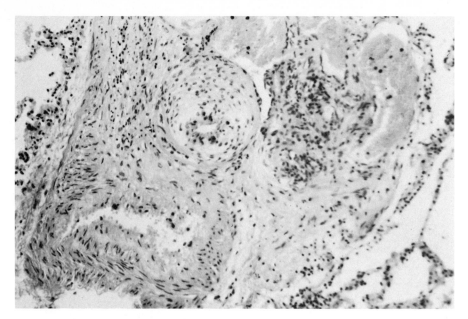

Figure 5-5. Branch of muscular pulmonary artery with concentric laminar intimal fibrosis and a plexiform lesion in its further course, in patient 1. The parent artery with mild intimal fibrosis in the lower left corner (H. and E., ×140).

PULMONARY ARTERIOVENOUS FISTULAE

Severe liver disease may be associated with pulmonary arteriovenous fistulae. Rydell and Hoffbauer (1956) demonstrated these first by postmortem injection of the lung in a young patient with hepatic cirrhosis in whom the pulmonary lesions were clinically undetected. Since then several cases have been reported (Bashour et al., 1961; Berthelot et al., 1966; El Gamal et al., 1970; Dalquen et al., 1974). Usually these patients have normal pulmonary arterial pressures although moderate pulmonary hypertension does occasionally occur (Murray et al., 1958).

These clumps of anastomotic channels usually are situated close to the pleura. They may even impress as pleural spider nevi and generally are associated with vascular spider nevi of the skin. Also coexistent aneurysms of the brain have been reported (Dalquen et al., 1974).

The pathogenesis of these vascular alterations is not clear. Vasodilatation on the basis of a humoral factor has been suggested (Berthelot et al., 1966).

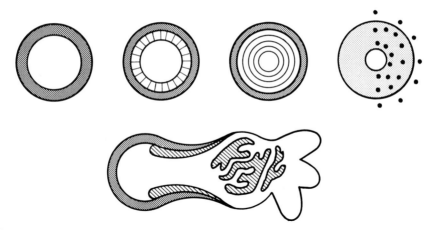

Plexogenic pulmonary arteriopathy: Arteries with medial hypertrophy, cellular intimal proliferation, concentric-laminar intimal fibrosis, fibrinoid necrosis without or with arteritis, plexiform lesions.

REFERENCES

Bayley, T. J., Segel, N., and Bishop, J. M.: The circulatory changes in patients with cirrhosis of the liver at rest and during exercise. *Clin. Sci.* **26:** 227, 1964.

Bashour, F. A., Miller, W. P., and Chapman, C. B.: Pulmonary venoarterial shunting in hepatic cirrhosis. Including a case with cirsoid aneurysm of the thoracic wall. *Amer. Heart J.* **62:** 350, 1961.

Berthelot, P., Walker, J. G., Sherlock, S., and Reid, L.: Arterial changes in the lungs in cirrhosis of the liver—lung spider nevi. *New Engl. J. Med.* **274:** 291, 1966.

Cohen, N., and Mendelow, H.: Concurrent "active juvenile cirrhosis" and "primary pulmonary hypertension." *Amer. J. Med.* **39:** 127, 1965.

Dalquen, P., Schmid, A. H., Ohnacker, H., and Rutishauser, M.: Multiple aneurysms of lung and brain in juvenile hepatic cirrhosis. *Vasa* **3:** 10, 1974.

El Gamal, M., Stoker, J. B., Spiers, E. M., and Whitaker, W.: Cyanosis complicating hepatic cirrhosis. Report of a case due to multiple pulmonary arteriovenous fistulas. *Amer. J. Cardiol.* **25:** 490, 1970.

Fishman, A. P.: Dietary pulmonary hypertension. *Circulation Res.* **35:** 657, 1974.

Grover, R. F., Vogel, J. H. K., Averill, K. H., and Blount, S. G.: Pulmonary hypertension: individual and species variability relative to vascular reactivity (editorial). *Amer. Heart J.* **66:** 1, 1963.

Heinemann, H. O.: Respiration and circulation in patients with portal cirrhosis of the liver. *Circulation* **22:** 154, 1960.

Jöbsis, A. C.: Twee gevallen van primaire pulmonale hypertensie gecombineerd met levercirrhose. *Nederl. Tijdschr. v. Geneesk.* **110:** 506, 1966.

Kerbel, N. C.: Pulmonary hypertension and portal hypertension. *Canad. Med. Ass. J.* **87:** 1022, 1962.

Lai, K. S., McFadzean, A. J. S., and Yeung, R.: Microembolic pulmonary hypertension in pyogenic cholangitis. *Brit. Med. J.* **1:** 22, 1968.

Lal, S., and Fletcher, E.: Pulmonary hypertension and portal venous system thrombosis. *Brit. Heart J.* **30:** 723, 1968.

Levine, O. R., Harris, R. C., Blanc, W. A., and Mellins, R. B.: Progressive pulmonary hypertension in children with portal hypertension. *J. Pediatr.* **83:** 964, 1973.

Mantz, F. A., and Craige, E.: Portal axis thrombosis with spontaneous portacaval shunt and resultant cor pulmonale. *Arch. Path.* **52:** 91, 1951.

Massumi, R. A., Rios, J. C., and Ticktin, H. E.: Hemodynamic abnormalities and venous admixture in portal cirrhosis. *Amer. J. Med. Sci.* **250:** 275, 1965.

Murray, J. F., Dawson, A. M., and Sherlock, S.: Circulatory changes in chronic liver disease. *Amer. J. Med.* **24**: 358, 1958.

Naeye, R. L.: "Primary" pulmonary hypertension with coexisting portal hypertension. A retrospective study of six cases. *Circulation* **22**: 376, 1960.

Owen, W. R., Thomas, W. A., Castleman, B., and Bland, E. F.: Unrecognized emboli to the lungs with subsequent cor pulmonale. *New Engl. J. Med.* **249**: 919, 1953.

Roberts, W. C., and Frederickson, D. S.: Gaucher's disease of the lung causing severe pulmonary hypertension with associated acute recurrent pericarditis. *Circulation* **35**: 783, 1967.

Rydell, R., and Hoffbauer, F. W.: Multiple pulmonary arteriovenous fistulas in juvenile cirrhosis. *Amer. J. Med.* **21**: 450, 1956.

Segel, N., Kay, J. M., Bayley, T. J., and Paton, A.: Pulmonary hypertension with hepatic cirrhosis. *Brit. Heart J.* **30**: 575, 1968.

Senior, R. M., Britton, R. C., Turino, G. M., Wood, J. A., Langer, G. A., and Fishman, A. P.: Pulmonary hypertension associated with cirrhosis of the liver and with portacaval shunts. *Circulation* **37**: 88, 1968.

Wagenvoort, C. A., Wagenvoort, N., and Dijk, H. J.: Effect of fulvine on pulmonary arteries and veins of the rat. *Thorax* **29**: 522, 1974.

CHAPTER SIX

Dietary Pulmonary Hypertension

The occasional occurrence of pulmonary hypertension in patients with severe hepatic injury, and the suggested explanation that this may be caused by intestinal metabolites, bypassing the liver and acting directly on the pulmonary vasculature (Chapter Five), has some bearing upon the subject discussed in this chapter.

Dietary pulmonary hypertension develops in response to ingested substances, whether taken as food, beverages, or medicines.

In recent years this form of hypertension has attracted a great deal of attention for two different reasons. The first was an explosion of cases of pulmonary hypertension in the period 1966 to 1968 in three European countries. This epidemic has been related to ingestion of appetite-suppressing drugs. Another circumstance focusing attention on dietary pulmonary hypertension, was the extensive experimental use made of the seeds of the plant genus Crotalaria or of the pyrrolizidine alkaloids derived from these plants which resulted in increased resistance in the pulmonary circulation of animals.

HERBAL TOXINS

We will discuss Crotalaria pulmonary hypertension first, since there can be no doubt that this is a genuine example of dietary pulmonary hypertension. The principle is not new. Kay and Heath (1969) relate that Stalker in 1884 described "crotalism" or "Missouri River bottom disease" in horses grazing on pastures where *Crotalaria sagittalis* was growing. The toxicity for horses of other Crotalaria species also has been recognized (Gardiner et al., 1965), and various reports indicate that the pyrrolizidine alkaloids contained in leaves and seeds of plants of this genus are toxic for cattle, pigs, and poultry. This poisonous action is not directed primarily against the lungs or the pulmonary circulation but particularly against the liver which usually shows hemorrhages and centrilobular necrosis. (Figure 6-1). In the older reports pulmonary hypertension or pulmonary vascular lesions generally have not even been mentioned.

Lalich and Merkow (1961) were the first to demonstrate lesions in the pulmonary vasculature of rats following a diet containing the ground seeds of *Crotalaria spectabilis*. The most striking change was pulmonary arteritis. In addition they found myocarditis and centrilobular hepatic necrosis.

Numerous studies have confirmed these observations. From these it has become clear that the pyrrolizidine alkaloids of Crotalaria, such as monocrotaline and fulvine, do not act directly on the pulmonary circulation but are converted in the liver, and that the metabolites exhibit a hepatotoxic effect (Mattocks, 1968) before they affect the pulmonary circulation. In keeping with these findings is the observation that rats poisoned with a single dose of fulvine become ill with weight loss during the first week after administration and may even die from hepatic necrosis after one week. Most animals, however, recover and gain weight again to experience a second episode of malaise and weight loss approximately 4 weeks after the application. Eventually, they all die from cardiopulmonary disease after 6 to 8 weeks (Barnes et al., 1964; Kay and Heath, 1969; Wagenvoort et al., 1974a).

The early lesions of the pulmonary vasculature of rats after feeding seeds of Crotalaria or after oral or intraperitoneal administration of the alkaloids are constriction and medial hypertrophy of muscular pulmonary arteries and arterioles. (Figure 6-2) This is borne out by morphometric assessment of these vessels (Kay and Heath, 1966; Kay et al., 1971; Wagenvoort et al., 1974a). Electron-microscopic observations are also indicative of vasoconstriction (Figure 6-3), which may become apparent after only one to 2 weeks (Kay et al., 1969; Wagenvoort et al., 1974b). Cartilage metaplasia in the media sometimes has been found (Turner and Lalich, 1965).

There is a concomitant increase in thickness of the walls of pulmonary trunk and right ventricle (Heath and Kay, 1967). Development of right ventricular hypertrophy also begins after one or 2 weeks (Wagenvoort et al., 1974a). That these morphologic alterations are indeed associated with elevation of pulmonary arterial pressure has been demonstrated by direct measurement (Carillo and Aviado, 1968; Kay and Heath, 1969).

Fibrinoid necrosis with or without arteritis (Figures 6-4 and 6-5) is a conspicuous finding in rats, 4 weeks or more after application of the drug (Lalich and Merkow, 1961; Kay et al., 1971; Stötzer et al., 1972). This is accompanied by swelling of the endothelium and marked deposition of fibrin (Figure 6-6) mainly in the interstitial spaces of the media, sometimes extending into the cytoplasm of the muscle cells, as shown by electron-microscopic studies. Also the adventitia may contain fibrin deposits. The smooth muscle cells of the media initially show increased cellular activity with increasing amounts of cytoplasmic organelles (Merkow and Kleinerman, 1966). Eventually the cells become desintegrated and necrotic (Wagenvoort et al., 1974b). Fibrin thrombi and aggregates of thrombocytes have been observed in the narrowed lumen (Allen and Carstens, 1970). Plexiform lesions or dilatation lesions never were demonstrated.

Crotalaria-induced alterations are not limited to arteries and arterioles. The pulmonary venules and veins also may be affected (Figures 6-7 and 6-8), in that these exhibit constriction and medial hypertrophy, intimal thickening with narrow-

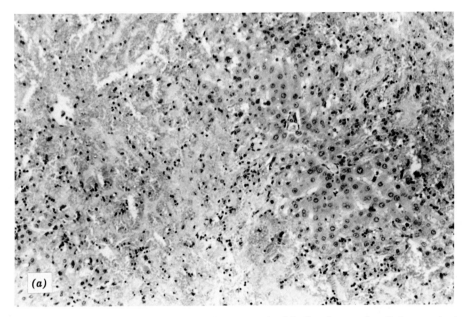

Figure 6-1. (*a*) Extensive centrilobular hemorrhagic necrosis of the liver in a rat that died one week after oral application of fulvine (H. and E., ×140).

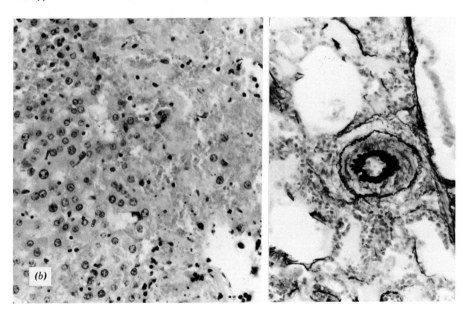

Figure 6-1. (*b*) Detail (H. and E., ×225).

Figure 6-2. Vasoconstriction and medial hypertrophy of muscular pulmonary artery in a rat that died 2 weeks after oral application of fulvine (El.v.G., ×350).

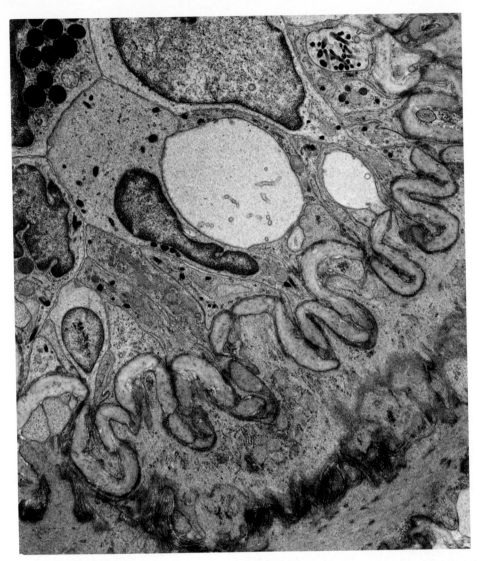

Figure 6-3.   Electron-micrograph of muscular pulmonary artery of a rat, 3 weeks after application of fulvine. Vasoconstriction is apparent by pronounced crenation of internal elastic lamina. The endothelial cells are swollen and contain some blebs in their cytoplasm. A mast cell (upper left corner) in the remnant of the lumen ($\times$11,500).

ing or obstruction of the lumen, and even fibrinoid necrosis, although the more severe changes are not as common as in the arteries (Wagenvoort et al., 1974a,b). This means that pulmonary arterial hypertension, produced by Crotalaria, may be complicated by pulmonary venous obstruction, which may impair its usefulness as a model for studying pulmonary hypertension in general.

Pulmonary vascular pathology, similar to that in rats, could be found in monkeys, particularly in young specimens. In the older animals hepatic disease and portal hypertension were more striking (Allen and Chessney, 1972; Chessney and Allen, 1973; Chessney et al., 1974).

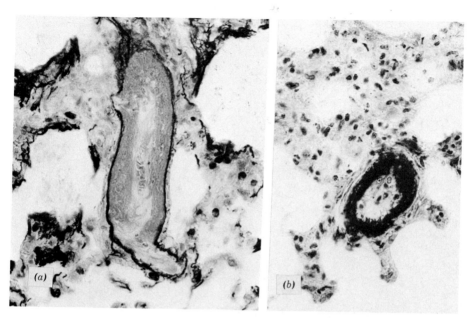

Figure 6-4. (*a*) Fibrinoid necrosis of muscular pulmonary artery in a rat, 5 weeks after application of fulvine. There is no inflammatory exudate. (*b*) Artery from the same rat stained to demonstrate fibrin (*a*: H. and E., ×225; *b*: Phosphotungstic acid hematoxylin, ×350).

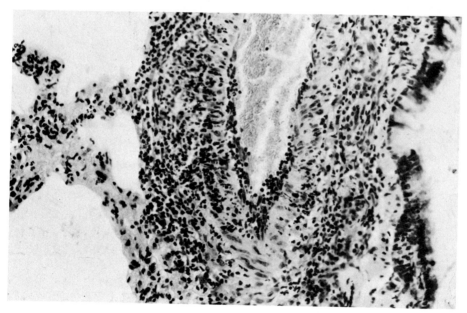

Figure 6-5. Muscular pulmonary artery from the same rat as Figure 6-4. There is a marked inflammatory exudate throughout the wall (H. and E., ×225).

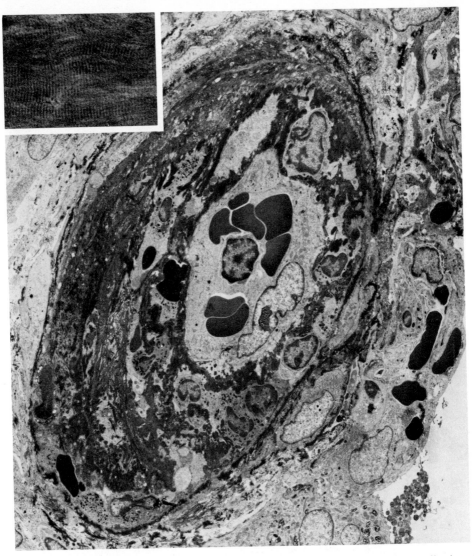

Figure 6-6. Electron-micrograph of muscular pulmonary artery of a rat, 4 weeks after application of fulvine. There is marked fibrin deposition within the media with desintegration and necrosis of muscle cells and with disappearance of the internal elastic lamina. The endothelium is swollen but intact. Erythrocytes have leaked out of the vessel (right) into the adventitia (×3050). (*Insert*) Detail of fibrin (×47,000).

Changes in the lung tissue included pulmonary and interstitial edema and hemorrhage (Valdivia et al., 1967), hemosiderosis, activity and swelling of pneumocytes and macrophages, and particularly accumulation of mast cells (Figure 6-9) not only in subpleural and peribronchial connective tissue but also in alveolar walls (Takeoka et al., 1962). The increase in the number of these cells starts abruptly around the third or fourth week after administration of the drug and may reach impressive proportions (Wagenvoort et al., 1974a). It is unknown whether there is a direct relation between mast cells and pulmonary hypertension. It has been suggested that the

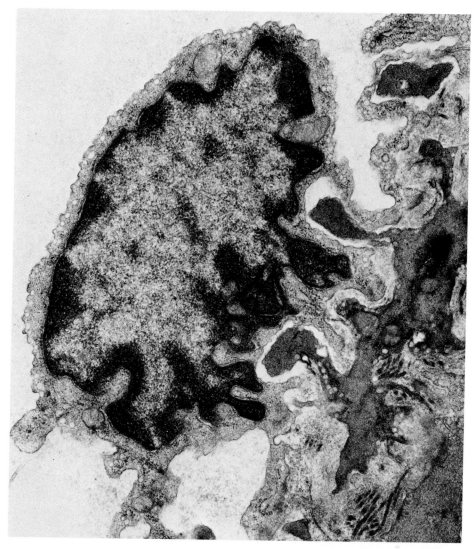

Figure 6-7. Electron-micrograph of pulmonary vein of a rat, 2 weeks after application of fulvine. Vaso-constriction is evident by cytoplasmic excrescences of smooth muscle cells (right) which penetrate into the endothelium and into the nucleus of an endothelial cell ($\times 21,000$).

effect is nonspecific and related to the exudative phenomena associated with cardiac insufficiency (Kay et al., 1967).

There are other plants besides those of the genus Crotalaria that contain pyrrolizi-dine alkaloids and may induce pulmonary hypertension following ingestion. The genera Senecio and Heliotropium, among others, are poisonous to rats and may lead to megalocytosis in the liver. *Senecio jacobaea* did not produce pulmonary vascular changes when fed to mice (Hooper, 1974), but it did in rats (Burns, 1972).

While the accidental or experimental ingestion of poisonous plants undoubtedly may produce dietary pulmonary hypertension in animals, the question has been

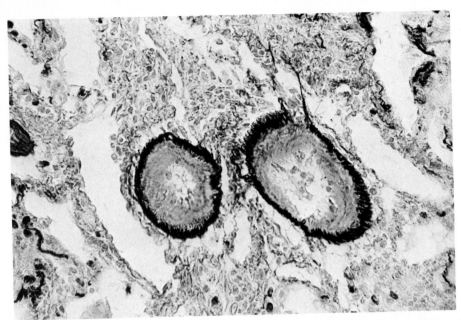

Figure 6-8. Pulmonary veins in a rat, 4 weeks after application of fulvine. There is vasoconstriction with marked crenation of internal elastic lamina and intimal thickening with narrowing of the lumen (El.v.G., ×350).

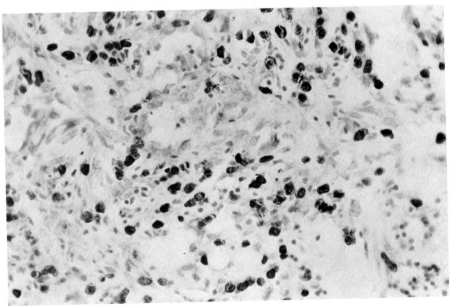

Figure 6-9. Accumulation of mast cells in perivascular interstitium and in pulmonary alveolar walls in a rat, 5 weeks after application of fulvine (Toluidine blue, ×350).

raised whether this sometimes may be responsible for the development of unexplained pulmonary hypertension in man. Schoental (1963) pointed out that *Senecio jacobaea* is available in some herbal medicines from health stores and (1972) that Senecio and similar plants are popular with the local "health doctors" in Africa. Kay and Heath (1969) suggested that in any case of so-called primary pulmonary hypertension a careful dietary history should be obtained from the patient, and Fishman (1974) warned against the unending stream of new drugs and "mysterious" herbal ingredients as possible causes for dietary pulmonary hypertension.

These admonitions should not be taken lightly. On the other hand, so far there has not been a single case of pulmonary hypertension in man that could be confidently attributed to the ingestion of herbs like Crotalaria or Senecio. Also, as far as we know, the incidence of primary pulmonary hypertension is generally not higher in those parts of the world where herbal medicines are very popular, such as Africa or the West Indies, than elsewhere. Moreover, in the rare accumulations of primary pulmonary hypertension, such as has been reported from Ceylon, no relation to the use of herbs could be established (Wallooppillai and Wagenvoort, 1976).

Particularly in the West Indies, Crotalaria intoxication has been recognized in man, mainly in children, less commonly in adults. Bras et al. (1954) described veno-occlusive disease of the liver in Jamaican children and later (1957) demonstrated conclusively that this was produced by Crotalaria ingredients contained in the so-called bush-tea, which is used as a beverage or for medicinal purposes. Intimal swelling followed by gradual fibrotic intimal thickening is responsible for the obstruction of small veins and venules in the liver. Thrombosis apparently plays no part in this occlusion. Cirrhosis of the liver and hemorrhage from esophageal varices frequently causes death. Although in the various case reports the interest clearly has been directed to the liver more than to the lungs, in none of these patients has there been evidence of pulmonary hypertension or pulmonary vascular disease.

Veno-occlusive disease of the lungs is known as a distinct, although rare, entity (Chapter Ten) but no relation to Crotalaria or other toxins is known, and it is unlikely that it is to be regarded as an example of dietary pulmonary hypertension.

ANOREXIGENS

We now come back to the role of anorexigens as a possible etiologic factor in the development of pulmonary hypertension.

In 1968, Gurtner and his coworkers reported a very dramatic increase of cases of primary pulmonary hypertension in Berne, Switzerland, which started in the second part of 1967. Before that time, primary pulmonary hypertension had been a rare disease that was diagnosed in only 0.87 percent of all adults in whom cardiac catheterization was performed. In the years 1967 and 1968 this incidence rose to 15.4 percent (Gurtner, 1969a). Since it appeared that many patients had used an appetite-suppressing drug, aminorex fumarate (Menocil), a causal relationship was accepted. Aminorex has a chemical structure (2-amino-5-phenyl-2-oxazoline) resembling that of amphetamine and epinephrine. By acting directly on the brain, it suppresses the appetite and may cause weight loss.

At approximately the same time as the epidemic in Berne, a markedly increased incidence of primary pulmonary hypertension was established in Austria (Kaindl, 1969; Schwingshackl et al., 1969) and to a lesser extent in West Germany (Hager et al., 1969; Lang et al., 1969; Steim, 1969). In these countries too anorexigenic drugs were implicated. Now that attention was aroused, reports on cases of primary pulmonary hypertension and its connection with aminorex multiplied. Numerous additional observations were published from clinical centers in Switzerland (Burkart et al., 1970; Gurtner, 1970; Nager and Bühlmann, 1970; Rivier, 1970; Wirz and Arbenz, 1970), Austria (Kaindl, 1970), and Germany (Gahl et al., 1970; Voss and Harms, 1970; Hager et al., 1971; Backmann et al., 1972). Rivier (1970) compared the incidence of primary pulmonary hypertension in five Swiss medical centers over the periods 1958 through 1965 and 1966 through 1969 and could trace 15 patients in the first period against 148 in the second. On a year basis this is a twentyfold increase.

Aminorex was introduced on the market in November 1965 in Switzerland, in April 1966 in West Germany, and in August 1966 in Austria. The drug was withdrawn in all three countries between September and December 1968. Shortly thereafter there was a distinct decline in the number of cases (Gurtner, 1969b; Blankart, 1970; Greiser, 1973). After the first rise in 1967 and the peak in 1969, the incidence was back to pre-epidemic proportions around 1972 (Greiser et al., 1975).

The time element, which was suggestive for a causal relationship between primary pulmonary hypertension and aminorex, was supported by the geographical distribution of the cases. The epidemic was limited to those countries where aminorex had been available. In the Netherlands, for instance, there was no increase in incidence (Wagenvoort, 1972), and the same applied to many other countries where aminorex was not introduced (Greiser et al., 1975).

The clinical course of the patients, who developed pulmonary hypertension following oral administration of anorexigenic drugs, is similar to that in other forms of severe pulmonary hypertension. It is a progressive and usually fatal disease. In some instances regression of pulmonary hypertension upon withdrawal of the drug has been reported (Gertsch and Stucki, 1970).

Women have been affected in a much higher proportion than men. Although this may be due to a higher susceptibility of the female in a similar way as in primary pulmonary hypertension (p. 120), it should be noted that anorexigenic drugs are taken particularly by women.

Appetite-suppressants other than aminorex also have been incriminated as acting upon the pulmonary vasculature. Phenformin and chlorphenformin among others have been reported to produce pulmonary hypertension (Fahlen et al., 1973; Greiser et al., 1975).

It is clear that the circumstantial evidence against aminorex is strong. Even so, some investigators have cautioned against accepting too easily the link between anorexigenic drugs and primary pulmonary hypertension (Kay et al., 1971; Fishman, 1974; W.H.O. Report, 1975).

In the first place there are obviously very few patients who have used anorexigens and who have developed pulmonary hypertension. It has been estimated that only 2 of 1000 individuals, who have been taking these drugs, develop pulmonary hypertension (Gahl et al., 1970). This is not necessarily a strong argument against a relationship, since it is very well possible that some persons have a higher susceptibility than others.

More disturbing was the fact that the dose of aminorex often had little relation to the risk of and the severity of the elevation of the pressure. Although Greiser et al. (1975) showed that the latent period for developing the disease was dose dependent, this dose was often minimal. Moreover, the very pronounced rise in the incidence of primary pulmonary hypertension could not be ascribed completely to the use of the drug, as the number of these patients who never had taken anorexigens rose as well (Rivier, 1970). Blankart (1970) stated that the fall in incidence of primary pulmonary hypertension after withdrawal of the drug started too early, although this was contradicted by later and larger studies (Greiser, 1973).

A distinct problem in establishing proof beyond doubt is the failure in many studies to induce pulmonary vascular disease in experimental animals with aminorex or other anorexigenic drugs. The earlier experiments seemed to lend some support to a relationship, since a slight and transient rise in pressure following intravenous infusion or oral application of aminorex in dogs was reported (Kraupp et al., 1969; Engelhardt et al., 1970). Many attempts have failed to produce pulmonary vascular lesions by administering aminorex to rats and dogs (Engelhardt et al., 1970; Kay et al., 1971; Will and Bisgard, 1972) and in monkeys (Smith et al., 1973). The results also were negative in cattle, even though chronic hypoxia was added as an extra stimulus by a high altitude environment (Byrne-Quinn and Grover, 1972).

We have administered aminorex fumarate to 20 rats as an oral dose of 20 mg/kg body weight for periods of 6 and 9 months. Morphometric assessment of the lung vessels could not detect any difference as compared to those in control animals. Also an intraperitoneal dose of 6 mg/kg body weight for the same periods of time had no effect. Similar negative results with regard to the lung vessels were obtained with chlorphentermine (Parwaresch et al., 1972).

This is in contrast to what is observed in patients who develop pulmonary hypertension after the use of aminorex. In most cases, severe pulmonary vascular disease of the plexogenic pulmonary arteriopathic type with concentric-laminar intimal fibrosis (Figure 6-10), necrotizing arteritis, and plexiform lesions develops (Figure 6-11) (Widgren and Kapanci, 1970; Kay et al., 1971, Obiditsch-Mayer and Kletter, 1972).

These vascular alterations are unlike those seen in chronic hypoxia. This is of importance since it might be argued that pulmonary hypertension following ingestion of anorexigens is not so much related to the drugs used as to the obesity that causes the patients to take these drugs. Severe obesity may cause pulmonary hypertension as seen in the Pickwickian syndrome (Chapter Eleven). Apart from the pulmonary vascular pathology being different, it is unlikely that obesity is responsible, since it appears that many patients who used aminorex and developed pulmonary hypertension, were only slightly overweight (Gurtner et al., 1968). Neither is there a correlation between the degree of obesity and the risk of developing pulmonary hypertension (Greiser and Gahl, 1970).

In evaluating the case against the appetite suppressants, it can be said that there are a number of strong arguments to link the recent outbreak of primary pulmonary hypertension to the use of aminorex and similar drugs. The proof of a direct causal relationship, however, is still lacking, with the failure of experimental reproducibility

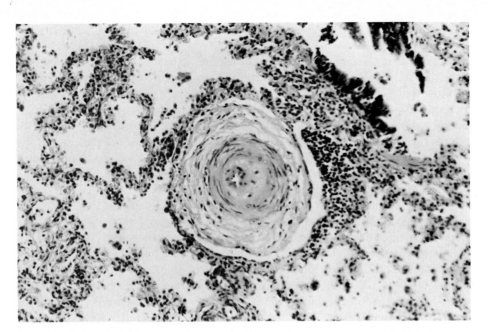

Figure 6-10. Muscular pulmonary artery with concentric laminar intimal fibrosis in a 56-year-old woman, who developed pulmonary hypertension following ingestion of aminorex (H. and E., ×125).

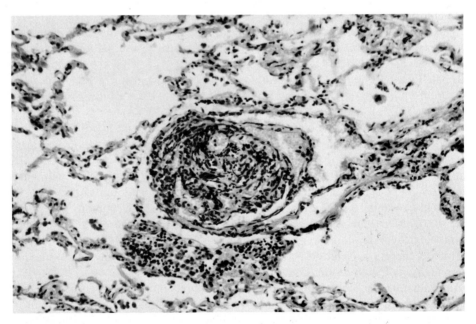

Figure 6-11. Plexiform lesion in muscular pulmonary artery from the same case as Figure 6-10 (H. and E., ×140).

as one of the most disturbing factors. It is true that the pulmonary circulation of animals may react differently from that in man. On the other hand, most forms of pulmonary hypertension, such as hyperkinetic, embolic, hypoxic, and congestive, can be produced at least in some animal species.

If aminorex should not be the culprit, the only other explanation at present, would be the coincidence of an epidemic of primary pulmonary hypertension with the aminorex episode. This possibility, though speculative, cannot be entirely dismissed since epidemics of this nature have been reported from Ceylon (Wagenvoort, 1973; Wallooppillai and Wagenvoort, 1976) and India, where appetite-suppressants certainly could not be blamed. Since further data are urgently needed, it is imperative to remain on the lookout for any side-effects of oral use of drugs on the pulmonary circulation and also for any epidemics of this nature, wherever they may occur.

In reviewing dietary pulmonary hypertension, the situation may be summed up in a few words. This form of pulmonary hypertension does occur in animals following ingestion of seeds or ingredients of Crotalaria, Senecio, and possibly other plants, although there is no proven case that this may happen in man. Anexorigens are under strong suspicion as causative agents of pulmonary hypertension in man. But, as Fishman (1974) predicted, it is unlikely that the saga of dietary pulmonary hypertension will end with the drugs we have mentioned.

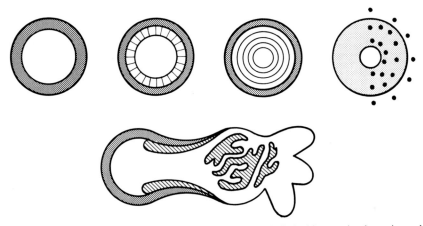

Dietary pulmonary hypertensive lesions: medial hypertrophy and fibrinoid necrosis of arteries and veins in animals and possibly plexogenic pulmonary arteriopathy in man.

REFERENCES

Allen, J. R., and Carstens, L. A.: Pulmonary vascular occlusions initiated by endothelial lysis in mono-crotaline-intoxicated rats. *Exp. Molec. Path.* 13: 159, 1970.

Allen, J. R., and Chessney, C. F.: Effect of age on development of cor pulmonale in non-human primates following pyrrolizidine alkaloid intoxication. *Exp. Molec. Path.* 17: 220, 1972.

Backmann, R., Dengler, H., Gahl, K., Greiser, E., Jesdinsky, H. J., and Loogen, F.: Primäre pulmonale Hypertonie. *Verh. Dtsch. Ges. Kreislaufforsch* 38: 134, 1972.

Barnes, J. M., Magee, P. N., and Schoental, R.: Lesions in the lungs and livers of rats poisoned with the pyrrolizidine alkaloid fulvine and its N-oxide. *J. Path. Bact.* 88: 521, 1964.

Blankart, R.: Der Zeitfaktor im Ablauf der primär vaskulären pulmonale Hypertonie. *Schweiz. Med. Wschr.* **100:** 2157, 1970.

Bras, G., Jelliffe, D. B., and Stuart, K. L.: Veno-occlusive disease of liver with nonportal type of cirrhosis, occurring in Jamaica. *Arch. Path.* **57:** 285, 1954.

Bras, G., Berry, D. M., and György, P.: Plants as aetiological factors in veno-occlusive disease of the liver. *Lancet* i: 960, 1957.

Burkart, F., Follath, F., and Jenzer, H. R.: Der Verlauf der obstruktiven pulmonale arteriellen Hypertension. *Schweiz. Med. Wschr.* **100:** 146, 1970.

Burns, J.: The heart and pulmonary arteries in rats fed on *Senecio jacobaea. J. Path.* **107:** 187, 1972.

Byrne-Quinn, E., and Grover, R. F.: Aminorex (Menocil) and amphetamine: acute and chronic effects on pulmonary and systemic haemodynamics in the calf. *Thorax* **27:** 127, 1972.

Carrillo, L., and Aviado, D. M.: Monocrotaline-induced pulmonary hypertension and p-chlorophenylalanine (PCPA). *Lab. Invest.* **20:** 243, 1968.

Chessney, C. F., and Allen, J. R.: Monocrotaline induced pulmonary vascular lesions in non-human primates. *Cardiovasc. Res.* **7:** 508, 1973.

Chessney, C. F., Allen, J. R., and Hsu, I. C.: Right ventricular hypertrophy in monocrotaline pyrrole treated rats. *Exp. Molec. Path.* **20:** 257, 1974.

Engelhardt, A., Kroneberg, G., Stoepel, K., and Stötzer, H.: On the effect of sympathomimetic substances on the systemic and pulmonary circulation following acute and chronic administration. *Proc. Meeting Europ. Soc. Study Drug Tox., Excerpta Medica,* Amsterdam, **12:** 110, 1970.

Fahlen, M., Bergman, H., Helder, G., Ryden, L., Wallentin, I., and Zettergren, L.: Phenformin and pulmonary hypertension. *Brit. Heart J.* **35:** 824, 1973.

Fishman, A. P.: Dietary pulmonary hypertension. *Circulation Res.* **35:** 657, 1974.

Gahl, K., Fabel, H., Greiser, E., Harmjanz, D., Ostertag, H., and Stender, H. S.: Primär vaskuläre pulmonale Hypertonie. *Z. Kreislaufforsch.* **59:** 868, 1970.

Gardiner, M. R., Royce, R., and Bokor, A.: Studies on *Crotalaria crispata,* a newly recognized cause of Kimberley horse disease. *J. Path. Bact.* **89:** 43, 1965.

Gertsch, M., and Stucki, P.: Weitgehend reversibele primär vaskuläre pulmonale Hypertonie bei einem Patienten mit Menocil-Einnahme. *Z. Kreislaufforsch.* **59:** 902, 1970.

Greiser, E.: Epidemiologische Untersuchungen zum Zusammenhang zwischen Appetitzüglereinnahme und primär vaskulärer pulmonaler Hypertonie. *Internist* **14:** 437, 1973.

Greiser, E., and Gahl, K.: Frequency estimations in ingestion of aminorex and incidence of primary pulmonary hypertension. *Proc. Meeting Europ. Soc. Study Drug Tox., Excerpta Medica,* Amsterdam, **12:** 89, 1970.

Greiser, E., Jesdinsky, H. J., Backmann, R., Both, A., Dengler, H. J., Gahl, K., and Loogen, F.: Primary pulmonary hypertension and Aminorex. Report on the epidemiological and statistical findings of the cooperative study of the association between ingestion of anorectic drugs and primary pulmonary hypertension, 1975.

Gurtner, H. P.: Ätiologie und Häufigkeit der primär vaskulären Formen des chronischen Cor pulmonale. *Dtsch. Med. Wschr.* **94:** 850, 1969a.

Gurtner, H. P.: Pulmonary hypertension produced by ingestion of substances. *Bull. Physio-Path. Resp.* **5:** 435, 1969b.

Gurtner, H. P.: Häufung der primär vaskulären pulmonale Hypertonie in der Schweiz, 1967–1970: Einleitung. *Schweiz. Med. Wschr.* **100:** 2144, 1970.

Gurtner, H. P., Gertsch, M., Salzmann, C., Stucki, P., and Wyss, F.: Häufen sich die primär vaskulären Formen des chronischen Cor pulmonale? *Schweiz. Med. Wschr.* **98:** 1579, 1695, 1968.

Hager, W., Wink, K., and Thiede, D.: Beobachtungen über die Zunahme der primär vasculären pulmonalen Hypertonie. *Verh. Dtsch. Ges. Inn. Med.* **75:** 436, 1969.

Hager, W., Thiede, D., and Wink, K.: Primär vaskuläre pulmonale Hypertonie und Appetitzügler. *Med. Klin.* **66:** 386, 1971.

Heath, D., and Kay, J. M.: Medial thickness of pulmonary trunk in rats with cor pulmonale induced by ingestion of Crotalaria seeds. *Cardiovasc. Res.* **1:** 74, 1967.

Hooper, P. T.: The pathology of *Senecio jacobaea* poisoning of mice. *J. Path.* **113**: 227, 1974.

Kaindl, F.: Primäre pulmonale Hypertension. *Wien. Zschr. Inn. Med.* **50**: 451, 1969.

Kaindl, F.: Pulmonale Hypertonie. *Wien. Med. Wschr.* **120**: 631, 1970.

Kay, J. M., and Heath, D.: Observations on the pulmonary arteries and heart weight of rats fed on *Crotalaria spectabilis* seeds. *J. Path. Bact.* **92**: 385, 1966.

Kay, J. M., Gillund, T. D., and Heath, D.: Mast cells in the lungs of rats fed on *Crotalaria spectabilis* seeds. *Amer. J. Path.* **51**: 1031, 1967.

Kay, J. M., and Heath, D.: *Crotalaria spectabilis. The Pulmonary Hypertension Plant.* Charles C Thomas, Springfield, Ill., 1969.

Kay, J. M., Smith, P., and Heath, D.: Electron microscopy of crotalaria pulmonary hypertension. *Thorax* **24**: 511, 1969.

Kay, J. M., Heath, D., Smith, P., Bras, G., and Summerell, J.: Fulvine and the pulmonary circulation. *Thorax* **26**: 249, 1971.

Kraupp, O., Stühlinger, W., Raberger, G., and Turnheim, K.: Die Wirkung von Aminorex (Menocil) auf die Hämodynamik des kleinen und grossen Kreislaufs bei i.v. Darreichung am Hund. *Arch. Exp. Path. Pharmak.* **264**: 389, 1969.

Lalich, J. J. and Merkow, L.: Pulmonary arteritis produced in rats by feeding *Crotalaria spectabilis. Lab. Invest.* **10**: 744, 1961.

Lang, E., Haupt, E. J., Köhler, J. A., and Schmidt, J.: Cor pulmonale durch Appetitzügler? *Münch. Med. Wschr.* **111**: 405, 1969.

Mattocks, A. R.: Toxicity of pyrrolizidine alkaloids. *Nature* **217**: 723, 1968.

Merkow, L., and Kleinerman, J.: An electron microscopic study of pulmonary vasculitis induced by monocrotaline. *Lab. Invest.* **15**: 547, 1966.

Nager, F., and Bühlmann, A.: Therapie und Prognose des chronischen Cor pulmonale. *Schweiz. Med. Wschr.* **100**: 135, 1970.

Obiditsch-Mayer, I. and Kletter, G.: Morphologische Untersuchungen an bioptischem und Sektionsmaterial bei pulmonaler Hypertonie nach "Menocil"-Medikation. *Verh. Dtsch. Ges. Path.* **56**: 509, 1972.

Parwaresch, M. R., Reil, G. H., and Seiler, K. U.: Organveränderungen nach chronischer Gabe von Appetitzüglern an Versuchstieren. *Verh. Dtsch. Ges. Path.* **56**: 513, 1972.

Rivier, J. L.: Hypertension artérielle pulmonaire primitive. *Schweiz. Med. Wschr.* **100**: 143, 1970.

Schoental, R.: Alkaloidal constituents of *Crotalaria fulva* Roxb., fulvine and its N-oxide. *Aust. J. Chem.* **16**: 233, 1963.

Schoental, R.: Herbal medicines to avoid. *Nature* **238**: 106, 1972.

Schwingshackl, H., Amor, H., and Dienstl, F.: Primäre pulmonale Hypertonie bei sieben jüngeren Frauen. *Dtsch. Med. Wschr.* **94**: 639, 1969.

Smith, P., Heath, D., Kay, J. M., Wright, J. S., and McKendrick, C. S.: Pulmonary arterial pressure and structure in the patas monkey after prolonged administration of aminorex fumarate. *Cardiovasc. Res.* **7**: 30, 1973.

Steim, H.: Primäre pulmonale Hypertonie. Klinische Beobachtungen an der medizinischen Universitätsklinik in Freiburg. *Wien. Zschr. Inn. Med.* **50**: 464, 1969.

Stötzer, H., Herbst, M., Reichl, R., and Köllmer, H.: Zur Pathogenese der experimentellen pulmonalen Hypertonie. Modellversuche mit *Crotalaria spectabilis* an Ratten. *Virch. Arch.* **356**: 331, 1972.

Takeoka, O., Angevine, D. M., and Lalich, J. J.: Stimulation of mast cells in rats fed various chemicals. *Amer. J. Path.* **40**: 545, 1962.

Turner, J. H., and Lalich, J. J.: Experimental cor pulmonale in the rat. *Arch. Path.* **79**: 409, 1965.

Valdivia, E., Sonnad, J., Hayashi, Y., and Lalich, J. J.: Experimental interstitial pulmonary edema. *Angiology* **18**: 378, 1967.

Voss, H., and Harms, H.: Epidemiologie und Klinik der primär vaskulären pulmonalen Hypertonie. Ein Bericht über 42 Fälle. *Z. Kreislaufforsch.* **59**: 887, 1970.

Wagenvoort, C. A.: Vasoconstrictive primary pulmonary hypertension and pulmonary veno-occlusive disease. *Cardiovasc. Clin.* **4**: 97, 1972.

Wagenvoort, C. A.: Primary pulmonary hypertension. *Lyon Médit. Méd.* **9:** 2717, 1973.

Wagenvoort, C. A., Wagenvoort, N., and Dijk, H. J.: Effect of fulvine on pulmonary arteries and veins of the rat. *Thorax* **29:** 522, 1974a.

Wagenvoort, C. A., Dingemans, K. P., and Lotgering, G. G.: Electron microscopy of pulmonary vasculature after application of fulvine. *Thorax* **29:** 511, 1974b.

Wallooppillai, N., and Wagenvoort, C. A.: Unpublished data, 1976.

World Health Organization: *Primary Pulmonary Hypertension. Report on a WHO Meeting.* S. Hatano, and T. Strasser (eds.), Geneva, 1975.

Widgren, S., and Kapanci, Y.: Menocilbedingte pulmonale Hypertonie. Vorläufige morphologische Ergebnisse über 8 pathologisch-anatomisch untersuchte Fälle. *Z. Kreislaufforsch.* **59:** 924, 1970.

Will, J. A., and Bisgard, G. E.: Haemodynamic effects of oral Aminorex and amphetamine in unanaesthetized beagle dogs. *Thorax* **27:** 120, 1972.

Wirz, P., and Arbenz, U.: Primär vaskuläre pulmonale Hypertonie in der Schweiz. *Schweiz. Med. Wschr.* **100:** 2147, 1970.

CHAPTER SEVEN

Unexplained Plexogenic Pulmonary Arteriopathy: Primary Pulmonary Hypertension

By their unique position in the circulation, the lungs often will show in their blood vessels or in their parenchyma the effects of processes elsewhere in the body. As a rule, a high pressure in the pulmonary circulation indicates a cardiac disorder or an embolic process, although the cause of the pulmonary hypertension also may be found in a disease of the lung tissue itself. Generally, the clinician will be able to diagnose an underlying heart or lung disease or to establish repeated thromboembolic events.

There are, however, patients in whom he will be unable to identify the etiology. These cases of pulmonary hypertension of unknown cause are relatively uncommon but present great difficulties in diagnosis and management to the clinician.

If patients with clinically unexplained pulmonary hypertension die and their lung tissue is studied morphologically, it appears that, with few exceptions, the lung vessels exhibit the features of one of three different pathologic entities (Wagenvoort, 1975).

In most of these instances the pulmonary arteries show a pattern of lesions, indicating that, in the course of time, repeated showers of usually small emboli have led to narrowing or obstruction of the vessels. This silent pulmonary embolism may go unnoticed for a long time until at last signs of right cardiac failure appear (Chapter Eight). These cases, although having remained unexplained during clinical observation, eventually should be classified in the category where they belong, that is, as embolic pulmonary hypertension.

Much rarer is the picture of obliteration of small pulmonary veins and venules with concomitant alterations in the lung tissue and to a lesser extent in the pulmonary arteries. This so-called pulmonary veno-occlusive disease, often difficult to diagnose during life and often confused with primary pulmonary hypertension (Wagenvoort, 1972), will be discussed in Chapter Ten.

There is a third and characteristic pattern of pulmonary vascular lesions, indicating another form of unexplained pulmonary hypertension. The lesions to be seen in this pattern are found exclusively in the pulmonary arteries. The veins as a rule are normal.

This form of unexplained pulmonary hypertension, to be dealt with in this chapter, is known under various names. The most commonly used terms are "primary" or "idiopathic" pulmonary hypertension, but the condition also has been designated as "solitary," "essential," or "of unknown etiology."

In the older literature the disease was known as "primary pulmonary vascular sclerosis," and the eponym "Ayerza's disease," although hardly justified (Wagenvoort et al., 1964), also was used to indicate the same condition.

In using the name "unexplained plexogenic pulmonary arteriopathy" for the underlying morphologic picture of the pulmonary vasculature, we conform to the terminology adopted by a World Health Organization committee (1975). This terminology relates to morphologic rather than clinical characteristics, and also stresses the identity of the pulmonary vascular pattern with that in cardiac disease with a shunt. The term "primary pulmonary hypertension," in conforming to the same report, will indicate the clinical picture of unexplained pulmonary hypertension.

While the causes of primary pulmonary hypertension are unknown, the recognizable alterations are primarily demonstrable in the lung vessels. Changes elsewhere, such as right ventricular hypertrophy or congestion of liver, are clearly secondary to the pulmonary vascular pathology.

This, of course, does not imply that factors outside the lung vessels may not be involved in the development of the pulmonary vascular disease. These factors, however, are obscure. In some instances a cause for pulmonary hypertension is suspected but not proven. This applies to patients with portal hypertension associated with pulmonary hypertension (p. 95) and also to patients who developed pulmonary hypertension following the ingestion of anorexigenic drugs (p. 111). It would be justifiable to speak of primary pulmonary hypertension in all these instances, as long as the etiology is not clarified, and this is what is done in most publications. For the sake of convenience we have discussed these conditions in Chapters Five and Six, respectively. If it should ever appear that the relation with hepatic injury or with appetite-suppressants is fortuitous, they should be placed under the heading of primary pulmonary hypertension.

Primary pulmonary hypertension is an uncommon disease but not as rare as often has been assumed. Since the first description by Romberg (1891), the number of cases reported in the literature, even without those associated with anorexigens, comes close to 1000, and although not all these are likely to be true examples, every pathologist may be expected to deal with such cases sooner or later.

The presence of an elevated pulmonary arterial pressure and resistance, at first only assumed on the basis of the pulmonary vascular lesions and right ventricular hypertrophy, was firmly established in later cases after the introduction of cardiac catheterization.

SEX INCIDENCE AND AGE

Primary pulmonary hypertension particularly affects young women, although neither men nor other age groups are exempt. Wood (1958) reported on a series of

26 patients, 21 of whom were female. Of 23 patients described by Walcott et al. (1970), 19 were female. This ratio of 5 to 1 was slightly lower in a larger series of 110 patients, in whom we have described the pathology (Wagenvoort and Wagenvoort, 1970a). There was an approximately equal sex ratio in children, but in the adult group of 71 patients, there were 56 females and 15 males—almost a 4 to 1 ratio.

The condition has been diagnosed in infants shortly after birth and in individuals over 60. The average age in our series was 23, and the great majority of the patients, known from the literature, were between 16 and 40.

FAMILIAL INCIDENCE

Familial occurrence of primary pulmonary hypertension was first reported by Clarke et al. (1927) and since then has been well established (Dresdale et al., 1954; Rogge et al., 1966; Delaye et al., 1969; Thompson and McRae, 1970). We found in the literature reports of 63 patients from 25 families. Usually the common occurrence concerns siblings but also parent-child and other relationships have been involved. Sometimes twins are affected (Porter et al., 1967; Czarnecki et al., 1968). This familial form of primary pulmonary hypertension does not have any distinctive features. Sex ratio, age, symptomatology, duration, and the pattern of pulmonary vascular lesions are all in the same range as found in the nonfamilial form.

EPIDEMICS

The most conspicuous accumulation of cases of primary pulmonary hypertension is that which occurred in the period 1967 to 1971 in three European countries. As we have noted in Chapter 6, this has been ascribed to the use of anorexigens, but as long as this relation is not clarified, it seems appropriate to designate these cases as primary pulmonary hypertension.

In approximately the same period there has been an accumulation of cases, if not an epidemic of this disease in Sri Lanka (Ceylon) from where 87 patients over an 8-year period have been recognized (Wallooppillai and Wagenvoort, 1976).

The cause of this epidemic remained unknown but appetite-suppressants most certainly were not involved. The accumulation of cases in this country had been attributed to infection with filarial worms (Obeyesekere and de Soysa, 1970), but later it appeared that the incidence of primary pulmonary hypertension was also high in areas where *Wuchereria bancrofti* is not endemic and that many patients had no eosinophilia (Wallooppillai and Wagenvoort, 1976). Moreover, it appeared that the pulmonary vasculature in those patients in whom a lung biopsy or autopsy material was available showed the picture of plexogenic pulmonary arteriopathy, while evidence for filariasis was found in none of them.

CLINICAL COURSE

In the established stage of the disease, the clinical signs and symptoms may suggest primary pulmonary hypertension, when the physical signs specific to primary heart or lung disease as a possible cause for the elevated pulmonary arterial pressure, are absent. Even so the definitive diagnosis depends on the data obtained from cardiac catheterization and angiography.

Diagnostic problems arise particularly when these cases must be differentiated from cases of pulmonary veno-occlusive disease and chronic embolic pulmonary hypertension (Fowler et al., 1966).

In effect, it is likely that numerous patients in whom a diagnosis of primary pulmonary hypertension has been made were actually suffering from other forms of pulmonary hypertension, most frequently from thromboembolism (Wagenvoort and Wagenvoort, 1970b).

Dyspnea on exertion and fatigue are the most common and usually the first symptoms. The history may further reveal in approximately half the cases (Yu, 1958) syncope, probably due to diminished cardiac output and cerebral blood flow (Dressler, 1952), and chest pain. Hemoptysis is less common but sometimes fatal (Forbes, 1958). Cyanosis is observed particularly in the later stages of the disease. Hoarseness, resulting from pressure on the left recurrent laryngeal nerve by the enlarged pulmonary artery is an occasional symptom (Soothill, 1951).

The physical and roentgenographic findings in patients with primary pulmonary hypertension are consistent with the elevation of pulmonary arterial pressure, right ventricular hypertrophy, and sometimes right heart failure (Sleeper et al., 1962; Fowler et al., 1966; Walcott et al., 1970) in the absence of signs of cardiac defects, vascular disease, or elevated left atrial pressure.

The duration of symptoms varies. The average period between the onset of the disease and death is between 2 to 3 years. A more precipitate course is not uncommon. Particularly in children death may follow the first symptoms within weeks. On the other hand, patients are known to have lived between 15 and 30 years with this disease (Charters and Baker, 1970; Wagenvoort and Wagenvoort, 1970a). It is possible that elevation of pulmonary arterial pressure starts long before the clinical signs become apparent (Shane et al., 1964). In some patients pulmonary hypertension was suspected 3 to 10 years before the first symptoms appeared (Ahlquist and Burstein, 1958; Stucki et al., 1963). In other cases such a long, silent course was unlikely (Durrance and Winchell, 1961).

Sudden death is not rare and particularly cardiac catheterization, angiocardiography, anesthesia, and surgical procedures have been reported not to be tolerated (Berthrong and Cochran, 1955; Cawley and Stofer, 1957; Caldini et al., 1959; Sleeper et al., 1962; Wagenvoort and Wagenvoort, 1970a). Also barbiturates have been deemed responsible for sudden death in these cases (Inkley et al., 1955).

There is no adequate therapy for primary pulmonary hypertension. Apart from symptomatic treatment, anticoagulants have been used but at best with very limited effect. Infusion with vasodilators such as acetylcholine (p. 4) may temporarily relieve the pulmonary vascular resistance but without arresting progression of the disease.

MORPHOLOGY

The morphologic alterations in primary pulmonary hypertension in principle are identical to those in congenital cardiac disease with a shunt and thus can be designated as plexogenic pulmonary arteriopathy. The differences, if any, are quantitative rather than qualitative (Wagenvoort and Wagenvoort, 1974). In a postmortem arteriogram the same dilatation of the larger arteries and the "pruned" and coiled appearance of the smaller ones to be observed in cardiac anomalies also is seen here (Figure 7-1). Therefore, we can confine ourselves to a short discussion, while referring to Chapter Four for a more detailed description.

Pulmonary Trunk, Main Arteries and Elastic Pulmonary Arteries

The pulmonary trunk is usually wider than the aorta with a thickness of its wall approximately the same as that of the aorta (Figure 7-2). Although the media is hypertrophied, atherosclerosis may contribute to the thickness of its wall and that of the main arteries (Figure 7-3).

As has been discussed in Chapter Four, in congenital cardiac shunts pulmonary hypertension is present from birth and the pulmonary trunk and main arteries show an "aortic" configuration with regular and intact elastic laminae.

In most cases of primary pulmonary hypertension, the disease is acquired in later life. This is suggested by the late appearance of symptoms and by the occasional

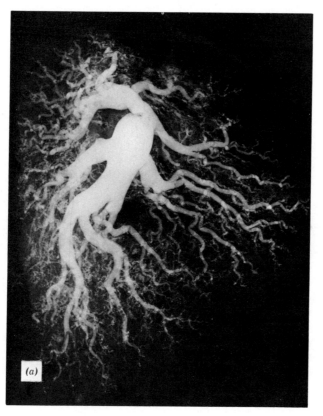

Figure 7-1. (a) Postmortem pulmonary arteriogram from an 18-year-old man with unexplained plexogenic pulmonary arteriopathy (primary pulmonary hypertension). The main branches are dilated.

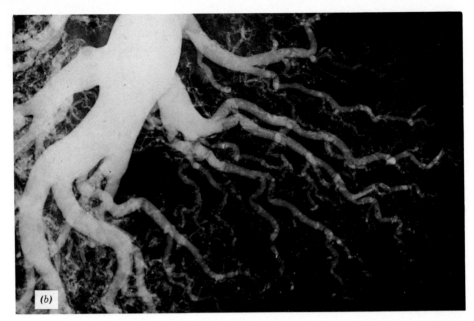

Figure 7-1. (*b*) Detail from Figure 7-1*a*. The peripheral pulmonary arteries are coiled and "pruned." There is little background filling.

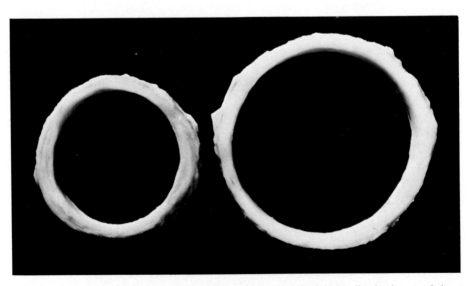

Figure 7-2. Transverse slices of aorta (*left*) and pulmonary trunk (*right*) after fixation in expanded state, in the same patient as in Figure 7-1. The pulmonary trunk is dilated and its wall thickness is at least equal to that of the aorta.

case of primary pulmonary hypertension in which previous study showed a normal pressure in the pulmonary arteries. Also the structure of the pulmonary trunk and main arteries usually suggests an acquired origin. Heath and Edwards (1960) demonstrated that in primary pulmonary hypertension the elastic configuration in these vessels is the same as in normal individuals with scarce and interrupted elastic laminae (Figure 7-4).

Occasionally, and then usually in children, an "aortic" configuration is present (Figure 7-5). Roberts (1963) described this pattern in a 16-year-old girl. This would indicate that the pressure was raised before the elastic structure of the pulmonary trunk had an opportunity to change to the "adult" configuration, that is, within the first year of life. It does not necessarily mean that pulmonary hypertension was congenital. In some cases the interpretation of the structure of the pulmonary trunk is equivocal in this respect (Farrar et al., 1961).

Atherosclerosis of the large pulmonary arteries (Figure 7-6) including intrapulmonary elastic arteries (Figure 7-7) usually is marked. Saccular aneurysms of pulmonary trunk or of its main branches (Van Epps, 1957) have been described. Cystic medial necrosis of large pulmonary arteries was reported by Rawson (1958) and partial rupture of the pulmonary trunk by Aars (1965). Primary thrombosis of the large pulmonary arteries (Montgomery, 1935; Soustek, 1960) is rare. The presence of thrombi in the major pulmonary arteries may throw serious doubt on the diagnosis of primary pulmonary hypertension since the chances are that these are embolic in origin.

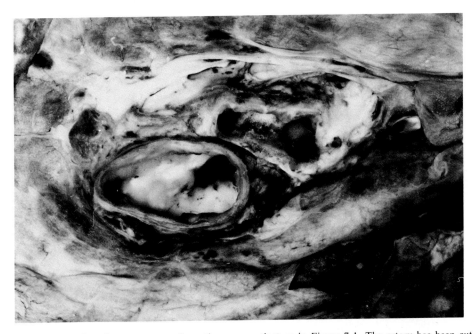

Figure 7-3. Main pulmonary artery from the same patient as in Figure 7-1. The artery has been cut close to the hilum of the lung. The orifices of its primary branches are narrowed by pronounced atherosclerosis.

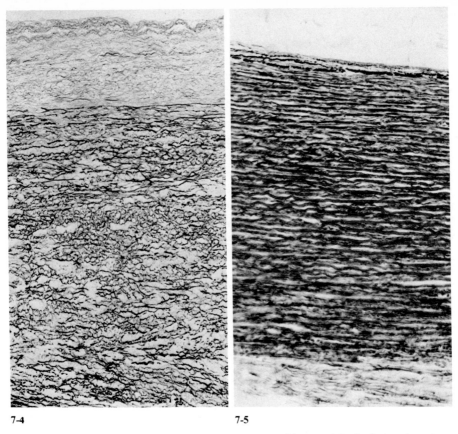

7-4   7-5

Figure 7-4. Pulmonary trunk in a 19-year-old woman with unexplained plexogenic pulmonary arteriopathy. There is an "adult" elastic configuration with interrupted and irregular elastic laminae and fibrous thickening of the intima (El.v.G., ×90).

Figure 7-5. Pulmonary trunk in a 2-year-old boy with unexplained plexogenic pulmonary arteriopathy. There is an "aortic" elastic configuration with regular intact elastic laminae (El.v.G., ×140).

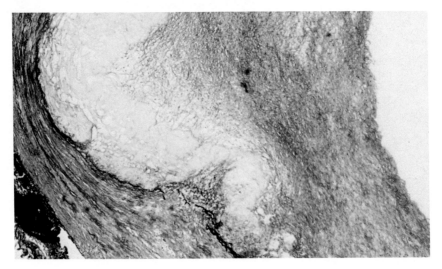

Figure 7-6. Main pulmonary artery with pronounced atherosclerosis in a 43-year-old man with unexplained plexogenic pulmonary arteriopathy (El.v.G., ×50).

126

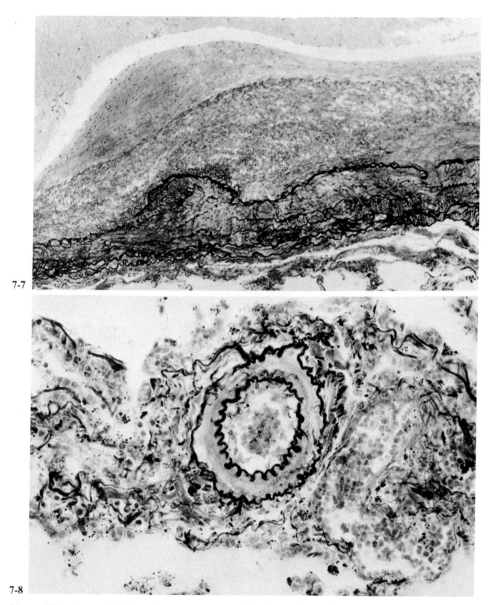

Figure 7-7. Large elastic pulmonary artery with atherosclerosis in a 22-year-old woman with unexplained plexogenic pulmonary arteriopathy (El.v.G., ×90).
Fig. 7-8. Muscular pulmonary artery with medial hypertrophy in a 44-year-old woman with unexplained plexogenic pulmonary arteriopathy (El.v.G., ×350).

Muscular Pulmonary Arteries and Arterioles

Medial hypertrophy of muscular pulmonary arteries (Figure 7-8) and muscularization of arterioles with extension of smooth muscle to peripheral segments of small branches is a constant feature of primary pulmonary hypertension. Even if it is masked by subsequent dilatation or by secondary atrophy of the media in the presence of severe intimal fibrosis, the average medial thickness, calculated from a large number of arteries, is in excess of normal limits.

The statement that in cases of primary pulmonary hypertension the wall of the pulmonary arteries may be entirely normal (De Navasquez et al., 1940; East, 1940; McKeown, 1952; McGuire et al., 1957) is unlikely and could be reputed in several instances (Wagenvoort and Wagenvoort, 1970a).

Cellular intimal proliferation may be present (Figure 7-9) as a lesion preceding concentric-laminar intimal fibrosis. The latter change is often widespread and obstructive (Figures 7-10 and 7-11). This form of intimal fibrosis is usually sharply demarcated from the excentric nonlaminar fibrotic patches due to organized thromboemboli.

It must be stipulated that the type of intimal fibrosis cannot be decided from a single artery or from a few arteries. The intimal fibrosis is not always purely concentric, and it may look distinctly excentric when it protrudes from a branch around its orifice into the lumen of the parent vessel (Figure 7-12). Also, one should keep in mind that an occasional thrombotic or thromboembolic intimal patch may be found in any lung even in normal individuals. The overall aspect of the arteries should be judged and will usually be conclusive.

Even so, in 6 of 110 cases of primary pulmonary hypertension, there were multiple or even numerous thrombotic or thromboembolic lesions in addition to widespread

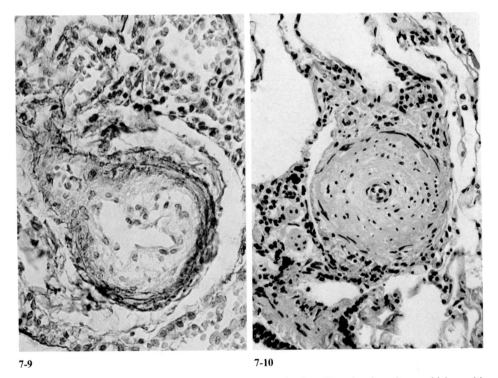

7-9   7-10

Figure 7-9. Muscular pulmonary artery with cellular intimal proliferation in a 2-year-old boy with unexplained plexogenic pulmonary arteriopathy (El.v.G., ×350).
Figure 7-10. Muscular pulmonary artery with concentric laminar intimal fibrosis in a 22-year-old woman with unexplained plexogenic pulmonary arteriopathy (H. and E., ×225).

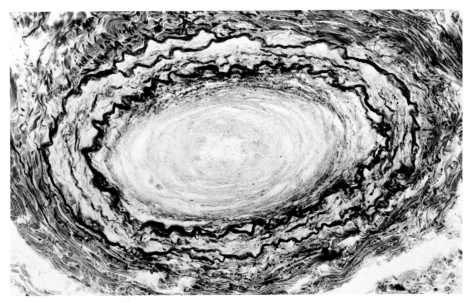

Figure 7-11. Muscular pulmonary artery with obliterating concentric laminar intimal fibrosis in a 2-year-old boy with unexplained plexogenic pulmonary arteriopathy (El.v.G., ×350).

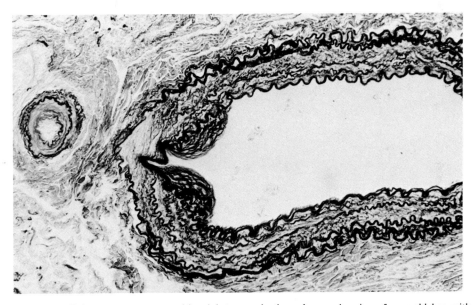

Figure 7-12. Pulmonary artery, transitional between elastic and muscular, in a 5-year-old boy with unexplained plexogenic pulmonary arteriopathy. At the site of origin of a branch (left) there are two cushion-like patches as part of concentric laminar intimal fibrosis protruding into the parent artery (El.v.G., ×140).

vasoconstrictive lesions including concentric laminar intimal fibrosis (Wagenvoort and Wagenvoort, 1970a). We will come back to the possible significance of the combination later (p. 133).

Necrotizing arteritis, plexiform lesions, and dilatation lesions are identical to the corresponding lesions in congenital heart disease, but their incidence in primary pulmonary hypertension is much higher. If enough blocks of lung tissue are studied, in our experience, necrotizing arteritis (Figure 7-13) is a fairly common finding, and plexiform lesions even may be found in approximately 70 percent of patients dying from primary pulmonary hypertension (Figures 7-14 and 7-15), although the number of these alterations in individual cases may vary considerably. This corresponds closely to the data reported by Walcott et al. (1970).

Postmortem angiography of the lungs of patients with primary pulmonary hypertension reveals the same "pruned tree" appearance as in congenital heart disease with pulmonary hypertension (p. 62). Microangiography also demonstrates the obstruction of the smallest arterial branches (Reeves and Noonan, 1973), and sometimes even plexiform lesions may show up by this method (Robertson, 1971).

Alveolar Capillaries

In some patients the capillaries are locally engorged but generally the alveolar walls, including the capillaries, are normal. Thickening of capillary basement membranes and of the endothelial layer in electron-microscopic preparations has been described (Meyrick et al., 1974). Although this observation rests on a single case, it would

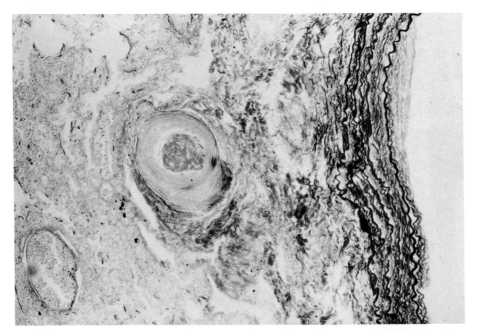

Figure 7-13. Fibrinoid necrosis in a muscular branch of an elastic pulmonary artery (right) in a 2-year-old boy with unexplained plexogenic pulmonary arteriopathy (El.v.G., ×90).

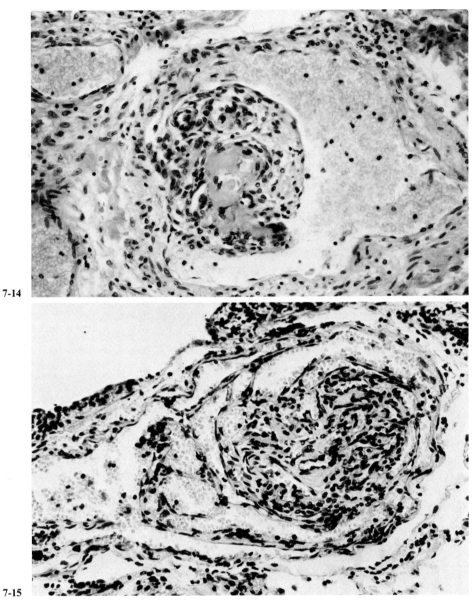

7-14

7-15

Figure 7-14. Early plexiform lesion in muscular pulmonary artery in a 13-year-old girl with unexplained plexogenic pulmonary arteriopathy. There is active proliferation of cells in a fibrin clot (H. and E., ×225).

Figure 7-15. Full-grown plexiform lesion in muscular pulmonary artery in a 28-year-old woman with unexplained plexogenic pulmonary arteriopathy (H. and E., ×225).

confirm what has been reported in patients with pulmonary hypertension due to congenital heart disease (p. 85). It certainly does not seem to be specific for primary pulmonary hypertension.

Pulmonary Veins and Venules

Primary pulmonary hypertension, in principle, affects only the arteries. The pulmonary veins and venules are normal. In the uncommon cases, exhibiting arterialization and increased thickness of venous walls, there is reason to believe that cardiac insufficiency is responsible for an elevated pressure in the left atrium and in the pulmonary venous system.

Hemosiderosis

Hemosiderosis, with iron pigment either free in the interstitium of the lung or within alveolar macrophages, is often present in cases of primary pulmonary hypertension, particularly when there are dilatation lesions. On the other hand, hemosiderosis is usually mild as compared to cases of increased pulmonary venous pressure. Its presence cannot be used as a diagnostic criterium for primary pulmonary hypertension nor is it a reliable feature for assessing the stage or severity of the disease.

PATHOLOGIC DIAGNOSIS

As we have seen, the pattern of the vascular lesions in primary pulmonary hypertension is essentially indistinguishable from that in congenital cardiac disease with a shunt and thus not pathognomonic (Heath et al., 1957). If, however, the pathologist can exclude the presence of such cardiovascular anomalies, the pulmonary vascular lesions are usually sufficiently characteristic to make an accurate morphologic diagnosis.

ETIOLOGY

As the cause of primary pulmonary hypertension is by definition unknown, it has long been regarded as a wastebasket diagnosis. Obviously, various cases of cardiac and pulmonary disease, leading to an elevated pulmonary arterial pressure and particularly thromboembolism, have been and still are thrown together under this ill-defined clinical diagnosis. There is no doubt that the total of published case reports forms a very heterogeneous collection.

With increasing numbers of reported cases it became clear that there was a group of patients in whom neither thromboembolism nor diseases of heart or lung tissue could be held responsible for the increased pressure. In these cases the changes apparently started in the vessels of the lung, even though the mechanism by which the lesions were brought about, remained a matter of speculation. Consequently the term "primary pulmonary hypertension" survived but, in view of the pattern of pulmonary vascular alterations in these cases, the diagnosis can now be narrowed down to "unexplained plexogenic pulmonary arteriopathy." Even though this is a morphologic entity, it is questionable whether all cases are based on a single etiologic factor. In the course of time the hypotheses for an etiologic explanation have multiplied. These various views will be discussed briefly.

Thromboembolism as Causative Factor

Thromboembolism has been suspected to be the cause in most, if not in all, cases of primary pulmonary hypertension (Owen et al., 1953; Thomas, 1955; Freilich and Szatkowski, 1961; Goodwin et al., 1963; Rosenberg, 1964; Dexter, 1965). Olsen (1973) believes that both thromboembolism and vasoconstriction contribute to the elevation of pressure. Chronic embolism may lead to pulmonary hypertension without clinical indication of embolic events ("silent" pulmonary embolism) and showers of minute emboli were thought to cause the elevation of pressure (Goodwin et al., 1963).

Even so it has been pointed out (Wood, 1958, 1959) that an embolic origin of primary pulmonary hypertension would not concur with its predominant occurrence in women nor would it explain its frequent occurrence in children. The epidemic of primary pulmonary hypertension in Sri Lanka (p. 121) also would be very difficult to explain on a thromboembolic basis since thromboembolism is there, as in most Asian countries, very rare.

Clotting disorders in patients with primary pulmonary hypertension are usually not demonstrable. In one family with the familial form, several members had an abnormal fibrinolysis but the lung vessels contained no microemboli (Inglesby et al., 1973).

In most autopsy cases a source for emboli was not found, even in cases in which an adequate search for venous thrombosis had been made. Recognizable thrombi in major or small pulmonary arteries are usually absent.

Also important is the fact that the morphologic alterations of the lung vessels in primary pulmonary hypertension differ from those in proven cases of chronic thromboembolism, as is revealed by a comparison of the pattern of these lesions in the two conditions (see also Chapter Eight).

There is no doubt that thromboembolic and primary pulmonary hypertension have often been confused not only by the clinician but also by the pathologist, who is not always aware of the characteristic pulmonary vascular pattern in these patients. In a series of 156 patients having died under the diagnosis of primary pulmonary hypertension, there were 31 in whom the elevation of pulmonary arterial pressure must have resulted from thromboembolism in view of the nature of the vascular changes (Wagenvoort and Wagenvoort, 1970a). It is, however, very likely that the number of embolic cases, misdiagnosed as "primary," is in fact much greater than reflected by the ratio to be derived from this series, since there was obviously selection in the way this material was composed.

Of 110 out of the 156 patients, who were considered true examples of primary pulmonary hypertension on the basis of pulmonary vascular pathology, there were 6 in whom the characteristic lesions of primary pulmonary hypertension were combined with vascular changes clearly due to thromboembolism. This may be coincidence or an expression of an increased risk for venous thrombosis in a late stage of the disease. On the other hand, the possibility that in certain cases vasoconstriction is elicited by pulmonary emboli can not be ruled out, although then apparently it must be very uncommon and certainly not a major cause for producing the disease.

Amniotic Fluid Embolism

The high incidence of primary pulmonary hypertension in women and particularly its frequent onset or aggravation during pregnancy and following delivery have led to the supposition that nonfatal embolism of amniotic fluid might trigger the disease (Shepherd et al., 1957). This, at best, could mean—and it is difficult to exclude the possibility—that amniotic fluid embolism is responsible for some cases, since in the great majority there is no relation with pregnancy. On the other hand, it has been shown that various forms of pulmonary hypertension are influenced by pregnancy and delivery (Jewett and Ober, 1956; Wagenvoort and Wagenvoort, 1970a), and thus that this relation is not reserved for primary pulmonary hypertension.

There can be hardly any doubt that factors related to maturity in the female sex are involved in the development of primary pulmonary hypertension. Otherwise it would be difficult to explain the marked preponderance of the disease in adult females as contrasted to the equal sex ratio in children. The case for amniotic fluid embolism as a causative factor, however, is not convincing.

Generalized Arteriopathy

Although primary pulmonary hypertension is generally a disease confined to the pulmonary circulation, with only secondary effects on the heart, in a certain percentage of the cases there are also lesions in systemic arteries.

Concomitant pulmonary and systemic hypertension has been described (Evans, 1959; Innocenti and Toso, 1965), but it is so rare that it is likely to be a coincidence. This, however, can not be maintained for the association of primary pulmonary hypertension with Raynaud's phenomenon.

From an analysis of published cases it appears that Raynaud's phenomenon is fairly common in patients with primary pulmonary hypertension. In our series (Wagenvoort and Wagenvoort, 1970a) it occurred in over 7 percent and in that of Walcott and associates (1970) in 30 percent. Moreover, it appears that in families of patients with primary pulmonary hypertension, other members not affected by this disease suffered from Raynaud's phenomenon (Rawson and Woske, 1960; Seldin et al., 1962).

As Raynaud's phenomenon often is associated with autoimmune diseases, it is not surprising that several patients with primary pulmonary hypertension also were affected by conditions like polyarteritis nodosa (Rose and Spencer, 1957), scleroderma (Trell and Lindström, 1971), dermatomyositis (Caldwell and Aitchison, 1956), disseminated lupus erythematosus (Slama et al., 1967), rheumatoid arthritis (Gardner et al., 1957), Hashimoto's disease (Rawson and Woske, 1960), and primary biliary cirrhosis of the liver (Cohen and Mendelow, 1965). Allergic vasculitis was suspected in the cases of Barnard and Davel (1956) and Maekawa and Hayashi (1965).

It is important to realize that in several of these autoimmune diseases, arterial necrosis and arteritis of both systemic and pulmonary circulations may occur, closely resembling the necrotizing arteritis, observed in severe pulmonary hypertension. If these alterations are limited to the pulmonary vasculature in the presence of an elevated pressure, it is likely that they are caused by the pulmonary hypertension, rather than by, for instance, polyarteritis nodosa (Braunstein, 1955).

The association of primary pulmonary hypertension with autoimmune diseases is too common to be dismissed as coincidence. On the other hand, it is not common enough to accept without hesitation the view of Farrar and associates (1961, 1963) that primary pulmonary hypertension must necessarily be regarded as part of an autoimmune process. It also must be stressed that the correlation of primary pulmonary hypertension with Raynaud's phenomenon is much stronger than that with the total group of autoimmune diseases, particularly since most patients from the latter group also suffered from Raynaud's phenomenon.

The common association of plexogenic pulmonary arteriopathy with Raynaud's phenomenon suggests another possible mechanism for the development of pulmonary hypertension. Raynaud's phenomenon is an expression of vasospasms in digital arteries and this, as was pointed out by Walcott et al. (1970), may strengthen the contention that in these patients there are vasospasms of pulmonary arteries as well (p. 137).

Even so, the possibility that immunologic disorders are basic to the lesions of plexogenic pulmonary arteriopathy requires further consideration. The association of this condition with pulmonary schistosomiasis (p. 166) and hepatic cirrhosis (p. 95) which often follows a virus hepatitis might suggest an immunologic reaction involving the lung vessels. There are, however, as we have seen before, also several examples of hepatic injury which were certainly not of an infectious nature, so that all we can say is that the immunologic theory awaits more substantiation.

James (1962) attributed the syncopal attacks, often occurring in patients with primary pulmonary hypertension, to lesions in the sinus node and in the sinus node artery and postulated that the hypertensive changes in the lung vessels were part of a generalized degenerative arterial disease. His findings in three patients, however, have not been confirmed by others (Blount, 1967). In six patients in whom we had an opportunity to study this aspect, the sinus node and sinus node artery were normal.

Congenital Vascular Disease

Lesions like medial hypertrophy, medial "hypoplasia," (Gilmour and Evans, 1946; Evans et al., 1957), and plexiform lesions (Hufner and McNicol, 1958; Moschcowitz et al., 1961; Masshoff and Röher, 1964) have been considered congenital malformations of the arteries and arterioles. If this supposition were correct, it might imply that primary pulmonary hypertension is a congenital pulmonary vascular disorder. In Chapter Four, however, we have demonstrated that these alterations are reactive to the hemodynamic situation and thus are acquired, even though medial hypertrophy is present immediately after or even at the time of birth.

The vast majority of patients with primary pulmonary hypertension acquired the condition during later life but some infants apparently have the elevation of pressure from birth. Even then this is unlikely to result from vascular anomalies. Rather the alterations should be regarded either as a response to abnormal functional stimuli or secondary to the increased pressure.

Genetic factors in the etiology of primary pulmonary hypertension, at least in some instances, are suggested by the fairly common familial incidence (p. 121).

Vasoconstriction

Pharmacologic agents like acetylcholine and tolazoline (priscoline) may have a vasodilatative effect on the pulmonary arteries in cases of primary pulmonary hypertension and thereby lower the pulmonary arterial pressure and resistance (Marshall et al., 1959). Unfortunately these drugs have no lasting effect (Yu, 1958; Marshall et al., 1959; Charms, 1961; Robertson et al., 1969; Rao et al., 1969). In other instances there is no effect at all (Rudolph et al., 1958). However, in view of the high incidence of intimal changes in the pulmonary arteries, it is hardly to be expected that all patients would react in the same way, since a decrease in vascular tone with subsequent dilatation presupposes a reactive, if hypertrophic, media. Severe narrowing or obstruction of arteries by intimal fibrosis will forestall the dilatory effect of pharmacologic agents. In this respect it is important to note that a patient with primary pulmonary hypertension who reacted strongly to an infusion of acetylcholine showed no effect three years later when the procedure was repeated (Samet et al., 1960; Samet and Bernstein, 1963).

One of the most potent pulmonary vasoconstrictors is hypoxia while oxygen acts as a vasodilator. We do not know by what mechanism these effects are brought about but there is no reason to suppose that hypoxia alone is basic to primary pulmonary hypertension. The morphologic picture of the lung vessels in primary pulmonary hypertension is different from that in hypoxic pulmonary hypertension at high altitude. In people living at high altitude there is medial hypertrophy, particularly of the smallest pulmonary arteries. The intima may contain longitudinal muscle fibers (p. 239) but the characteristic lesions of plexogenic pulmonary arteriopathy are absent.

On the other hand, there may be some indication that the incidence of primary pulmonary hypertension is higher in high altitude regions, where hypoxia prevails, than at sea level. Exact epidemiologic data are lacking but Blount (1967) mentioned his experience with cardiac catheterization in "approximately 50 patients" from the Denver area. Berthrong et al. (1965) stipulated that of 30 patients studied at autopsy, 18 were living at an altitude of 4500 to 7000 feet and 5 at altitudes of 8000 to 10,000 feet. In view of the relatively small population at the latter altitudes, this is suggestive of a remarkably high incidence. Khoury and Hawes (1963) reported on 11 children with primary pulmonary hypertension from high altitude regions. Some of their cases have been criticized as not being true examples of primary pulmonary hypertension (Blount, 1963). Even so, two of their patients died of pulmonary hypertension, while the majority was symptomatic. Epidemiologic data on the incidence of the disease in high altitude as compared to sea level areas, are clearly indicated.

If primary pulmonary hypertension should have a higher incidence at high altitude, it must be caused by a factor other than hypoxia, although the threshhold for this unknown factor may have been influenced by the high altitude environment.

As we have seen, the striking relation between primary pulmonary hypertension and Raynaud's phenomenon also draws attention to a possible vasoconstrictive action in the lung vessels, even though the link with the spasms in the systemic arteries remains enigmatic.

The morphology of the pulmonary arteries in cases of primary pulmonary hypertension lends further support to the concept of vasoconstriction and to spasms of the arterial muscle in particular. A sustained increase of arterial muscular tone will lead to medial hypertrophy of the muscular pulmonary arteries. Although this feature is conspicuous in early cases of primary pulmonary hypertension, particularly in children, it is little helpful since all forms of pulmonary hypertension will show some degree of medial hypertrophy.

Fibrinoid necrosis and an inflammatory reaction in the muscular pulmonary arteries, however, may well be related to severe vasoconstriction or even more likely to bouts of arterial spasms (p. 75). This is also known in the systemic circulation. Moreover, in rats exposed to a single intraperitoneal injection of fulvine, intense vasoconstriction of the pulmonary arteries can be produced, demonstrable by histologic and electron-microscopic techniques and followed by medial hypertrophy and fibrinoid necrosis of pulmonary arteries. As we have seen (p. 78), there is evidence that in the human the plexiform lesions develop on the basis of this necrotizing arteritis.

While vasoconstriction apparently plays an important part in the pathogenesis of plexogenic pulmonary arteriopathy, this has not helped us significantly in clarifying the etiology of the disease. The most potent vasoconstrictive factor, we know, that affects many individuals, is hypoxia; but as a sole factor this appears not to produce primary pulmonary hypertension, although at best, it may influence the incidence in an indirect way.

Why does the condition occur more in women than in men, at least after sexual maturity is reached? What is the exact role of portal hypertension (p. 95) and eventually of anorexigens (p. 111) in the development of plexogenic pulmonary arteriopathy? Is there a similar pathogenesis in patients with pulmonary schistosomiasis (p. 166) as in those with primary pulmonary hypertension, since schistosomiasis of the lungs also is characterized by the morphologic features of plexogenic arterial disease? These questions and many others have remained unanswered in spite of numerous efforts. The sorely needed solution to the etiology of primary pulmonary hypertension also probably would have a great impact on our understanding of the pulmonary circulation in general.

Hyper-reactivity of Lung Vessels

If vasoconstriction is an important factor in the pathogenesis of the pulmonary arterial lesions and in the initial elevation of the pressure, it is hardly likely that there is one single factor that triggers the contraction of vascular smooth muscle.

Patients affected by this condition can be found all over the world. Apart from the occasional accumulation of cases and from some familial incidence, it concerns usually isolated cases. There is no clear common factor with regard to environment, social circumstances, living habits, or diet.

Therefore, it seems likely that multiple, possibly numerous factors may elicit this disease. Even then we must assume that only very few individuals exposed to these stimuli develop pulmonary hypertension and pulmonary vascular lesions.

This would be in keeping with the supposition that there is an individual hyperreactivity of the pulmonary arteries (p. 15). In animals, a great variability in pulmonary arterial reactivity has been demonstrated not only for various species but also for individuals within one species (Grover et al., 1963; Wagenvoort et al., 1969; Weir et al., 1974).

Years ago, Snellen (1960, personal communication) expressed the opinion that the uncommon patient with atrial septal defect associated with severe pulmonary hypertension, in fact is suffering from primary pulmonary hypertension in conjunction with his cardiac anomaly. Recently, Bessinger et al. (1975) also suggested the possibility that primary vascular disease was involved in their patient, a male infant with a patent ductus arteriosus. It is certainly possible that "hyper-reactive" individuals develop severe and irreversible plexogenic pulmonary arteriopathy in the presence of a pre- or post-tricuspid shunt which in the majority of the patients thus affected, would not lead to pronounced elevation of pulmonary arterial pressure. At the end of the line, the rare individual with extreme hyperreactivity may in the absence of any cardiac shunt, develop unexplained plexogenic pulmonary arteriopathy in response to even more subtle stimuli, of which the nature may escape us.

This could lead to the hypothesis that primary pulmonary hypertension is a disease of individuals with hyper-reactive lung vessels, in whom various stimuli may initiate vasoconstriction with subsequent development of the characteristic vascular lesions. More intensive study of cases of primary pulmonary hypertension and of eventual causative factors is urgently needed.

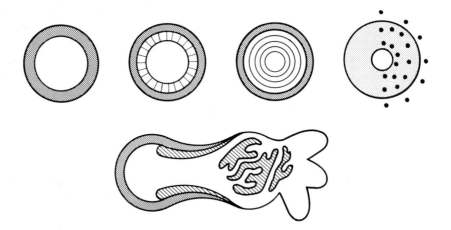

Plexogenic pulmonary arteriopathy: Arteries with medial hypertrophy, cellular intimal proliferation, concentric-laminar intimal fibrosis, fibrinoid necrosis without or with arteritis, plexiform lesions.

REFERENCES

Aars, H.: Plexiform lesions of pulmonary arteries. *Acta Path. Microbiol. Scand.* **64:** 401, 1965.

Ahlquist, J., and Burstein, J.: A case of idiopathic pulmonary hypertension. *Acta Med. Scand.* **160:** 1, 1958.

Barnard, P. J., and Davel, J. G. A.: Primary pulmonary vascular disease with cor pulmonale. Report of three cases in children, one with congenital hypertension and two siblings with allergic vasculitis and disorders of skeletal epiphyses. *Amer. J. Dis. Child.* **92:** 115, 1956.

Berthrong, M., and Cochran, T. H.: Pathological findings in nine children with "primary" pulmonary hypertension. *Bull. Johns Hopk. Hosp.* **97:** 69, 1955.

Berthrong, M., Blount, S. G., and Robinson, J. C.: Pulmonary vascular lesions in "primary" pulmonary hypertension. *Amer. J. Path.* **46:** 31a, 1965.

Bessinger, F. B., Blieden, L. C., and Edwards, J. E.: Hypertensive pulmonary vascular disease associated with patent ductus arteriosus: primary or secondary? *Circulation* **52:** 157, 1975.

Blount, S. G.: Primary pulmonary hypertension at high altitude. *Pediatrics* **63:** 1053, 1963.

Blount, S. G.: Primary pulmonary hypertension. *Mod. Conc. Cardiovasc. Dis.* **36:** 67, 1967.

Braunstein, H.: Periarteritis nodosa limited to the pulmonary circulation. *Amer. J. Path.* **31:** 837, 1955.

Caldini, P., Gensini, G. G., and Hoffman, M. S.: Primary pulmonary hypertension with death during right heart catheterization. *Amer. J. Cardiol.* **4:** 519, 1959.

Caldwell, I. W., and Aitchison, J. D.: Pulmonary hypertension in dermatomyositis. *Brit. Heart J.* **18:** 273, 1956.

Cawley, L. P., and Stofer, B. E.: Pulmonary arteriosclerosis of unknown etiology. *Arch. Path.* **64:** 270, 1957.

Charms, B. L.: Primary pulmonary hypertension. Effect of unilateral pulmonary artery occlusion and infusion of acetylcholine. *Amer. J. Cardiol.* **8:** 94, 1961.

Charters, A. D., and Baker, W. de C.: Primary pulmonary hypertension of unusually long duration. *Brit. Heart J.* **32:** 130, 1970.

Clarke, R. C., Coombs, C. F., Hadfield, G., and Todd, A. T.: On certain abnormalities, congenital and acquired of the pulmonary artery. *Quart. J. Med.* **21:** 51, 1927.

Cohen, N., and Mendelow, H.: Concurrent "active juvenile cirrhosis" and "primary pulmonary hypertension." *Amer. J. Med.* **39:** 127, 1965.

Czarnecki, S. W., Rosenbaum, H. B., and Wachtel, H. L.: The occurrence of primary pulmonary hypertension in twins with a review of etiological considerations. *Amer. Heart J.* **75:** 240, 1968.

Delaye, J., Loire, R., Brune, J., Dalloz, C., Delahaye, J. P., and Gonin, A.: L'hypertension artérielle pulmonaire primitive familiale. Histoire de deux familles et revue de la littérature. *Coeur et Méd. Int.* **8:** 31, 1969.

De Navasquez, S., Forbes, J. R., and Holling, H. E.: Right ventricular hypertrophy of unknown origin: so-called pulmonary hypertension. *Brit. Heart J.* **2:** 177, 1940.

Dexter, L.: Thromboemboli as a cause of cor pulmonale. *Bull. N. Y. Acad. Med.* **41:** 981, 1965.

Dresdale, D. T., Michtom, R. J., and Schultz, M.: Recent studies in primary pulmonary hypertension including pharmacodynamic observation on pulmonary vascular resistance. *Bull. N. Y. Acad. Med.* **30:** 195, 1954.

Dressler, W.: Effort syncope as an early manifestation of primary pulmonary hypertension. *Amer. J. Med. Sci.* (n.s.) **223:** 131, 1952.

Durrance, F. Y., and Winchell, P.: Pulmonary hypertension of unknown cause. *Dis. Chest* **39:** 452, 1961.

East, T.: Pulmonary hypertension. *Brit. Heart J.* **2:** 189, 1940.

Evans, W.: The less common forms of pulmonary hypertension. *Brit. Heart J.* **21:** 197, 1959.

Evans, W., Short, D. S., and Bedford, D. E.: Solitary pulmonary hypertension. *Brit. Heart J.* **19:** 93, 1957.

Farrar, J. F.: Idiopathic pulmonary hypertension. *Amer. Heart J.* **66:** 128, 1963.

Farrar, J. F., Reye, R. D. K., and Stuckey, D.: Primary pulmonary hypertension in childhood. *Brit. Heart J.* **23:** 605, 1961.

Forbes, I. J.: Primary pulmonary arteritis with fatal haemoptysis. *J. Path. Bact.* **76:** 288, 1958.

Fowler, N. O., Black-Schaffer, B., Scott, R. C., and Gueron, M.: Idiopathic and thromboembolic pulmonary hypertension. *Amer. J. Med.* **40:** 331, 1966.

Freilich, J. K., and Szatkowski, J.: Pelvic vein thrombosis with pulmonary vascular lesions simulating primary pulmonary hypertension. *Amer. J. Cardiol.* **7:** 297, 1961.

Gardner, D. L., Duthie, J. J. R., MacLeod, J., and Allan, W. S. A.: Pulmonary hypertension in rheumatoid arthritis: Report of a case with intimal sclerosis of the pulmonary and digital arteries. *Scot. Med. J.* **2:** 183, 1957.

Gilmour, J. R., and Evans, W.: Primary pulmonary hypertension. *J. Path. Bact.* **58:** 687, 1946.

Goodwin, J. F., Harrison, C. V., and Wilcken, D. E. L.: Obliterative pulmonary hypertension and thrombo-embolism. *Brit. Med. J.* **i:** 701, 1963.

Grover, R. F., Vogel, J. H. K., Averill, K. H., and Blount, S. G.: Pulmonary hypertension. Individual and species variability relative to vascular reactivity. *Amer. Heart J.* **66:** 1, 1963.

Heath, D., Whitaker, W., and Brown, J. W.: Idiopathic pulmonary hypertension. *Brit. Heart J.* **19:** 83, 1957.

Heath, D., and Edwards, J. E.: Configuration of elastic tissue of pulmonary trunk in idiopathic pulmonary hypertension. *Circulation* **21:** 59, 1960.

Hufner, R. F., and McNicol, C. A.: The pathologic physiology of microscopic pulmonary vascular shunts. *Arch. Path.* **65:** 554, 1958.

Inglesby, T. V., Singer, J. W., and Gordon, D. S.: Abnormal fibrinolysis in familial pulmonary hypertension. *Amer. J. Med.* **55:** 5, 1973.

Inkley, S. R., Gillespie, L., and Funkhouser, R. K.: Two cases of primary pulmonary hypertension with sudden death associated with the administration of barbiturates. *Ann. Int. Med.* **43:** 396, 1955.

Innocenti, P., and Toso, M.: Ipertensione pulmonare idiopatica con ipertensione arteriosa sistemica. *Cuore e Circ.* **49:** 283, 1965.

James, T. N.: On the cause of syncope and sudden death in primary pulmonary hypertension. *Ann. Int. Med.* **56:** 252, 1962.

Jewett, J. F., and Ober, W. B.: Primary pulmonary hypertension as a cause of maternal death. *Amer. J. Obst. Gynec.* **71:** 1335, 1956.

Khoury, G. H., and Hawes, C. R.: Primary pulmonary hypertension in children living at high altitude. *J. Pediatr.* **62:** 177, 1963.

Maekawa, M., and Hayashi, K.: Malignant pulmonary hypertension. *Jap. Med. J.* **4:** 41, 1965.

Marshall, R. J., Helmholtz, H. F., and Shepherd, J. T.: Effect of acetylcholine on pulmonary vascular resistance in a patient with idiopathic pulmonary hypertension. *Circulation* **20:** 391, 1959.

Masshoff, W., and Röher, H. D.: Pulmonaler Hochdruck bei Glomangiose der Lungen. *Klin. Wschr.* **42:** 655, 1964.

McGuire, J., Scott, R. C., Helm, R. A., Kaplan, S., Gall, E. A., and Biehl, J. P.: Is there an entity primary pulmonary hypertension. *Arch. Int. Med.* **99:** 917, 1957.

McKeown, F.: The pathology of pulmonary heart disease. *Brit. Heart J.* **14:** 25, 1952.

Meyrick, B., Clarke, S. W., Symons, C., Woodgate, D. J., and Reid, L.: Primary pulmonary hypertension: a case report including electron-microscopic study. *Brit. J. Dis. Chest* **68:** 11, 1974.

Montgomery, G. L.: A case of pulmonary artery thrombosis with Ayerza's syndrome. *J. Path. Bact.* **41:** 221, 1935.

Moschcowitz, E., Rubin, E., and Strauss, L.: Hypertension of the pulmonary circulation due to congenital glomoid obstruction of the pulmonary arteries. *Amer. J. Path.* **39:** 75, 1961.

Obeyesekere, I., and de Soysa, N.: "Primary" pulmonary hypertension, eosinophilia, and filariasis in Ceylon. *Brit. Heart J.* **32:** 524, 1970.

Olsen, E. G. J.: *The Pathology of the Heart.* Georg Thieme Publishers, Stuttgart, 1973.

Owen, W. R., Thomas, W. A., Castleman, B., and Bland, E. F.: Unrecognized emboli to the lungs with subsequent cor pulmonale. *New Engl. J. Med.* **249:** 919, 1953.

Porter, C. M., Cruech, B. J., and Billings, T.: Primary pulmonary hypertension occurring in twins. *Arch. Int. Med.* **120:** 224, 1967.

Rao, B. N. S., Moller, J. H., and Edwards, J. E.: Primary pulmonary hypertension in a child. Response to pharmacologic agents. *Circulation* **40:** 583, 1969.

Rawson, A. J.: Incomplete rupture of the pulmonary artery based on cystic medionecrosis. *Amer. Heart J.* **55:** 766, 1958.

Rawson, A. J., and Woske, H. M.: A study of etiologic factors in so-called primary pulmonary hypertension. *Arch. Int. Med.* **105:** 233, 1960.

Reeves, J. T., and Noonan, J. A.: Microarteriographic studies of primary pulmonary hypertension. *Arch. Path.* **95:** 48, 1973.

Roberts, W. C.: The histologic structure of the pulmonary trunk in patients with "primary" pulmonary hypertension. *Amer. Heart J.* **65:** 230, 1963.

Robertson, B.: Idiopathic pulmonary hypertension in infancy and childhood. Microangiographic and histological observations in five cases. *Acta Path. Microbiol. Scand. A.* **79:** 217, 1971.

Robertson, B., Rosenhamer, G., and Lindberg, J.: Idiopathic pulmonary hypertension in two siblings. *Acta Med. Scand.* **186:** 569, 1969.

Rogge, J. D., Mishkin, M. E., and Genovese, P. D.: The familial occurrence of primary pulmonary hypertension. *Ann. Int. Med.* **65:** 672, 1966.

Romberg, E.: Ueber sklerose der Lungenarterie. *Dtsch. Arch. Klin. Med.* **48:** 197, 1891.

Rose, G. A., and Spencer, H.: Polyarteritis nodosa. *Quart. J. Med.* **24** (n.s.), 43, 1957.

Rosenberg, S. A.: A study of the etiological basis of primary pulmonary hypertension. *Amer. Heart J.* **68:** 484, 1964.

Rudolph, A. M., Paul, M. H., Sommer, L. S., and Nadas, A. S.: Effects of tolazoline hydrochloride (priscoline) on circulatory dynamics of patients with pulmonary hypertension. *Amer. Heart J.* **55:** 424, 1958.

Samet, P., Bernstein, W. H., and Widrich, J.: Intracardiac infusion of acetylcholine in primary pulmonary hypertension. *Amer. Heart J.* **60:** 433, 1960.

Samet, P., and Bernstein, W. H.: Loss of reactivity of the pulmonary vascular bed in primary pulmonary hypertension. *Amer. Heart J.* **66:** 197, 1963.

Seldin, D. W., Ziff, M., DeGraff, A. C., Fallis, B. D., and Burns, R. R.: Raynaud's phenomenon associated with pulmonary hypertension. *Texas J. Med.* **58:** 654, 1962.

Shane, S. J., Atermann, K., Roy, D. L., and Chandler, B. M.: Primary pulmonary hypertension: A review, and report of five cases. *Canad. Med. Ass. J.* **91:** 145, 1964.

Shepherd, J. T., Edwards, J. E., Burchell, H. B., Swann, H. J. C., and Wood, E. H.: Clinical, physiological, and pathological considerations in patients with idiopathic pulmonary hypertension. *Brit. Heart J.* **19:** 70, 1957.

Slama, R., Crevelier, A., Coumel, P., and Snanoudj, S.: Hypertension artérielle pulmonaire primitive et lupus érythemateux disséminé. *Presse Méd.* **75:** 961, 1967.

Sleeper, J. C., Orgain, E. S., and McIntosh, H. D.: Primary pulmonary hypertension. Review of clinical features and pathologic physiology with a report of pulmonary hemodynamics derived from repeated catheterization. *Circulation* **26:** 1358, 1962.

Soothill, J. F.: A case of primary pulmonary hypertension with paralysed left vocal cord. *Guy's Hosp. Reports* **100:** 232, 1951.

Soustek, Z.: Eigenartige Veränderungen an den Lungengefässen bei angeborener Hypertonie im kleinen Kreislauf. *Zbl. Allg. Path. u. Path. Anat.* **101:** 425, 1960.

Stucki, P., Bürki, K., and Baumgartner, U.: Über primäre pulmonale Hypertonie. *Schweiz. Med. Wschr.* **93:** 1823, 1963.

Thomas, W. A.: Clinico-pathologic conference: Right-sided heart failure occurring during successive pregnancies, polycythemia and sudden peripheral vascular collapse. *Amer. J. Med.* **19:** 126, 1955.

Thompson, P., and McRae, C.: Familial pulmonary hypertension. Evidence of autosomal dominant inheritance. *Brit. Heart J.* **32:** 758, 1970.

Trell, E., and Lindström, C.: Pulmonary hypertension in systemic sclerosis. *Ann. Rheum. Dis.* **30**: 390, 1971.

Van Epps, E. F.: Primary pulmonary hypertension in brothers. *Amer. J. Roentg.* **78**: 471, 1957.

Wagenvoort, C. A.: Vasoconstrictive primary pulmonary hypertension and pulmonary veno-occlusive disease. *Cardiovasc. Clin.* **4**: 97, 1972.

Wagenvoort, C. A.: Unexplained pulmonary hypertension. *Pathol. Microbiol.* **43**: 239, 1975.

Wagenvoort, C. A., Heath, D., and Edwards, J. E.: *The Pathology of the Pulmonary Vasculature.* Charles C Thomas, Springfield, Ill., 1964.

Wagenvoort, C. A., Wagenvoort, N., and Vogel, J. H. K.: The pulmonary vasculature in cattle at an altitude of 1600 metres with and without one-sided pulmonary arterial ligation. *J. Comp. Path.* **79**: 517, 1969.

Wagenvoort, C. A., and Wagenvoort, N.: Primary pulmonary hypertension: a pathologic study of the lung vessels in 156 clinically diagnosed cases. *Circulation* **42**: 1163, 1970a.

Wagenvoort, C. A., and Wagenvoort, N.: A classification of "primary pulmonary hypertension." *Progr. Resp. Res.* **5**: 17, 1970b.

Wagenvoort, C. A., and Wagenvoort, N.: Pathology of the Eisenmenger syndrome and primary pulmonary hypertension. *Adv. Cardiol.* **11**: 123, 1974.

Walcott, G., Burchell, H. B., and Brown, A. L.: Primary pulmonary hypertension. *Amer. J. Med.* **49**: 70, 1970.

Wallooppillai, N. J., and Wagenvoort, C. A.: Unpublished data, 1976.

Weir, E. K., Tucker, A., Reeves, J. T., Will, D. H., and Grover, R. F.: The genetic factor influencing pulmonary hypertension in cattle at high altitude. *Cardiovasc. Res.* **8**: 745, 1974.

Wood, P.: Pulmonary hypertension with special reference to the vasoconstrictive factor. *Brit. Heart J.* **20**: 557, 1958.

Wood, P.: Pulmonary hypertension. *Mod. Conc. Cardiovasc. Dis.* **28**: 513, 1959.

World Health Organization: *Primary Pulmonary Hypertension. Report on a WHO Meeting.* S. Hatano, and T. Strasser (eds.), Geneva, 1975.

Yu, P. N.: Primary pulmonary hypertension: report of six cases and review of literature. *Ann. Int. Med.* **49**: 1138, 1958.

CHAPTER EIGHT

Embolic Pulmonary Hypertension

Emboli, lodged in the pulmonary arteries, may be a cause of increased pulmonary arterial resistance and pressure, if by their size and numbers, they produce a considerable obstruction to the vascular bed of the lungs. With few exceptions, embolic pulmonary hypertension is caused by thromboemboli. In the various other forms of embolism an elevation of pressure in the pulmonary circulation, if it occurs at all, is usually temporary. Sustained pulmonary hypertension in these instances is very rare.

THROMBOEMBOLISM

Pulmonary thromboembolism undoubtedly is a frequent phenomenon and a common cause of disability and death (Sasahara, 1974), but there is still much confusion about its pathogenesis, clinical picture, and incidence. The statement made by De Bakey in 1954, that "The need for closer scrutiny and more critical evaluation of the problem is as great today as it was over 20 years ago," could be repeated now, over 20 years later.

The incidence of thromboembolism appears difficult to establish. In part this is due to problems of clinical diagnosis. Embolic events often do not produce clinical symptoms, and if they do, these symptoms may be difficult to interpret. But even in autopsy studies there is a wide variation in reported incidence. Belt (1936) found recent or organized thromboemboli to the lungs in 14.6 percent of 1094 autopsies on adult patients, Chomette et al. (1966) in 24 percent of 1800 routine autopsies, and Brenner (1935) in 28 percent of 100 consecutive autopsies. In a prospective study of a small series of 61 routine autopsies on adult patients, Freiman et al. (1965) found old or recent emboli to the lungs in 64 percent. In patients with recent embolism, older organized thrombi were detected in nearly 80 percent (Smith et al., 1964).

The marked discrepancy in the reported percentage is not difficult to explain. To some extent the incidence depends on the degree in which medical, surgical, urological, and gynecological departments contribute to the autopsy material (Fowler and Bollinger, 1954). Moreover, it depends on the accuracy used in the search for emboli in the lungs, or maybe even better on the size of thromboembolus the pathologist is looking for. If an adequate amount of lung tissue is studied, occasional small emboli, either recent or organized, can be found in muscular pulmonary arteries in the majority of all autopsy cases. Obviously, the incidence falls when larger emboli or larger numbers of emboli are used as a criterium for the diagnosis.

The origin of pulmonary emboli is mainly from thrombi developed in the veins of the leg (Marshall, 1965), often originating in the sinus of venous valves (Beckering and Titus, 1969). To a lesser extent the pelvic veins and the heart are the sites of primary thrombosis, while other locations are rare.

Massive Pulmonary Embolism

Pulmonary embolism may be massive and is then often fatal. It has been found to be the cause of death in between 4 to 7 percent of all autopsy cases (Hartmann, 1963; Hackl, 1967; Kaufmann and Keresztes, 1971).

The thromboemboli may be scattered over various intrapulmonary elastic arteries or may fill one or both main pulmonary arteries, the pulmonary trunk, or even the right cardiac ventricle (Figure 8-1). Massive pulmonary embolism may occur in previously healthy individuals (Fleming and Bailey, 1966). These may survive obstruction of at least 50 percent of the pulmonary vascular bed. On the other hand, sudden death sometimes results from embolic obstruction of one main pulmonary artery. This brings up the possibility of reflex vasospasm of the arterial bed in response to the embolic occlusion of a main branch (p. 149). It is, however, important to realize that thromboembolism is not commonly confined to a single event and tends to consist of multiple episodes. This means that many branches in both lungs may have been obstructed prior to the final attack.

The immediate hemodynamic effect of massive pulmonary embolism is an elevation of pulmonary arterial pressure proximal to the site of obstruction, eventually with shock and death as a result.

If enough blood can be forced by the right ventricle along the remaining pathway to keep the patient alive, an embolic mass in one of the main pulmonary arteries or even in the pulmonary trunk may be organized (Figure 8-2), but this is not a common occurrence. In these instances chronic pulmonary hypertension may develop. Occasionally silent massive obstruction of the extrapulmonary arteries is found, without a distinct history of an embolic event (Behrendt, 1963). It is likely, however, that in these cases, which may be diagnosed as primary pulmonary hypertension, propagation of the thrombus mass with gradual narrowing of the arterial lumen or repeated embolic events, account for the eventual massive obstruction (Figure 8-3).

Pulmonary Infarcts

The consequences of thromboemboli obstructing secondary or tertiary pulmonary arterial branches are less severe. As long as the bronchial circulation is intact, the

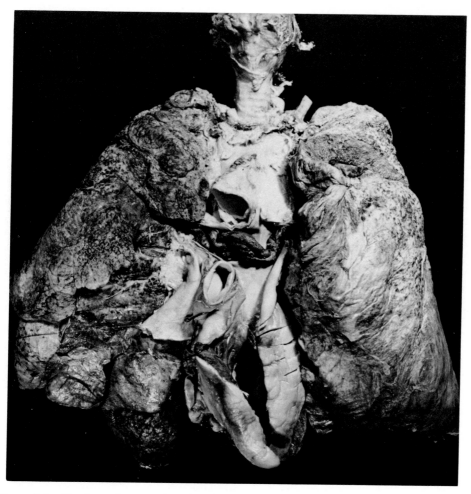

Figure 8-1. Massive pulmonary thromboembolism obstructing pulmonary trunk and both main pulmonary arteries in a 63-year-old man who died 2 weeks after traffic accident. The right ventricle, which showed acute dilatation, also contains some emboli.

area of lung tissue that is now deprived of its pulmonary arterial blood supply, may remain vital since some blood is provided by way of the bronchial arteries. Particularly in young individuals with an adequate cardiovascular circulation, such an area may remain intact, although there is often hemorrhage. A hemorrhagic pulmonary infarct (Figure 8-4) with necrosis of lung tissue (Figure 8-5), is observed especially in patients who are in cardiac failure or in whom the circulation is impaired. Infarcts are often multiple and more common in the lower than in the upper lobes. Their incidence is low as compared to that of thromboembolism.

Chronic Thromboembolic Pulmonary Hypertension

Embolic obstruction of small elastic or of muscular pulmonary arteries often will remain clinically unnoticed and is of little consequence unless numerous arteries are

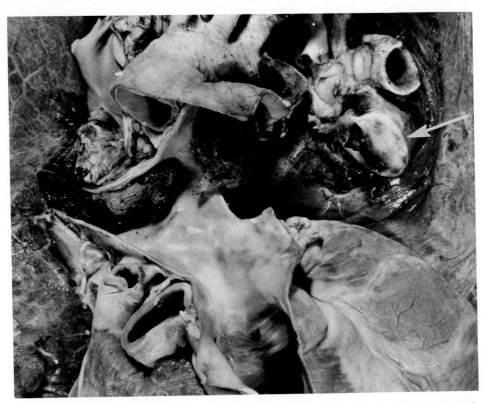

Figure 8-2. Massive pulmonary thromboembolism simulating primary pulmonary hypertension in a 22-year-old man who exhibited clinical symptoms of pulmonary hypertension for 2 years. Both main pulmonary arteries were severely narrowed by old organized thromboemboli, as shown in cross section of the left main pulmonary artery (arrow). The immediate cause of death was multiple recent emboli obstructing both main pulmonary arteries and pulmonary trunk. There was severe right ventricular hypertrophy.

involved. This may happen particularly in recurrent pulmonary embolism, when repeated showers of small emboli gradually block a large proportion of the pulmonary vascular bed. Each of these episodes may be clinically difficult to recognize or even remain undetected (Wilhelmsen et al., 1963).

It is likely that in this "silent" thromboembolism the action of the first showers of emboli with resulting blockage of arteries is easily overcome by the physiologic reserve of the pulmonary vasculature. After subsequent events the hemodynamic effect will be obvious only during exercise. Finally, sustained pulmonary hypertension at rest develops (Wilhelmsen et al., 1970).

Incidence

Chronic embolic pulmonary hypertension is not a common disease but its incidence is difficult to assess. Recurrent pulmonary embolism is fairly common in bedridden patients with serious conditions such as malignant disease or cardiovascular or pulmonary disorders. Often the underlying disease causes death before pulmonary hypertension sets in or, if this develops, it may remain unnoticed as it is overshadowed by the general deterioration of the patient.

There is, however, a group of seemingly healthy, sometimes young individuals in whom silent pulmonary embolism in the absence of obvious reasons may occur and may give rise to pulmonary hypertension. Such cases, although not common, are probably not rare either (Wilhelmsen et al., 1963).

Clinical Course

The clinical course in patients with chronic embolic pulmonary hypertension may be protracted and last as long as 9 years (Castleman and Bland, 1946). On the basis of the clinical picture it is possible to divide these patients into two groups (Goodwin et al., 1963; Wilhelmsen et al., 1963; Fleischner, 1967). In one group there is generally a history of an acute onset with chest pain, acute dyspnea, and sometimes, although uncommonly, hemoptysis. There may be a history of previous thrombotic episodes but signs of leg vein thrombosis are seldom noticed at the time of the acute attack, which is often mistaken for myocardial infarction or pneumonia.

The other group, consisting mainly of women (Goodwin et al., 1963), is characterized by an insidious course without previous signs of embolism. There is a slowly progressive dyspnea on exertion with tachycardia and fatigue. Signs of right cardiac failure not uncommonly form the first indication of this, presumably microembolic, type of the disease. It is particularly in these instances that the clinical recognition of thromboembolic pulmonary hypertension may be very difficult or impossible.

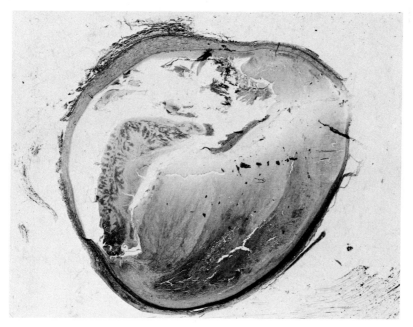

Figure 8-3.   Left main pulmonary artery in cross section from the same case as Figure 8-2. Layers of old organized thromboemboli cause narrowing of the lumen, suggesting repeated embolic events or propagation of the thrombus mass. The lumen is further obstructed by a recent embolus (H. and E., ×25).

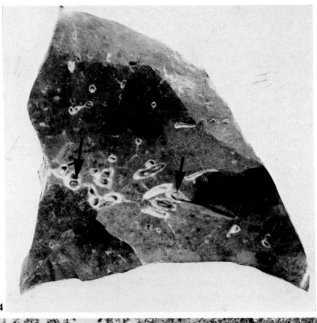

8-4

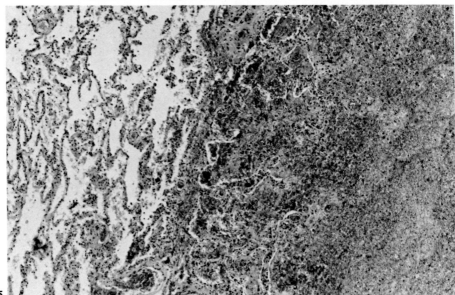

8-5

Figure 8-4. Cut surface of lung with multiple hemorrhagic infarcts in a 39-year-old man with recurrent thromboembolism. Thromboemboli in pulmonary arteries are indicated by arrows.

Figure 8-5. Lung tissue with hemorrhagic infarct in a 55-year-old woman with recurrent thromboembolism. There is extensive necrosis (to right) separated from intact lung tissue by a hemorrhagic zone (H. and E., ×55).

Hemodynamic studies in patients with chronic embolic pulmonary hypertension reveal an elevated pulmonary arterial pressure and normal wedge and left atrial pressures (Wilhelmsen et al., 1970).

The condition is often confused with primary pulmonary hypertension. It has been suggested, as we have seen in Chapter Seven, that most cases of primary pulmonary hypertension are in fact embolic and then particularly microembolic, in origin (Goodwin et al., 1963).

Once pulmonary hypertension is established, the benefit of anticoagulant therapy is reduced and the prognosis is poor. When a large proportion of the pulmonary vascular bed has become obliterated, right cardiac failure and death usually result.

Mechanisms

Recovery from pulmonary embolism may be complete without clinically demonstrable sequelae (Brantigan et al., 1966). Chronic pulmonary hypertension develops in a minority of these cases, although it is impossible to give exact numbers. It is likely that in many patients, who experienced one or more embolic episodes, the compensatory mechanisms of the pulmonary vascular bed were sufficient to counterbalance the vascular obstruction so that elevation of the pulmonary arterial pressure did not occur.

Thrombolysis is another mechanism that may account for the restitution of the available vascular bed in the lungs. Although there is probably considerable individual variation in this respect, it is likely that many small emboli can be dissolved by lysis (Wilhelmsen et al., 1970). Moreover, there is evidence that sometimes fairly large emboli may undergo lysis and may disappear in part or completely (Sautter et al., 1964).

The usual fate of small and large emboli is organization and recanalization. Both processes contribute somewhat to the restitution of the blood flow. Shrinkage during organization and incorporation of the organized embolus into the pulmonary arterial wall will often lead to widening of the remaining lumen, while recanalization may provide some additional channels. Usually, however, the effect of these processes is limited.

Several studies have suggested that vasoconstriction either by humoral (Comroe et al., 1953; Halmagyi et al., 1964; Hyman et al., 1964; Levy et al., 1969) or by reflex mechanisms (Niden and Aviado, 1956; Weidner and Light, 1958; Parmley et al., 1962) would be responsible or at least contribute to the increased pulmonary vascular resistance and pressure.

Comroe and coworkers (1953) suggested that serotonin liberated from the platelets in a blood clot in a pulmonary artery might produce widespread vasoconstriction. This vasoconstriction would appear only if the emboli are lodged in vessels of a caliber smaller than $250\,\mu$ (Galland et al., 1964). Others pointed out that the amount of serotonin that could become active in this way was too low to account for a vasoconstrictive effect (Sanders et al., 1959; Dexter, 1965).

Experimental embolization of a variety of substances to the lung is believed to release prostaglandins from the lung tissue. In this way prostaglandin $F_{2\alpha}$, for instance, could increase pulmonary vascular resistance (Lindsey and Wyllie, 1970; Piper and Vane, 1971). However, prostaglandins are inactivated rapidly, while it also appeared that indomethacin, which has an inhibitory effect on prostaglandins did not prevent the rise in pulmonary arterial pressure following microembolization of barium sulphate to the lungs (Nakano and McCloy, 1973).

The results of embolization in experimental animals are controversial. Many authors reported that they were unable to demonstrate vasoconstriction and that mechanical blockage alone could account for the rise in pressure (Courtoy and Salonikides, 1956; Williams, 1956; Weidman et al., 1963; Gurewich et al., 1968; Williams et al., 1969). In vivo observation of embolized and nonembolized arteries in the same lung did not reveal a decrease in vascular diameter (Knisely et al., 1957).

In the human, the significance of vasoconstriction for the development of pulmonary hypertension in response to acute pulmonary embolism is equally doubtful (Dexter, 1965). In recurrent pulmonary embolism it is even very unlikely that humoral or reflexogenic factors are involved. There is little or no effect of vasodilatory substances like priscoline and acethylcholine or of oxygen inhalation (Wilhelmsen et al., 1963, 1970; Widimsky et al., 1965). As we will see, the morphology in these cases also supports mechanical obstruction as the main cause of pulmonary hypertension.

Morphology

Pulmonary Trunk and Main Arteries. In massive pulmonary thromboembolism the lumen of the pulmonary trunk and main arteries is filled to a varying degree by long, often folded, recent thrombi. Although this is often the final event, it appears that in these cases, with very few exceptions, there are numerous and usually older embolic lesions in the smaller branches of the pulmonary arteries in both lungs. This indicates that in the vast majority of the cases, the fatal attack has not been the first. It may also explain that occlusion of a single main pulmonary artery is often fatal, while ligation during pneumonectomy, as a rule, is well sustained.

If, however, the patient survives, the embolus may become organized and incorporated into the arterial wall. There are uncommon cases in which the pulmonary trunk or both main arteries are severely narrowed by organized clot. It is likely that survival of these patients was due to incomplete occlusion by the embolic mass. It is also possible that in some instances severe narrowing was brought about gradually by propagating thrombosis on top of an embolus, so that adaptation was possible. In these cases marked right ventricular hypertrophy will reflect the increased pressure in the right ventricle.

Primary thrombosis of the pulmonary trunk and main arteries is probably rare and unlikely if there is no underlying alteration in the walls of these vessels to be held responsible for the development of a thrombus at that site.

In some instances of massive thromboembolism to main pulmonary arteries, recanalization of the organized clot occurs to such an extent that fibrous strands and networks are formed, spread out in the lumen of the artery (Figure 8-6). These "bands and webs" were first described by Zahn (1889) who took them for congenital malformations of the artery. In fact, they are a distinct sign of previous thromboembolism (Vanek, 1961; Korn et al., 1962). Such fibrous strands also have been produced in experimental thromboembolism (Dunnill, 1968). The bands are formed by paucicellular fibrous tissue (Figure 8-7), consisting of collagen with occasional

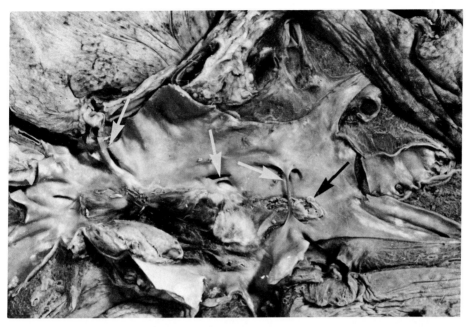

Figure 8-6. Main pulmonary artery with some bands (arrows) due to organized thromboembolus in an 81-year-old woman with embolic pulmonary hypertension. A later embolus has been caught by one of these bands and is subsequently organized (black arrow).

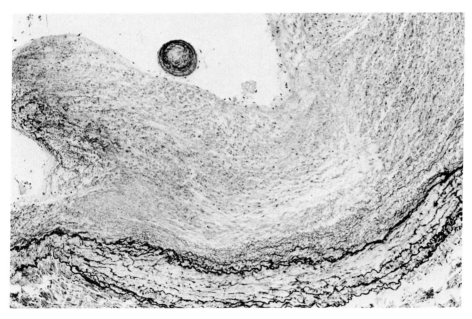

Figure 8-7. Section of main pulmonary artery with bands and webs in a 62-year-old man with embolic pulmonary hypertension. One of the bands, shown in cross section, contains elastic fibers (El.v.G., ×90).

elastic fibers. An endothelial lining is sometimes present but more often not apparent.

In thromboembolic pulmonary hypertension the wall of the pulmonary trunk and main arteries usually exhibits hypertrophy of the media (Figure 8-8) and atherosclerotic plaques in the intima (Figure 8-9).

Elastic Pulmonary Arteries. Recent and old thromboemboli often are present in various elastic arteries within the same lung. Organization may be apparent in successive stages. In the early stages the thrombus is still recognizable. Later, an usually excentric fibrous mass (Figure 8-10) may narrow or even totally obstruct the vascular lumen. Recanalization with the formation of "bands and webs" is commonly observed in these vessels (Figures 8-11 and 8-12).

Muscular Pulmonary Arteries and Arterioles. Widespread involvement of muscular pulmonary arteries and to a lesser extent of arterioles, in cases of chronic embolic pulmonary hypertension, proves that numerous emboli entering the pulmonary circulation in these cases are of small size or, more likely, have been fragmented at the time of impact. As in elastic arteries, the emboli may be recent (Figure 8-13) but most are organized. In early stages fibroblasts grow into the clot

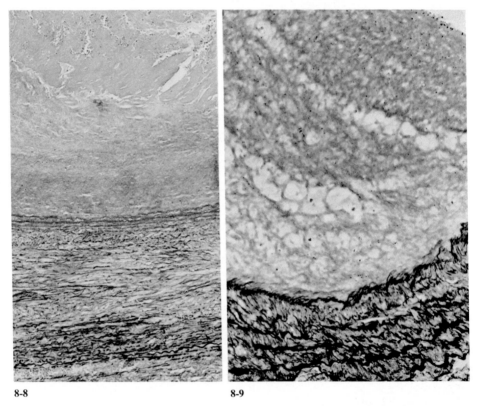

8-8   8-9

Figure 8-8. Main pulmonary artery in a 22-year-old man with embolic pulmonary hypertension. There is a partly organized thrombus and marked medial hypertrophy with an "adult" elastic configuration (El.v.G., ×55).

Figure 8-9. Main pulmonary artery with atheromatous plaque in a 35-year-old woman with recurrent pulmonary embolism (El.v.G., ×90).

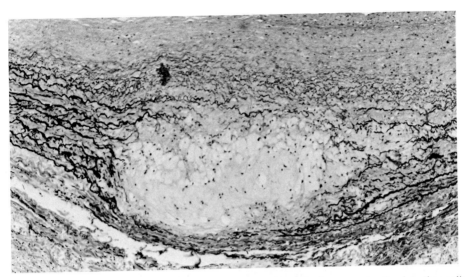

Figure 8-10. Elastic pulmonary artery with organized embolus and atheroma extending into the media in a 62-year-old man with embolic pulmonary hypertension (El.v.G., ×150).

which is often lined by a layer of endothelial cells (Figure 8-14). Gradually the embolus is replaced by proliferating fibroblasts with subsequent deposition of collagen and elastic fibers.

In cross section, there is usually some lumen left in these obstructed arteries. In most instances this is an eccentric, or less commonly a central, channel. This remaining lumen is an expression of the fact that not all emboli are occlusive, certainly not over their whole length. Furthermore it may result form retraction of the thrombotic mass or from recanalization.

The process of embolization and its consequences for the muscular pulmonary arteries have been studied extensively in experimental animals, particularly in rabbits (Harrison, 1948, 1951) and rats (Barnard, 1953).

Fibrinolysis accounts for the disappearance of large numbers of emboli, predominantly the smaller ones (Heard, 1952; Stringate et al., 1962), although there is a species variability. Invasion of blood clot by polymorphonuclear and mononuclear cells respectively and endothelization precedes the ingrowth of fibroblasts in the thrombus (Ardlie and Schwarz, 1968). Complete organization results in patches of intimal fibrosis.

In principle, the fate of thromboemboli in the human lung is much the same as in animals. Organization with incorporation into the pulmonary arterial wall, (Figure 8-15) leads to the development of cushion-like patches of intimal fibrosis protruding into the lumen (Wagenvoort, 1975). These patches are usually eccentric (Figure 8-16) and often irregular in shape. Central recanalization produces circumferential intimal fibrosis (Figure 8-17). Although less common than the eccentric patches, at least in man, circumferential intimal fibrosis may be observed particularly in vessels of small caliber. This may explain why lesions of this type are relatively more common and may outnumber eccentric changes in experimental animals, like the rabbit, when these animals are submitted to embolization (Barnard, 1954; Olsen, 1975).

Even then the type of intimal fibrosis can usually be differentiated from that in

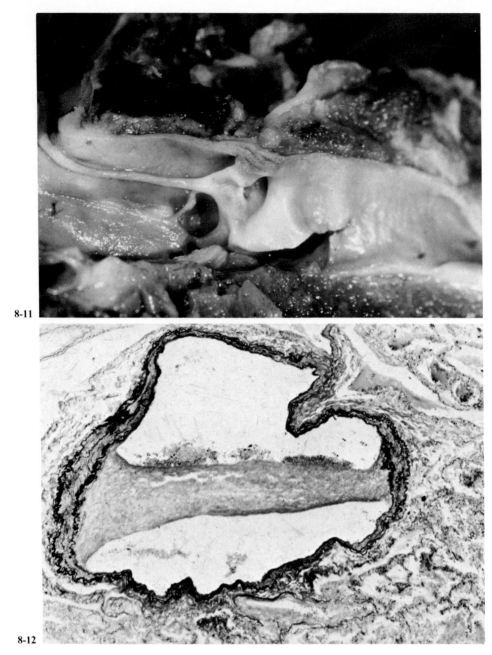

Figure 8-11. Elastic pulmonary artery with web-like structure due to organization of emboli in a 76-year-old woman with recurrent pulmonary embolism.

Figure 8-12. Section of elastic pulmonary artery with a fibrous band in a 66-year-old woman with recurrent pulmonary embolism (El.v.G., ×50).

154

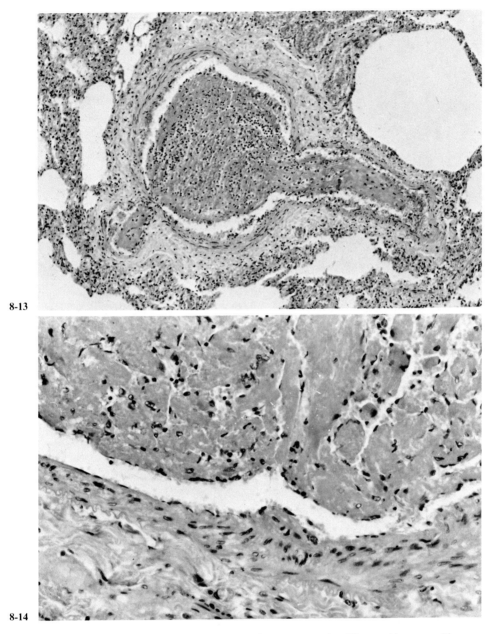

8-13

8-14

Figure 8-13. Recent thromboembolus in muscular pulmonary artery in a 75-year-old woman with recurrent pulmonary embolism (H. and E., ×90).

Figure 8-14. Early organization and endothelization of a thromboembolus in a large muscular pulmonary artery in a 72-year-old woman with recurrent pulmonary embolism (H. and E., ×230).

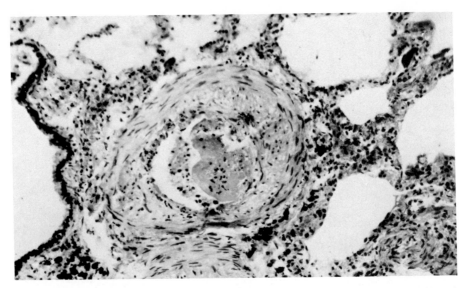

Figure 8-15. Muscular pulmonary artery with a recent thromboembolus on top of an organized patch of eccentric intimal fibrosis in a 62-year-old woman with recurrent pulmonary embolism (H. and E., ×140).

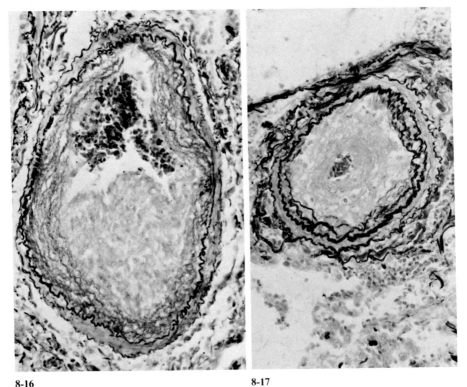

8-16   8-17

Figure 8-16. Muscular pulmonary artery with an eccentric and irregular patch of intimal fibrosis due to organization of thromboembolus in a 62-year-old man (El.v.G., ×230).
Figure 8-17. Circumferential intimal fibrosis due to central recanalization of an organized thromboembolus in a 66-year-old woman (El.v.G., ×230).

vasoconstrictive pulmonary hypertension, since it lacks the laminar, onionskin arrangement.

It is not always appreciated, as we have pointed out before (Wagenvoort, 1973), that in an elastic stain the elastic fibers may tend to be parallel, thus sometimes imitating in circumferential intimal lesions a concentric-laminar intimal fibrosis. A laminar arrangement, however, can be recognized in an hematoxylin stained section. Therefore, we cannot accept Olsen's (1975) interpretation of embolic lesions in the pulmonary arteries of rabbits as concentric-laminar intimal fibrosis.

In dogs, Geer and coworkers (1965) demonstrated that the pulmonary arterial lesions in thromboembolism are distinctly different from those in hyperkinetic pulmonary hypertension. Their description corresponds to the classical picture of thromboembolic lesions. If hyperkinetic pulmonary hypertension is produced in dogs by ligation of pulmonary arteries with subsequent experimental thromboembolism, this does not change the process of organization of emboli (Downing and Vidone, 1967).

Recanalization may present itself in various forms. Initially there may be a single channel (Figure 8-18) or multiple small capillary-like spaces (Figure 8-19). The latter may widen to such an extent that the lumen is divided in several compartments by intra-arterial septa. These form the counterpart of the bands and webs in the larger arteries. They are more often coarse and thick (Figure 8-20) but sometimes consist of lattices of delicate trabeculae (Figures 8-21 and 8-22).

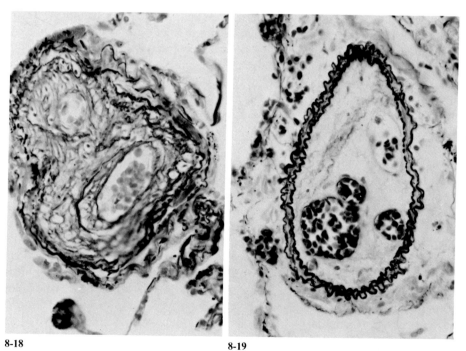

8-18

8-19

Figure 8-18. Muscular pulmonary artery obstructed by organized embolus with a single recanalization channel which extends into a branching arteriole in a 59-year-old woman (El.v.G., ×350).

Figure 8-19. Muscular pulmonary artery with multiple small channels of recanalization in a 17-year-old girl (El.v.G., ×350).

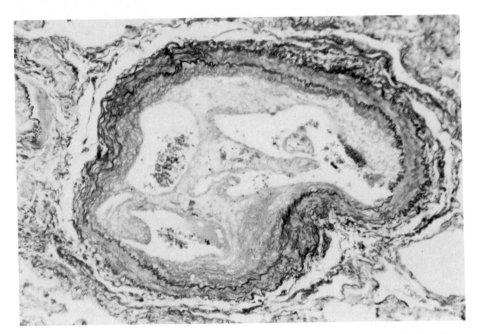

Figure 8-20. Large muscular pulmonary artery with recanalization of organized embolus in a 66-year-old woman. Multiple coarse intraluminal fibrous septa are formed (El.v.G., ×140).

Iron pigment can be found in organized emboli, particularly in those with the earlier stages of organization and recanalization, but the view, sometimes expressed, that hemosiderosis must be present in order to decide on the thrombotic nature of an intimal plaque, cannot be upheld. Hemosiderin apparently is washed out very soon, since it is absent in the great majority of older patches of embolic intimal fibrosis.

The media of the artery at the site of the intimal plaque is usually intact but thinning of the media sometimes with destruction of the internal elastic lamina does occur (Figure 8-23).

On the other hand, the media is often thicker at the site of obstruction than elsewhere (Figure 8-24), and this may have led to the concept that marked medial hypertrophy is one of the characteristic features of embolic pulmonary hypertension. In general, however, this is incorrect. There are cases with marked chronic elevation of pulmonary arterial pressure with generalized medial hypertrophy of the muscular pulmonary arteries, but in most instances the overall medial thickness is no more than mildly increased or even within normal limits.

In 20 patients in whom the clinical diagnosis of chronic embolic pulmonary hypertension was morphologically confirmed, we determined the thickness of media and intima of muscular pulmonary arteries expressed as percentages of external and internal vascular diameter (Wagenvoort and Wagenvoort, 1970). The mean medial thickness of the pulmonary arteries in this group was 7.7 percent, and this constitutes only mild medial hypertrophy.

If vasoconstriction by reflex or by humoral means, such as serotonin released from emboli, is responsible for the elevated pressure, as has been suggested (p. 149), in most instances this is not reflected by marked medial hypertrophy. Moreover,

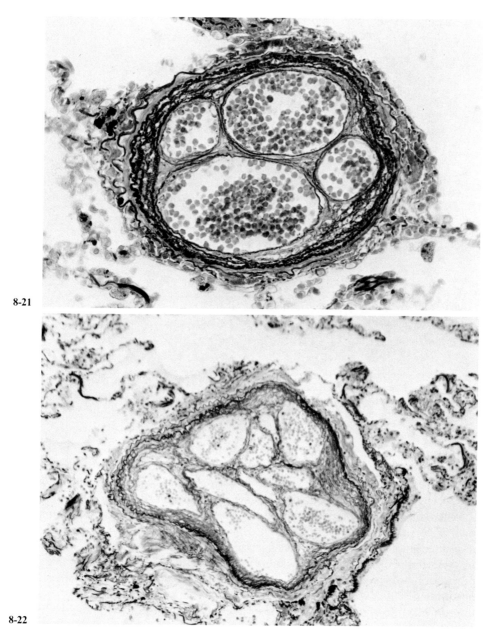

8-21

8-22

Figure 8-21. Muscular pulmonary artery with four channels of recanalization producing intraluminal fibrous septa. Same case as Figure 8-20 (El.v.G., ×350).
Figure 8-22. Muscular pulmonary artery with multiple recanalization channels and lattices of delicate trabeculae. Same case as Figure 8-20 (El.v.G., ×140).

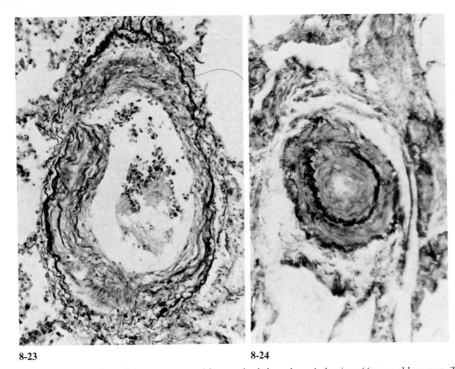

8-23   8-24

Figure 8-23. Muscular pulmonary artery with organized thromboembolus in a 66-year-old woman. The media is thin and the internal elastic lamina largely destroyed (El.v.G., ×140).
Figure 8-24. Muscular pulmonary artery with very thick media at the site of obstruction by intimal fibrosis due to chronic thromboembolism in a 55-year-old woman (El.v.G., ×140).

there was no striking difference between muscular pulmonary arteries of larger and smaller caliber as far as their relative medial thickness was concerned. In this respect it may be significant that medial hypertrophy was absent in rabbits following embolization, whether cor pulmonale had developed or not (Barnard, 1954).

When, on the other hand, embolic pulmonary hypertension is caused entirely or mainly by mechanical obstruction, it is necessary that there is a considerable impediment to the pulmonary vascular pathway. In the group of 20 patients just mentioned, the overall intimal thickness was 21.3 percent. This is less than in several other forms of pulmonary hypertension, but one should realize that the vascular obstruction is almost always sharply localized, as becomes clear when serial sections are studied. In a single histologic section the lumen of most arteries may be patent at this level. Still the same arteries often are occluded or narrowed at a different level and this may not be reflected by the average degree of intimal fibrosis.

Pulmonary arteritis (Figure 8-25) sometimes does occur in embolic pulmonary hypertension and then most probably as a result of infected emboli. Fibrinoid necrosis with subsequent inflammation of the arterial wall is exceedingly rare in these cases. Dilatation lesions or plexiform lesions do not occur. The intra-arterial septa, due to recanalization, may sometimes mimic plexiform lesions, but study of serial sections will reveal the true nature of the lesions. The possibility that thromboembolism may complicate a case of primary pulmonary hypertension has been discussed in Chapter Seven (p. 133).

Pulmonary Capillaries and Veins. Pulmonary capillaries and pulmonary venules and veins are generally normal in chronic embolic pulmonary hypertension. Sometimes, particularly in older patients, the veins exhibit lesions indicative of increased pulmonary venous pressure, such as arterialization and thickening of the venous wall, but this is observed especially in patients with left heart failure.

Bronchial Vessels and Anastomoses. Bronchial arteries, mainly those that are lying close to obstructed pulmonary arteries, undergo distinct alterations in pulmonary thromboembolism (Smith et al., 1964; Spencer, 1968). Dilatation and hypertrophy of the media along with varying degrees of intimal fibrosis are observed in these bronchial arteries that also provide anastomoses with pulmonary arterial branches (Heath and Thompson, 1969). There is also an increased number of other systemic collateral arteries from the thoracic cage and the diaphragm, contributing to the systemic pulmonary anastomoses. Dilated vasa vasorum in the walls of obstructed and recanalized pulmonary arteries form connections with the recanalized channels.

If time permits, the collateral circulation in patients with thromboembolism may become very extensive and may prevent infarction and permit survival even after complete occlusion of a main pulmonary artery (Smith et al., 1964).

Shunting of blood in the involved areas from pulmonary arteries to pulmonary veins has been reported in experimental animals (Tobin and Zariquiey, 1950). Wilhelmsen and coworkers (1970) expressed the opinion that the wide, thin-walled vessels often found around obstructed pulmonary arteries, are pulmonary veins, engorged as a result of shunting from the bronchial circulation.

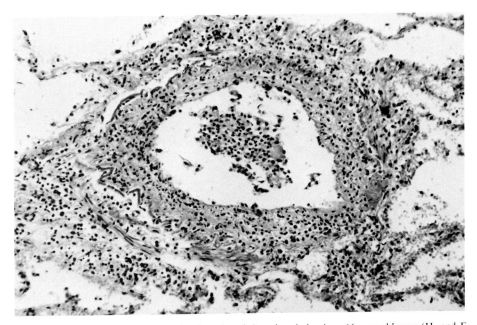

Figure 8-25.   Pulmonary arteritis at the site of an infected embolus in a 66-year-old man (H. and E., ×140).

OTHER FORMS OF EMBOLISM

The vast majority of pulmonary emboli are thrombotic. Nonthrombotic emboli are relatively infrequent. Although they may sometimes give rise to an acute and temporary elevation of pulmonary arterial pressure, a sustained pulmonary hypertension caused by emboli other than thrombi is very rare. Even if it occurs, it is likely that obstruction of the pulmonary vascular bed is only partly due to emboli such as clumps of tumor cells or foreign body material alone but that local thrombosis at the site of lodging of these emboli, contributes significantly to the arterial blockage.

Fat Embolism

If fat embolism in itself is fatal, it causes death because of obstruction of cerebral vessels rather than of pulmonary arteries (Sevitt, 1960). Sudden death due to obstruction of pulmonary arteries by fat is probably exceedingly rare, although its occurrence has been suggested (Robb-Smith, 1941) and although numerous and even large vessels may be occluded (Figures 8-26 and 8-27). Sustained pulmonary hypertension based on fat embolism, to our knowledge has not been described.

In dogs, experimental fat embolism produced either a temporary increase in pulmonary arterial pressure (Hecht and Korb, 1960) or no increase at all (Jaques and Saini, 1962).

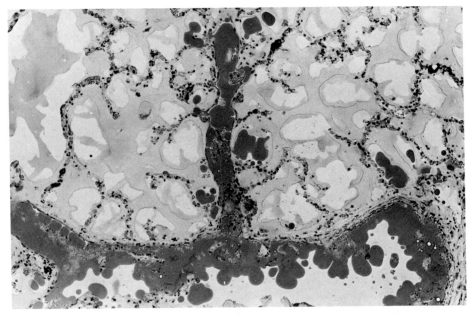

Figure 8-26. Elastic pulmonary artery with its muscular branches filled with multiple fat droplets in a 21-year-old woman who died one and a half days after a traffic accident (Frozen section. Sudan III-stain, ×90).

Air and Gas Embolism

Although air and gas embolism can be responsible for a brief period of elevation of pressure in the pulmonary circulation, there is no evidence that it ever induces chronic pulmonary hypertension in man.

In experimental animals and particularly in rabbits intravenous injections of air or gas, repeated over a long period, eventually lead to pulmonary hypertension and marked intimal proliferation and fibrosis of pulmonary arteries (Barnard, 1957; Wright, 1962; Boerema, 1965). Pulmonary hypertension also has been produced in this way in the dog (Gilbert et al., 1968). It appears, however, that when the injections are discontinued, both the elevation of pressure and the vascular alterations are reversible (Wright, 1962; Boerema, 1965).

Amniotic Fluid Embolism

Infusion of amniotic fluid may cause obstruction of small pulmonary arteries by lanugo hairs, keratotic squames, and amorphous and mucous components of the amniotic fluid. Sudden death in these cases originally was attributed to mechanical obstruction by this form of embolism, but it has become clear that pulmonary arterial blockage is rarely, if ever, caused by these constituents but results from the accompanying intravascular clotting (Reid et al., 1953).

As has been discussed before (p. 134), amniotic fluid embolism has been implicated in the etiology of primary pulmonary hypertension, but there is no evidence that it ever leads to sustained elevation of the pulmonary arterial pressure.

In dogs, infusion of amniotic fluid gives rise to an acute elevation of pressure, followed by a decrease within 2 or 3 hours. During the next few months the pulmonary arterial pressure may still be slightly raised but sustained pulmonary hypertension has not been observed (Jaques et al., 1960).

Tumor Embolism

All sorts of cells and fragments of tissue, when detached from their original site, usually by trauma, may enter the pulmonary circulation and may obstruct pulmonary arteries or arterioles. Such tissue or cell embolism almost always has no effect on the hemodynamics of the pulmonary circulation. Only very rarely has right ventricular dilatation been attributed to such a mechanism as in a case of massive embolism of megakaryocytes to the lungs (Bettendorf and Meyer Breiting, 1974).

The only form of tissue embolism in which pulmonary hypertension has been described fairly regularly is tumor embolism (Figures 8-28 and 8-29). In patients with malignant tumors, particularly of stomach and breast, embolism of tumor tissue to the lung vessels has been demonstrated in 26 percent of the cases (Winterbauer et al., 1968). In most instances the underlying disease will be fatal before cardiac failure develops or becomes a major problem.

However, pulmonary hypertension leading to right cardiac failure has been described in patients with various tumors, notably in gastric carcinoma (Morgan, 1949; Lignac, 1951; Schumann, 1962) and mammary carcinoma (Lignac, 1951; Ihr-

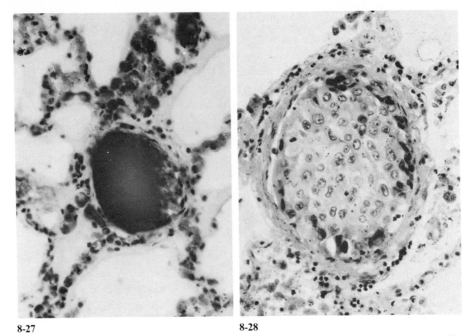

8-27   8-28

Figure 8-27. Pulmonary arteriole and alveolar capillaries containing fat emboli. Same case as Figure 8-26 (Frozen section. Sudan III-stain, ×230).

Figure 8-28. Muscular pulmonary artery obstructed by tumor embolus in a 59-year-old man with a hepatocellular carcinoma of the liver and right ventricular hypertrophy (H. and E., ×230).

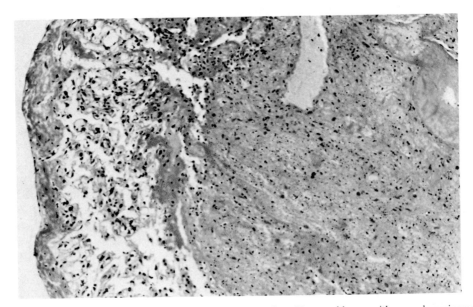

Figure 8-29. Clot removed from main pulmonary artery in a 71-year-old man with a renal carcinoma and right ventricular hypertrophy. The clot consists partly of pale tumor cells (left) and partly of thrombus (H. and E., ×90).

164

inger, 1953; Cain, 1958) and also in ovarian carcinoma (Kuhlman, 1934), cervical carcinoma (Barger et al., 1948), myxoma of the right atrium (Schweizer, 1953; Heath and McKinnin, 1964), and hydatidiform mole (Fahrner) et al., 1959; Lipp et al., 1962).

Foreign Body Embolism

Extraneous matter may be introduced in the bloodstream by intravenous injections, cardiac catheterization, or other intravascular procedures. Emboli of cotton-wool or gauze particles within pulmonary arteries or arterioles are commonly observed (Figure 8-30) but have no clinical significance.

In recent years an increasing number of cases have been reported in which intravenous injection of various drugs in narcotic addicts has caused pulmonary hypertension. These drugs, intended for oral use, are dissolved in a medium containing talcum or starch particles. After embolization to the pulmonary arterioles, these particles cause a granulomatous reaction (Figure 8-31) with obstruction of the vascular lumen (Krainer et al., 1962; Puro and Wolf, 1964; Szwed, 1970; Zientara and Moore, 1970; Groth et al., 1972; Hopkins, 1972; Lamb and Roberts, 1972;

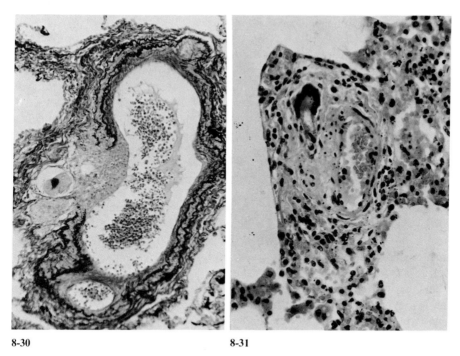

8-30   8-31

Figure 8-30. Muscular pulmonary artery, from a 40-year-old woman with rheumatic mitral stenosis with granuloma in response to embolized cotton-wool fiber. Some foreign body giant cells are present. The arterial wall is interrupted (El.v.G., ×140).

Figure 8-31. Muscular pulmonary artery with granuloma in its wall in a 21-year-old male drug addict with pulmonary hypertension due to intravenous heroin injection. The granuloma contains a foreign body giant cell around a birefringent talcum particle (H. and E., ×230).

Lewman, 1972; Siegel, 1972; Byers et al., 1975). With polarized light the birefringent talcum particles can be easily detected. When the cause of the pulmonary hypertension in these cases is recognized, it is too late and the fatal outcome cannot be avoided.

Embolism by Parasites

Parasites may enter the systemic veins and may reach the pulmonary circulation and become lodged in the pulmonary arteries or arterioles. Parasites causing pulmonary embolism, are almost always helminths, although in monkeys a lung mite (*Pneumonyssus simicola*) is known to enter the lumina of pulmonary arteries and to cause changes in these vessels (Woodard, 1968; Knezevich and McNulty, 1970).

In helminthic infections either the adult worms or their ova or larvae may lodge in the pulmonary arteries. The passage to the lungs is sometimes accidental but may be part of the life cycle of the parasite.

The consequences of parasitic embolism to the lungs vary widely. In some cases no clinical symptoms are produced, so that a granuloma with calcified remnants of the parasite may be an incidental autopsy finding. In ascariasis multiple lung abcesses have been reported (Broz et al., 1960), while in filariasis pulmonary infarction has been described (Beaver et al., 1971; Beaver and Cran, 1974) and also, although rarely, pulmonary hypertension (Obeyesekere and Peiris, 1974).

Another nematode, *Dirofilaria immitis,* well known as a cause for pulmonary hypertension and cardiac failure in the dog, now also has been identified as a human lung parasite responsible for coin lesions and infarcts (Goodman and Gore, 1964; Harrison and Thompson, 1965; Navarete-Reyna and Noon, 1968; Neafie and Piggott, 1971; Hendricks et al., 1973) but not as yet for pulmonary hypertension.

Massive and even fatal embolization to the lungs of membranes and contents of ruptured hepatic Echinococcus cysts occurs rarely (Richmond and Bernstein, 1968).

Pulmonary Schistosomiasis

Schistosomiasis is a parasitic infection of tropical areas produced by one of the following species of schistosomes or blood flukes, which are parasitic in man: *Schistosoma haematobium, mansoni,* and *japonicum.* While in other forms of parasitic embolism, pulmonary hypertension is, at best, a rare and haphazard complication, in schistosomiasis it is fairly common.

Shaw and Ghareeb (1938) in their classical description of schistosomiasis of the lungs in Egypt, indicate that in bilharzial infection 33 percent of the patients had pulmonary involvement and that in 2 percent the pulmonary lesions were the immediate cause of death. The ova of *Schistosoma haematobium* were more often found in the lungs but pulmonary vascular lesions were caused more often by those of *Schistosoma mansoni.*

The adult worms live in the human host. Their eggs escape with feces and urine and mature into larval forms or miracidiae as soon as they are deposited in fresh water. Here they penetrate into certain species of snails in which they develop into a second larval form, the cercariae, which are highly infective to man. The cercariae penetrate the skin, enter the capillaries and small venules, and pass along the bloodstream as metacercariae through the heart and the lungs, where they may produce a Löffler's syndrome (Cortes and Winters, 1961), to reach eventually the portal circulation.

In the intrahepatic branches of the portal veins, they mature to adult flukes that migrate to the large bowel (*S. mansoni*), the small bowel (*S. japonicum*) or the pelvic organs including the urinary bladder (*S. haematobium*). The adult parasites copulate within the veins. The ova may penetrate the wall of bowel or urinary bladder and leave the body with feces and urine.

A large proportion of the ova is carried with the blood to other organs, notably the liver, where they may cause hepatic cirrhosis. From here ova may embolize to the lungs where they become lodged in pulmonary arterioles. In endemic areas occasional ova are commonly found in lung vessels of carrier-patients without apparent clinical significance (Chaves, 1966).

The pulmonary vascular pathology in schistosomal pulmonary hypertension is complex and not clearly defined. Apparently several mechanisms are involved. In part the pulmonary vascular alterations in pulmonary schistosomiasis are due to obstruction of the vessels by ova or by the accompanying thrombotic and granulomatous reaction related to the ova (Shaw and Ghareeb, 1938; Marchand et al., 1957; Garcia-Palmieri, 1964).

When schistosome ova become impacted in the pulmonary arterioles they either remain in the lumen causing a granulomatous reaction within the vessel or, more often, they penetrate the arterial wall so that a granuloma is formed outside the artery (Naeye, 1961; Wagenvoort et al., 1964), sometimes at some distance in the pulmonary parenchyma (Figure 8-32). Their migration outside the vessels sometimes results in focal interstitial fibrosis of the lungs (Zaky et al., 1968). In the granulomas, which may contain some foreign body giant cells, mononuclear cells, and eosinophils, the ova (Figure 8-33) or their calcified remnants (Figure 8-34) usually can be recognized. Thrombi in pulmonary arterioles, often described as hyalin or fibrin thrombi, have been reported in varying numbers (De Faria, 1954a; Chaves, 1966; Berkman et al., 1974).

If many lung vessels are blocked by ova or by the accompanying reactions, it is conceivable that the pulmonary arterial pressure will be raised. This would be a clear example of embolic pulmonary hypertension, but it is questionable whether the mechanical factor plays a predominant part in the production of the elevated pressure (Cavalcanti et al., 1962).

A peculiar necrotizing arteritis is one of the most common changes in pulmonary schistosomiasis. It may occur in the immediate vicinity of impacted ova (Figure 8-35). The arteritis most likely results from an allergic reaction to the ovum or its products (De Faria, 1954a; Marchand et al., 1957; Garcia-Palmieri, 1964) rather than to the mechanical damage inflicted on the vascular wall, since necrotizing arteritis is commonly seen in the absence of ova. Also the granulomas are considered to result from an immunologic reaction of the delayed hypersensitivity type and differences in granuloma formation have been described in response to various species of Schistosoma (Warren et al., 1975).

The example of necrotizing arteritis shows that there are vascular lesions in pulmonary schistosomiasis not directly caused by the ova of the parasite. There are other changes in the pulmonary arteries and arterioles that are unrelated to a local action of the ova. Marked medial hypertrophy, concentric-laminar intimal fibrosis,

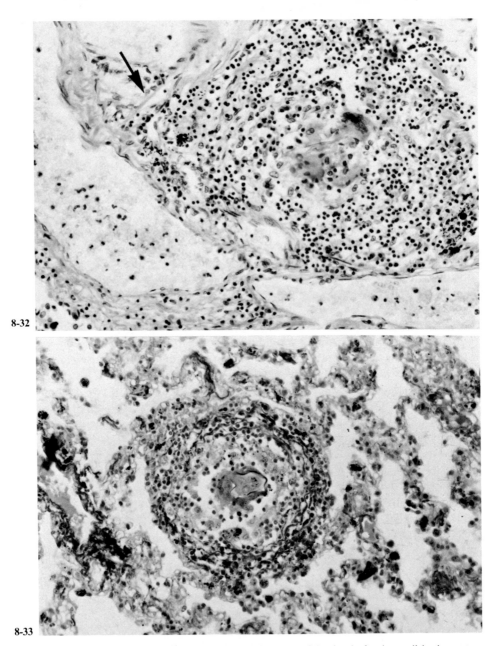

Figure 8-32. Schistosome granuloma with remnant of ovum and foreign body giant cell in the center. The granuloma is adjacent to a muscular pulmonary artery. The point where the ovum probably penetrated the arterial wall is indicated by an arrow. Woman aged 27 years with pulmonary schistosomiasis (H. and E., ×230).

Figure 8-33. Schistosome granuloma in lung tissue containing the remnant of an ovum in an 11-year-old boy with pulmonary schistosomiasis (El.v.G., ×230).

168

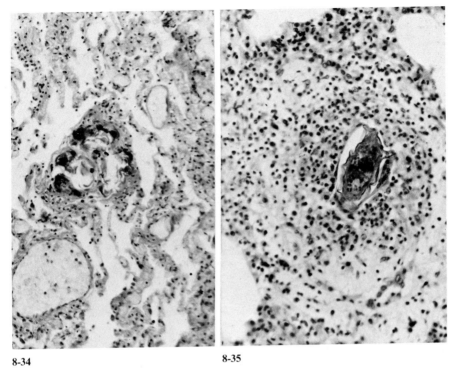

8-34   8-35

Figure 8-34.   Lung tissue with calcified ova of *Schistosoma mansoni* within some fibrous tissue. Same case as Figure 8-32 (H. and E., ×140).

Figure 8-35.   Pulmonary arteriole in which an impacted ovum with lateral spine (*S. mansoni*) has caused necrotizing arteritis with virtually complete destruction of its wall. Same case as Figure 8-33 (H. and E., ×230).

and plexiform lesions (Figure 8-36), and angiomatoids have been regularly reported (Shaw and Ghareeb, 1938; Marchand et al., 1957; Wagenvoort et al., 1964; Al Naaman et al., 1967). In other words, pulmonary schistosomiasis may be complicated by plexogenic pulmonary arteriopathy.

It has been suggested that lesions not directly caused by ova are to a larger extent responsible for increased pulmonary vascular resistance and right cardiac failure (De Faria, 1954b; Naeye, 1961).

The question may be raised whether the plexiform and angiomatoid lesions to be found in these patients are identical to those observed in congenital cardiac shunts. Many descriptions and illustrations leave in abeyance the decision whether we are dealing with plexiform lesions or with granulomas of a dumbbell type within a pseudoaneurysm of a muscular pulmonary artery (Marchand et al., 1957), which may mimic plexiform lesions. Moreover, these structures have been interpreted as arteriovenous anastomoses (De Faria, 1954b).

On the other hand, careful reconstructions of the lesions have shown that at least some of them did not differ in structure from the well-known plexiform lesions in congenital heart disease (Brewer, 1955; Naeye, 1961). Naeye (1961) believes that true plexiform lesions do not contain ova. Others have reported ova in plexiform

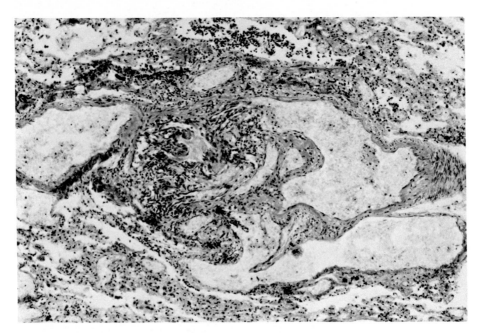

Figure 8-36. Plexiform lesion in a muscular pulmonary artery from a 27-year-old woman with pulmonary schistosomiasis (H. and E., ×90).

lesions (Shaw and Ghareeb, 1938; Liebow, 1960). Even if the confusing similarity between plexiform lesions and the granulomatous reaction to the ova does not play a part in this observation, it does not necessarily indicate a direct causal relationship. In patients with hepatic involvement, numerous ova are continuously shedded to the pulmonary circulation, and if plexiform lesions have developed in the pulmonary arteries, ova may subsequently be trapped by them.

If severe pulmonary hypertension has developed, the clinical picture resembles that of primary pulmonary hypertension. Hemoptysis is a fairly frequent symptom (Cavalcanti et al., 1962). Aneurysms of pulmonary trunk or main pulmonary arteries have sometimes been described (Al-Naaman, 1967; Zaky et al., 1967). The clinical course is irreversible and the patients die in cardiac failure.

It is unknown what causes plexogenic pulmonary arteriopathy in patients with schistosomiasis. The presence of a vasoconstrictive factor has been suggested (Cavalcanti et al., 1962). Simultaneous involvement of the lungs with vasoconstrictive lesions in pulmonary arteries and in the liver in these patients may be significant.

Schistosomal pulmonary hypertension and cardiac failure are associated with hepatic cirrhosis, portal hypertension, and porto-systemic anastomoses in the great majority of the cases (Garcia-Palmieri, 1964; Chaves, 1966). The condition, therefore, has been termed "porto-pulmonary schistosomiasis" (Zaky et al., 1968) and "schistosomal porto-pulmonary obstruction" (Rodriguez et al., 1963). Naeye (1961) has speculated that thromboemboli may reach the lungs along these collateral pathways, but this, as we have seen (p. 97), would not explain the development of plexogenic pulmonary arteriopathy.

It is, however, very possible that in many patients the pipestem cirrhosis of the liver and the associated collateral circulation are basic to the development of pulmonary hypertension and plexogenic pulmonary arteriopathy in the same way as this is known to happen in other instances of hepatic injury (Chapter Five).

This would explain the presence of such changes as concentric intimal fibrosis and plexiform lesions in arteries without ova and also the occasional development of severe pulmonary hypertension in patients with schistosomal cirrhosis of the liver in whom there were no parasites or ova in the lungs (Rodriguez et al., 1963).

Thus it is likely that pulmonary hypertension in this condition may be caused by at least three different mechanisms, which may operate alone or in combination with the others. These are embolic obstruction, allergic arteritis with obliteration, and vasoconstriction followed by plexogenic pulmonary arteriopathy in association with hepatic injury.

Embolic hypertensive vascular lesions: Arteries with mild medial hypertrophy, eccentric intimal fibrosis, and intravascular fibrous septa.

REFERENCES

Al-Naaman, Y. D., Shamma, A. M., Damluji, S. F., and El-Sayed, H. M.: Angiologic manifestation of cardiopulmonary schistosomiasis "Bilharziasis." *Angiology* **17:** 40, 1967.

Ardlie, N. G., and Schwartz, C. J.: A comparison of the organization and fate of autologous pulmonary emboli and of artificial plasma thrombi in the anterior chamber of the eye, in normocholesterolaemic rabbits. *J. Path. Bact.* **95:** 1, 1968.

Barger, J. D., Edwards, J. E., Parker, R. L., and Dry, T.: Cardiac clinics. Atrial septal defect: Presentation of a case with obstructive pulmonary vascular lesions caused by metastatic carcinoma. *Proc. Mayo Clin.* **23:** 182, 1948.

Barnard, P. J.: Experimental fibrin thrombo-enbolism of the lungs. *J. Path. Bact.* **65:** 129, 1953.

Barnard, P. J.: Pulmonary arteriosclerosis and cor pulmonale due to recurrent thromboembolism. *Circulation* **10:** 343, 1954.

Barnard, P. J.: Pulmonary arteriosclerosis due to oxygen, nitrogen, and argon embolism. Experimental study. *Arch. Path.* **63:** 322, 1957.

Beaver, P. C., Fallon, M., and Smith, G. H.: Pulmonary nodule caused by a living Brugia malayi like filaria in an artery. *Amer. J. Trop. Med. Hyg.* **20:** 661, 1971.

Beaver, P. C., and Cran, I. R.: Wuchereria like filaria in an artery associated with pulmonary infarction. *Amer. J. Trop. Med. Hyg.* **23:** 869, 1974.

Beckering, R. E., and Titus, J. L.: Femoral-popliteal venous thrombosis and pulmonary embolism. *Amer. J. Clin. Path.* **52:** 530, 1969.

Behrendt, W.: Die massive "stumme" Lungenembolie. *Münch. Med. Wschr.* **105:** 2216, 1963.

Belt, T. H.: Demonstration of small pulmonary emboli at autopsy. *J. Techn. Methods* **15:** 39, 1936.

Berkman, M., Akoun, G., Lancastre, F., Brocard, H., and Chiche, P.: Le coeur pulmonaire chronique d'origine bilharzienne. *Sem. Hôp.* Paris **50:** 143, 1974.

Bettendorf, U., and Meyer Breiting, E.: Massive Megakaryozytenembolie der Lungen. *Dtsch. Med. Wschr.* **99:** 1918, 1974.

Boerema, B.: Appearance and regression of pulmonary arterial lesions after repeated intravenous injection of gas. *J. Path. Bact.* **89:** 741, 1965.

Brantigan, O. C., Kress, M. B., and Goco, R. B.: Pulmonary emboli; A factor in the etiology and pathogenesis of pulmonary emphysema. *Dis. Chest* **49:** 491, 1966.

Brenner, O.: Pathology of the vessels of the pulmonary circulation. Part V. *Arch. Int. Med.* **56:** 1189, 1935.

Brewer, D. B.: Fibrous occlusion and anastomosis of the pulmonary vessels in a case of pulmonary hypertension associated with patent ductus arteriosus. *J. Path. Bact.* **70:** 299, 1955.

Broź, O., Trinh, P., and Cong, T. C.: Complications cardio-pulmonaires rares et fatales de l'ascaridiose: ascaris dans le coeur et pneumonite par embolisation de leurs oeufs. *Path. Microbiol.* **23:** 36, 1960.

Byers, J. M., Soin, J. S., Fisher, R. S., and Hutchins, G. M.: Acute pulmonary alveolitis in narcotics abuse. *Arch. Path.* **99:** 273, 1975.

Cain, H.: Hämatogene Geschwulstzellenausbreitung in der Lunge, unter besondere Berücksichtigung sog. regelwidriger Fälle. *Z. Krebsforsch.* **62:** 323, 1958.

Castleman, B., and Bland, E. F.: Organized emboli of the tertiary pulmonary arteries. An unusual cause of cor pulmonale. *Arch. Path.* **42:** 581, 1946.

Cavalcanti, I. de L., Tompson, G., De Souza, N., and Barbosa, F. S.: Pulmonary hypertension in schistosomiasis. *Brit. Heart J.* **24:** 363, 1962.

Chaves, E.: The pathology of the arterial pulmonary vasculature in Manson's schistosomiasis. *Dis. Chest* **50:** 72, 1966.

Chomette, G., Pinaudeau, Y., Auriol, M., Brocheriou, C., and Daddi, G.: Les embolies pulmonaires. Etude statistique de 1800 nécropsies systématiques. *Laval Méd.* **37:** 584, 1966.

Comroe, J. H., Van Linge, B., Stroud, R. C., and Roncoroni, A.: Reflex and direct cardiopulmonary effects of 5-OH-tryptamine (serotonin): their possible role in pulmonary embolism and coronary thrombosis. *Amer. J. Physiol.* **173:** 379, 1953.

Cortes, F. M., and Winters, W. L.: Schistosomiasis cor pulmonale. *Amer. J. Med.* **31:** 808, 1961.

Courtoy, P., and Salonikides, N.: Acute experimental pulmonary hypertension by pulmonary embolization. I. Circulatory dynamics. *Acta Cardiol.* **11:** 52, 1956.

De Bakey, M. E.: Critical evaluation of the problem of thromboembolism. *Surg. Gyn. Obst.* **98:** 1, 1954.

De Faria, J. L.: Pulmonary vascular changes in schistosomal cor pulmonale. *J. Path. Bact.* **68:** 589, 1954a.

De Faria, J. L.: Cor pulmonale in Manson's schistosomiasis. I. Frequency in necropsy material; pulmonary vascular changes caused by schistosome ova. *Amer. J. Path.* **30:** 167, 1954b.

Dexter, L.: Thromboemboli as a cause of cor pulmonale. *Bull. N. Y. Acad. Med.* **41:** 981, 1965.

Downing, S. E., and Vidone, R. A.: Pulmonary vascular responses to embolization with autologous thrombi. *Surg. Gyn. Obst.* **125:** 269, 1967.

Dunnill, M. S.: The pathology of pulmonary embolism. *Brit. J. Surg.* **55:** 790, 1968.

Fahrner, R. J., McQueeney, A. J., Mosely, J. M., and Petersen, R. W.: Trophoblastic pulmonary thrombosis with cor pulmonale. Report of a case due to malignant hydatiform mole of five years' duration. *J.A.M.A.* **170:** 1898, 1959.

Fleischner, F. G.: Recurrent pulmonary embolism and cor pulmonale. *New Engl. J. Med.* **276:** 1213, 1967.

Fleming, H. A., and Bailey, S. M.: Massive pulmonary embolism in healthy people. *Brit. Med. J.* **1:** 1322, 1966.

Fowler, E. F., and Bollinger, J. A.: Pulmonary embolism: a clinical study of ninety-seven fatal cases. *Surgery* **36:** 650, 1954.

Freiman, D. G., Suyemoto, J., and Wessler, S.: Frequency of pulmonary thromboembolism in man. *New Engl. J. Med.* **272:** 1278, 1965.

Galland, F., Maldonado, G., Medrano, G., and Cimta, M.: Acute pulmonary hypertensive heart disease: Pathophysiology. *Dis. Chest* **45:** 515, 1964.

Garcia-Palmieri, M.: Cor pulmonale due to *Schistosoma mansoni.* Amer. Heart J. **68:** 714, 1964.

Geer, J. C., Glass, B. A., and Albert, H. M.: Pulmonary vascular lesions in the dog produced by autogenous clot embolism. *Exp. Molec. Path.* **4**: 391, 1965.

Gilbert, J. W., Berglund, E., Dahlgren, S., Ovenfors, C. O., and Barnes, R.: Experimental pulmonary hypertension in the dog. A preparation involving repeated air embolism. *J. Thor. Cardiov. Surg.* **55**: 565, 1968.

Goodman, M. L., and Gore, I.: Pulmonary infarct secondary to dirofilaria larvae. *Arch. Int. Med.* **113**: 702, 1964.

Goodwin, J. F., Harrison, C. V., and Wilcken, D. E. L.: Obliterative pulmonary hypertension and thrombo-embolism. *Brit. Med. J.* **i**: 701, 1963.

Groth, D. H., Mackay, G. R., Crable, J. V., and Cochran, T. H.: Intravenous injection of talc in a narcotics addict. *Arch. Path.* **94**: 171, 1972.

Gurewich, V., Cohen, M. L., and Thomas, D. P.: Humoral factors in massive pulmonary embolism. An experimental study. *Amer. Heart J.* **76**: 784, 1968.

Hackl, H.: Über das Vorkommen von Pulmonalembolien. *Med. Klin.* **62**: 44, 1967.

Halmagyi, D. F. J., Starzecki, B., and Horner, G. J.: Humoral transmission of cardiorespiratory changes in experimental lung embolism. *Circ. Res.* **14**: 546, 1964.

Harrison, C. V.: Experimental pulmonary arteriosclerosis. *J. Path. Bact.* **60**: 289, 1948.

Harrison, C. V.: Experimental pulmonary hypertension. *J. Path. Bact.* **63**: 195, 1951.

Harrison, E. G., and Thompson, J. H.: Dirofilariasis of human lung. *Amer. J. Clin. Path.* **43**: 224, 1965.

Hartmann, H.: Analyse von 500 Lungenembolien. *Zbl. Allg. Path. Path. Anat.* **104**: 567, 1963.

Heard, B. E.: An experimental study of thickening of the pulmonary arteries of rabbits produced by the organisation of fibrin. *J. Path. Bact.* **64**: 13, 1952.

Heath, D., and MacKinnon, J.: Pulmonary hypertension due to myxoma of the right atrium. With special reference to the behavior of emboli of myxoma in the lung. *Amer. Heart J.* **68**: 227, 1964.

Heath, D., and Thompson, I. M.: Bronchopulmonary anastomoses in sickle-cell anaemia. *Thorax* **24**: 232, 1969.

Hecht, A., and Korb, G.: Vergleichende Untersuchungen über pathologisch-anatomische und funktionelle Veränderungen bei der Lungenfettembolie. *Verh. Dtsch. Ges. Path.* **44**: 184, 1960.

Hendricks, G. L., Berness, W. T., and Larman, D. S.: Dirofilaria immitis: a cause of pulmonary coin lesions in human beings. *Amer. J. Thor. Surg.* **16**: 526, 1973.

Hopkins, G. B.: Pulmonary angiothrombotic granulomatosis in drug offenders. *J.A.M.A.* **221**: 909, 1972.

Hyman, A. L., Myers, W. D., and Meyer, A.: The effect of acute pulmonary embolus upon cardiopulmonary hemodynamics. *Amer. Heart J.* **67**: 313, 1964.

Ihringer, G.: Über das Schicksal embolisierter Tumorzellen in den Lungen. *Zbl. Allg. Path. Path. Anat.* **90**: 123, 1953.

Jaques, W. E., Hampton, J. W., Bird, R. M., Bolten, K., and Randolph, B.: Pulmonary hypertension and plasma thromboplastin-antecedent deficiency in dogs. Experimental induction by infusion of amniotic fluid. *Arch. Path.* **69**: 248, 1960.

Jaques, W. E., and Saini, N.: A physiologic and anatomic study of experimental fat embolism in dogs. *Exp. Molec. Path.* **1**: 57, 1962.

Kaufmann, F., and Keresztes, A.: Bericht über die fulminante, tödliche Lungenembolie des Obduktionsmaterials der Jahre 1952 bis 1965. *Wiener Klin. Wschr.* **79**: 155, 1967.

Knezevich, A. L., and McNulty, W. P.: Pulmonary acariasis (*Pneumonyssus simicola*) in colony-bred *Macaca mulatta*. *Lab. Animal Care* **20**: 693, 1970.

Knisely, W. H., Wallace, J. M., Mahaley, M. S., and Satterwhite, W. M.: Evidence, including in vivo observation, suggesting mechanical blockage rather than reflex vasospasm as the cause of death in pulmonary embolization. *Amer. Heart J.* **54**: 483, 1957.

Korn, D., Gore, I., Blenke, A., and Collins, D. P.: Pulmonary arterial bands and webs: an unrecognized manifestation of organized pulmonary emboli. *Amer. J. Path.* **40**: 129, 1962.

Krainer, L., Berman, E., and Wishnick, S. D.: Parenteral talcum granulomatosis. A complication of narcotic addiction. *Lab. Invest.* **11**: 671, 1962.

Kuhlman, F.: Miliarcarcinoma and Lungenstauung. *Klin. Wschr.* **13:** 770, 1934.

Lamb, D., and Roberts, G.: Starch and talc emboli in drug addicts. *J. Clin. Path.* **25:** 876, 1972.

Levy, S. E., Shapiro, B. J., and Simmons, D. H.: Pulmonary hemodynamics after autologous in vivo pulmonary thromboembolism. *J. Amer. Physiol.* **22:** 53, 1969.

Lewman, L. V.: Fatal pulmonary hypertension from intravenous injection of methylphenidate (Ritalin) tablets. *Human Path.* **3:** 67, 1972.

Liebow, A. A. Cardiopulmonary disease. In Gould, *Pathology of the Heart,* 2nd ed. Charles C Thomas, Springfield, Ill., 1960.

Lignac, G. O. E.: Waaraan is de patient eigenlijk overleden. *Nederl. Tschr. v. Geneesk.* **95:** 2454, 1951.

Lindsey, H. E., and Wyllie, J. H.: Release of prostaglandins from embolized lungs. *Brit. J. Surg.* **57:** 738, 1970.

Lipp, R. G., Kinschi, J. D., and Schmitz, R.: Death from pulmonary embolism associated with hydatidiform mole. *Amer. J. Obst. Gyn.* **83:** 1644, 1962.

Marchand, E. J., Marcial-Rojas, R. A., Rodriguez, R., Polanco, G., and Diaz-Rivera, R. S.: The pulmonary obstruction syndrome in *Schistosoma mansoni* pulmonary endarteritis. *Arch. Int. Med.* **100:** 965, 1957.

Marshall, R.: *Pulmonary Embolism. Mechanism and Management.* Charles C Thomas, Springfield, Ill., 1965.

Morgan, A. D.: The pathology of subacute cor pulmonale in diffuse carcinomatosis of the lungs. *J. Path. Bact.* **61:** 75, 1949.

Naeye, R. L.: Advanced pulmonary vascular changes in schistosomal cor pulmonale. *Amer. J. Trop. Med. Hyg.* **10:** 191, 1961.

Nakano, J., and McCloy, R. B.: Effects of indomethacin on the pulmonary vascular and air way resistance responses to pulmonary microembolization. *Proc. Soc. Exp. Biol. Med.* **143:** 218, 1973.

Navarete-Reyna, A., and Noon, G.: Pulmonary dirofilariasis manifested as a coin lesion. *Arch. Path.* **85:** 266, 1968.

Neafie, R. C., and Piggott, M. A. J. J.: Human pulmonary dirofilariasis. *Arch. Path.* **92:** 342, 1971.

Niden, A. H., and Aviado, D. M.: Effects of pulmonary embolism on the pulmonary circulation with special reference to arteriovenous shunts in the lung. *Circ. Res.* **4:** 67, 1956.

Obeyesekere, I., and Peiris, D.: Pulmonary hypertension and filariasis. *Brit. Heart J.* **36:** 676, 1974.

Olsen, E. G. J.: Repeated pulmonary thromboembolism in rabbits. *Lab. Invest.* **32:** 323, 1975.

Parmley, L. F., North, R. L., and Ott, B. S.: Hemodynamic alterations of acute pulmonary thromboembolism. *Circ. Res.* **11:** 450, 1962.

Piper, P. J., and Vane, J. R.: The release of prostaglandins from lung and other tissues. *Ann. N. Y. Acad. Sci.* **180:** 363, 1971.

Puro, H. E., and Wolf, P. L.: Angiothrombotic pulmonary hypertension in paregoric-pyribenzamine addicts. *Lab. Invest.* **13:** 946, 1964.

Reid, D. E., Weiner, A. E., and Robby, C. C.: I. Intravascular clotting and afibrinogenemia, the presumptive lethal factors in the syndrome of amniotic fluid embolism. *Amer. J. Obst. Gyn.* **66:** 465, 1953.

Richmond, D. R., and Bernstein, L.: Hydatid pulmonary embolism. *Austr. Ann. Med.* **17:** 270, 1968.

Robb-Smith, A. H. T.: Pulmonary fat-embolism. Lancet **i,** 135, 1941.

Rodriguez, H. F., Fernandez-Duran, A., Garcia-Moliner, L. and Rivera, E.: Cardiopulmonary schistosomiasis. *Amer. Heart J.* **65:** 253, 1963.

Sanders, R., Waalkes, T. P., Gilbert, G. W. and Terry, L. L.: Serotonin (5-hydroxytryptamine) and pulmonary thromboembolism. *Surg. Gyn. Obst.* **109:** 455, 1959.

Sasahara, A. A.: Current problems in pulmonary embolism: Introduction. *Progr. Cardiovasc. Dis.* **17:** 161, 1974.

Sautter, R. D., Fletcher, F. W., Emmanuel, D. A., Lawton, B. R., and Olsen, T. G.: Complete resolution of massive pulmonary thromboembolism. *J.A.M.A.* **189:** 948, 1964.

Schumann, H.-J.: Ungewöhnliche tödliche Kreislauffolgen bei rezidivierender Tumorzellembolie der Lungen. *Frankf. Z. Path.* **71**: 569, 1962.

Schweizer, W.: Die pulmonäre arterielle Hypertension. *Schweiz. Med. Wschr.* **83**: 1055, 1953.

Sevitt, S.: The significance and classification of fat-embolism. *Lancet* **ii**: 825, 1960.

Shaw, A. F. B., and Ghareeb, A. A.: The pathogenesis of pulmonary schistosomiasis in Egypt with special reference to Ayerza's disease. *J. Path. Bact.* **44**: 401, 1938.

Siegel, H.: Human pulmonary pathology associated with narcotic and other addictive drugs. *Human Path.* **3**: 55, 1972.

Smith, G. T., Hyland, J. W., Piemme, T., and Wells, R. E.: Human systemic-pulmonary arterial collateral circulation after pulmonary thromboembolism. *J.A.M.A.* **188**: 452, 1964.

Spencer, H.: *Pathology of the Lung*, 2nd ed. Pergamon Press, London, 1968.

Stringate, C. S., Fechner, R. E., Scott, R. C., Jystad, G. R., and O'Neal, R. M.: Disappearance of clot-emboli in rabbits. *Arch. Path.* **73**: 407, 1962.

Szwed, J. J.: Pulmonary angiothrombosis caused by blue velvet addiction. *Ann. Int. Med.* **73**: 771, 1970.

Tobin, C. E., and Zariquiey, M. O.: Arteriovenous shunts in the human lung. *Proc. Soc. Exp. Biol. Med.* **75**: 827, 1950.

Vanek, J.: Fibrous bands and networks of postembolic origin in the pulmonary arteries. *J. Path. Bact.* **81**: 537, 1961.

Wagenvoort, C. A.: Hypertensive pulmonary vascular disease complicating congenital heart disease: A review. *Cardiovasc. Clinics* **5**: 43, 1973.

Wagenvoort, C. A.: Editorial. The pathology of the pulmonary vasculature in various forms of pulmonary hypertension. *Giorn. Ital. Card.* **5**: 1, 1975.

Wagenvoort, C. A., Heath, D., and Edwards, J. E.: *The Pathology of the Pulmonary Vasculature.* Charles C Thomas, Springfield, Ill., 1964.

Wagenvoort, C. A., and Wagenvoort, N.: Primary pulmonary hypertension. A pathologic study of the lung vessels in 156 clinically diagnosed cases. *Circulation* **42**: 1163, 1970.

Warren, K. S., Boros, D. L., Le Minh Hang, and Mahmoud, A. F.: The *Schistosoma japonicum* egg granuloma. *Amer. J. Path.* **80**: 279, 1975.

Weidman, W. H., Marshall, R. J., Wagenvoort, C. A., and Shepherd, J. T.: Relation in dogs of pulmonary vascular obstruction to pulmonary vascular resistance. *Lab. Invest.* **12**: 821, 1963.

Weidner, M. G., and Light, R. A.: Role of the autonomic nervous system in the control of the pulmonary vascular bed. *Ann. Surg.* **147**: 895, 1958.

Widimsky, J., Kasalický, J., Přerovsky, I., and Dejdar, R.: Central hemodynamics in recurrent embolism. *Amer. Heart J.* **71**: 206, 1966.

Wilhelmsen, L., Selander, S., Söderholm, B., Paulin, S., Varnauskas, E., and Werkö, L.: Recurrent pulmonary embolism. *Medicine* **42**: 335, 1963.

Wilhelmsen, L., Bjure, J., Korsgren, M., and Zettergren, L.: Pathophysiology of pulmonary embolism with special reference to recurrent embolism. *Bull. Physio-Path. Resp.* **6**: 99, 1970.

Williams, H.: Mechanical vs. reflex effects of diffuse pulmonary embolism in anesthesized dogs. *Circ. Res.* **4**: 325, 1956.

Williams, G. D., Westbrook, K. C., and Campbell, G. S.: Reflex pulmonary hypertension and systemic hypotension after microsphere pulmonary embolism: a myth. *Amer. J. Surg.* **118**: 925, 1969.

Winterbauer, R. H., Elfenbein, I. B., and Ball, W. C.: Incidence and clinical significance of tumor embolization to the lungs. *Amer. J. Med.* **45**: 271, 1968.

Woodard, J. C.: Acarous (*Pneumonyssus simicola*) arteritis in rhesus monkeys. *J. Amer. Vet. Med. Ass.* **153**: 905, 1968.

Wright, R. R.: Experimental pulmonary hypertension produced by recurrent air emboli. *Med. Thorac.* **19**: 231, 1962.

Zahn, W.: Ueber ein eigenthümliches congenitales Netzwerk in der linken Pulmonalarterie. *Virch. Arch. Path. Anat.* **115**: 58, 1889.

Zaky, H. A., El Heneidy, A. R., Foda, M., Khalil, M., and Tarabeih, A. A.: Cardio-pulmonary bilharzia. In Mostofi, F. K., *Bilharziasis. Internat. Acad. Path. Spec. Monogr.* Springer Verlag, Berlin, 1967, p. 30.

Zaky, H. A. El Heneidy, A. R., and Tarabeih, A. A.: Hyperventilation and effort dyspnea in porto-pulmonary bilharziasis. *Dis. Chest* **53:** 162, 1968.

Zientara, M., and Moore, S.: Fatal talc embolism in a drug addict. *Human Path.* **1:** 423, 1970.

CHAPTER NINE

Pulmonary Venous Hypertension

Elevation of pressure in the pulmonary veins usually results from processes outside the lungs, particularly in the heart, causing obstruction to the pulmonary venous flow. Even so, the lungs usually are involved to a considerable extent so that, if one's attention should be directed mainly to the lungs, one could regard the condition as a pulmonary disorder (Arnott, 1963).

Although pulmonary venous hypertension is common, and in spite of extensive studies in this field, many of its hemodynamic and morphologic aspects are largely unsolved. A significant rise in pulmonary venous pressure is observed particularly in cases of mitral valve disease and most of the data and considerations discussed in this chapter are derived from patients with mitral stenosis or incompetence.

HEMODYNAMICS

Left Atrial and Pulmonary Venous Pressure

Except in rare cases of obstruction of pulmonary veins or of cor triatriatum, the impediment to the pulmonary venous flow is located at, or distal to, the mitral valve. If it is distal to the mitral valve, elevated left atrial and pulmonary venous pressures can be expected only in the presence of mitral incompetence or left ventricular failure.

A raised left atrial pressure is transmitted directly to the pulmonary veins and alveolar capillaries and to the pulmonary arteries. Under normal circumstances, at least in experimental animals, this may result in a decrease in the pulmonary vascular resistance by distension of the lung vessels (Carlill et al., 1957). As we will see, this does not apply to patients with pulmonary venous hypertension.

Pulmonary Edema

The pulmonary capillary bed can withstand a mild increase in pressure, but when the hydrostatic pressure exceeds the osmotic pressure of the blood, which is in the range of 25mmHg, fluid will leak from the capillaries with the risk of pulmonary edema.

Since in mitral valve disease, left atrial and pulmonary arterial wedge pressures in excess of 25mmHg are common, particularly during exercise, pulmonary edema with its consequences of impairment of gas exchange through the capillary-alveolar walls, theoretically would take a high toll in these patients. It appears that the pulmonary arterial pressure rises proportionally with the wedge pressure up to a value of the latter of approximately 25mmHg. Thereafter, however, there is a disproportionate increase of the pulmonary arterial pressure so that slight increases of wedge pressure produce gradually more marked elevations of the pressure in the pulmonary arteries (Dexter et al., 1950; Harris and Heath, 1962; Arnott, 1963).

That pulmonary edema actually occurs much less often than one would expect, is probably due to a number of mechanisms that can be considered protective or compensatory, although it often is not clear exactly how these mechanisms work, while their results also are not solely beneficial.

There is no doubt that a markedly increased drainage of fluid by way of the pulmonary lymphatics diminishes considerably the risk of pulmonary edema. Direct evidence of this has been obtained from experiments (Rabin and Meyer, 1960; Uhley et al., 1962). In patients it is also witnessed by the dilatation of the lymphatic system in histologic sections (p. 201). Distension of lymphatics together with edema of the connective tissue septa of the lungs, produce the so-called Kerley B-lines (Kerley, 1951) in the chest roentgenogram (Figure 9-1). These lines disappear after recovery from pulmonary edema.

A diminished permeability of the capillary-alveolar barrier may be another factor in keeping pulmonary edema in check. Although morphologic evidence of thickening of the layer between capillary lumen and alveolar space has been put forward, as discussed later (p. 205), its significance with regard to diminishing permeability and the risk for pulmonary edema, is still under discussion (Lucas, 1972).

Pulmonary Arterial Pressure

We have just seen that the increased pressure in left atrium and pulmonary veins will be transmitted not only to the pulmonary capillary bed but also to the pulmonary arteries. In cases of chronic pulmonary venous hypertension, however, the pressure in the pulmonary artery may rise to very high levels, approaching systemic pressure. Since the pulmonary arterial blood flow usually is reduced somewhat in these patients, the high pressure results from the marked increase in pulmonary vascular resistance which in turn may reduce the right ventricular output, particularly during exercise (Dexter, 1952, 1956; Harris and Heath, 1962).

It is believed that this increase in resistance is, at least in part, due to vasoconstriction. The evidence for this has been derived mainly from hemodynamic data (Dexter et al., 1950; Davies et al., 1954; Goodale et al., 1955; Dexter, 1956; Yu et al., 1956; Doyle et al., 1957; Evans and Short, 1957; Wood et al., 1957; Charms et

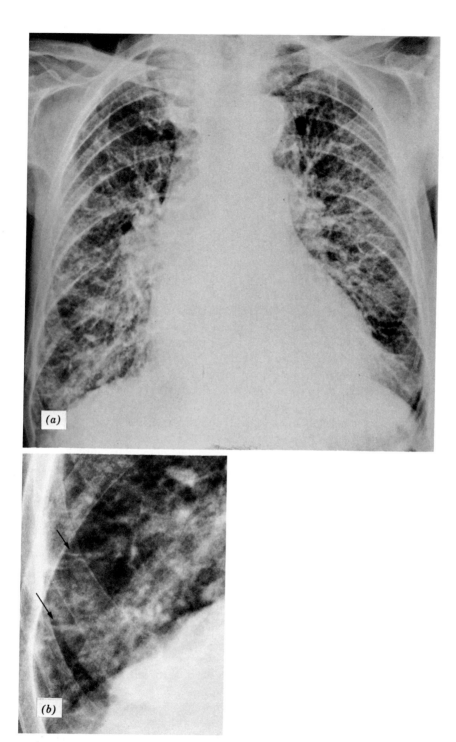

Figure 9-1. Chest roentgenogram of a 52-year-old man with aortic and mitral incompetence and chronic congestion of the lungs. There is a prominent vasculature. Kerley B-lines can be recognized in the detail (arrows).

al., 1959; Selzer, 1959; Meszaros, 1973). There has also been supporting evidence from roentgenologic (Davies et al., 1953; Thomas et al., 1962) and experimental findings (Silove et al., 1972).

To what extent constriction of muscular pulmonary arteries and arterioles is instrumental in bringing about the increase of resistance is not decided nor whether it is of equal importance in early and late stages of the underlying disease.

Even if vasoconstriction acts as a protective mechanism, in the sense that it might help to prevent pulmonary edema, it will increase the workload of the right ventricle and the risk of cardiac failure, while the left ventricular output diminishes.

How vasoconstriction in these instances is brought about is not clear. A neuro-reflex mechanism was suggested by Sanger et al. (1959) and Yoshida (1969) and hypoxia by Bader et al. (1955), Donald (1959), and Jordan (1965), while Harris (1955) supposed that a slight rise in pressure in the pulmonary arteries would provide a stimulus for the arterial smooth muscle cells to increase their tone. This myogenic theory, initially developed with regard to pulmonary arterial hypertension as in patent ductus arteriosus, was later expanded to include pulmonary hypertension in mitral stenosis (Harris and Heath, 1962).

The observations of Edwards and Burchell (1951) and Inkley and Abbott (1961) that medial hypertrophy of pulmonary arteries is limited to those lungs or parts of lungs in which the veins are narrowed could indicate that the mechanism causing constriction of arteries is a localized one.

During exercise, both the pulmonary arterial pressure and the wedge pressure usually rise considerably, even in those patients in whom these pressures were not elevated, or only mildly so, at rest (Harris and Heath, 1962). The rise in cardiac output, on the other hand, is usually less than in normal individuals during exercise. In the more severe cases it may not increase at all.

The possibility that increased resistance in the pulmonary circulation also is influenced by vasomotor activity at the venous level, either by general vasoconstriction of the pulmonary veins or by a sphincter-like mechanism at the pulmonary vein-left atrial junction, has been suggested (Rudolph, 1962; Braun and Stern, 1967).

Regional Pulmonary Flow

While in the normal lungs the pulmonary flow is mainly through the lower parts of the lung whereas the apices are hardly perfused (p. 2), in patients with mitral stenosis this flow pattern is reversed so that much more of the flow is directed to the upper parts and less to the lower parts (Dollery and West, 1960; West and Dollery, 1960; Friedman and Braunwald, 1966; Jebavý et al., 1970; Stanek et al., 1971).

An increased vascular resistance in the lower parts of the lungs in mitral stenosis has been explained by West et al. (1964) on the basis of perivascular cuffs of edema, supposedly causing compression of the vessels, but their explanation has been criticized (Ritchie et al., 1969). Donald (1959) and Jordan (1965) have put forward the hypothesis that uneven ventilation and alveolar hypoxia, as a result of thickening of alveolar membranes, produce constriction of the muscular pulmonary arteries in patients with mitral stenosis. According to Stanek et al. (1971) the hydrostatic pressure in the lower parts of the lungs, coming on top of an increased left atrial pressure, may reach a critical level and thus trigger an autonomous myogenic mechanism in the arteries of these areas.

CAUSES OF CHRONIC PULMONARY VENOUS HYPERTENSION

The most common causes of pulmonary venous hypertension are acquired rheumatic mitral stenosis and mitral incompetence or the combination of both. Mitral incompetence also may be brought about by bacterial endocarditis causing damage to the valve or rupture of the chordae. Moreover, it may result from rupture or dysfunction of the papillary muscle consequent to myocardial infarction. A left atrial myxoma may simulate mitral stenosis by its effect on the pulmonary circulation.

Congenital cardiac malformations which give rise to chronic pulmonary congestion, include cor triatriatum, congenital mitral stenosis and atresia, congenital mitral incompetence, and total anomalous pulmonary venous connection. Congenital stenosis of pulmonary veins is another, although uncommon cause (Edwards, 1960).

Moreover, left ventricular failure caused by severe systemic hypertension, myocarditis, myocardial fibrosis (Heath et al., 1957), myocardial infarction, or aortic valve disease usually will lead to chronic pulmonary venous hypertension. Sometimes in patients with for instance aortic stenosis, the lung vessels may reveal hypertensive lesions in the absence of clinical signs of pulmonary hypertension.

Other causes include narrowing or obstruction of pulmonary venous trunks by processes in the immediate vicinity of the veins such as fibrous mediastinitis (Edwards and Burchell, 1951; Andrews, 1957; Inkley and Abbott, 1961; Botticelli et al., 1966; Yacoub and Thompson, 1971).

In all these instances there is an elevated pressure in the pulmonary veins and the result with regard to the pulmonary vasculature and parenchyma is therefore the same, irrespective of the underlying disease. There remains of course the possibility that other vascular lesions are superimposed on the pulmonary vascular pattern of chronic congestion, for instance, when this is complicated by pulmonary thromboembolism or by a coexistent congenital cardiac shunt.

When the pulmonary veins and venules are primarily affected, and not as a result of an increased pressure, the morphology of the vascular lesions can be entirely different. For this reason the rare condition, known as pulmonary veno-occlusive disease, is not discussed here but in Chapter Ten.

MORPHOLOGY

In pulmonary venous hypertension, in contrast to most other forms of pulmonary hypertension, pulmonary arteries as well as pulmonary veins are affected. Moreover, the lung tissue reacts with various alterations to the elevation of pressure. In the long run the gross appearance of the lung may be characterized by the term "brown induration." In these instances the lungs show little tendency to collapse when the thorax is opened. They are firm and easily cut. Pulmonary edema is not an outstanding feature. More often the cut surface is dry and areas of fibrosis, particularly perivascular fibrosis can be recognized grossly.

The cut surface is darker than normal and often patchy with areas of recent hemorrhage amid fields that are colored rusty-brown as a result of hemosiderosis.

Increased pressure in the pulmonary arteries has its impact on the tracheobronchial tree in the same way as in other forms of pulmonary hypertension. Indentation of the left side of the trachea by the aorta, which in turn is pushed upward and to the right by the distended left pulmonary artery, and indentations of bronchi by distended left and right pulmonary arteries are often observed in mitral valve disease. Moreover, pronounced dilatation of the left atrium in patients with pulmonary venous hypertension causes enlargement of the angle of the tracheal bifurcation, so that a normal angle in the range of 90° may increase to close to 180° (Edwards and Burchell, 1960).

Pulmonary Trunk and Main Arteries

As in all forms of pulmonary hypertension, the wall of the pulmonary trunk and of the main pulmonary arteries is generally thicker than normal (Figure 9-2) in spite of dilatation, which is usually apparent in roentgenograms. The weight of the extrapulmonary part of the pulmonary arteries often increases considerably as compared to that in normal situations (Meyer and Richter, 1956).

The elastic configuration is essentially the same as in normal individuals, when pulmonary venous hypertension is acquired, as it usually is (Figure 9-2). This implies that there is almost always an "adult" elastic configuration with scarce and interrupted elastic laminae (p. 21). Moreover, there is often a marked increase of mucopolysaccharides in the media of pulmonary trunk and main arteries (Tredal et

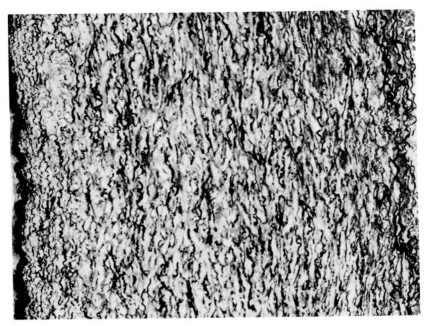

Figure 9-2. Wall of pulmonary trunk in a 69-year-old man with rheumatic mitral incompetence. The thickness of the media is increased but the configuration of the elastic tissue is normal (El.v.G., ×90).

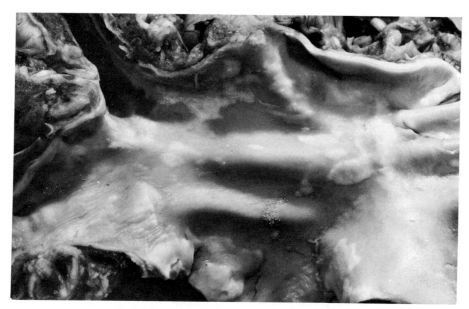

Figure 9-3. Pulmonary trunk and main artery cut open to show intimal atherosclerotic patches. Woman aged 59 years with rheumatic mitral stenosis.

al., 1974). The term "cystic medionecrosis" has been used with regard to this alteration, although the lesions are not cystic, nor the media necrotic.

In congenital mitral stenosis, when pulmonary hypertension is present from birth, the "aortic" type of elastic configuration is prevalent (Heath and Edwards, 1959).

Spontaneous rupture of the pulmonary trunk, either incomplete (Levy, 1961) or complete with fatal hemorrhage (Thomas et al., 1955; Madeloff and Rushton, 1956; Klos, 1969), occasionally may occur in mitral stenosis. Rupture shortly after commissurotomy also has been reported (Seidenberg et al., 1962).

Aneurysms of the pulmonary trunk or of the main pulmonary arteries have been described in rheumatic mitral stenosis, although uncommonly (Urbanek, 1945; Isemein et al., 1962).

Atherosclerosis of pulmonary trunk (Figure 9-3) and its main branches and of the larger intrapulmonary elastic arteries is common and sometimes severe, even with calcification (Wagenvoort et al., 1964). Primary thrombosis of the pulmonary trunk or its main branches has occasionally been reported in chronic pulmonary venous hypertension. In these instances however, it is, difficult to exclude thromboembolism as the cause for the thrombotic masses in pulmonary trunk and main arteries.

The elastic pulmonary arteries within the lungs do not differ from those in other forms of pulmonary hypertension. The medial thickness is increased while the intima may be thickened by intimal fibrosis or atherosclerotic patches (Figure 9-4). Sometimes there is calcification of the arterial wall (Figure 9-5).

Muscular Pulmonary Arteries and Arterioles

The morphology of the lung vessels in cases of chronic pulmonary venous hypertension has been studied extensively, particularly in patients with mitral stenosis. The

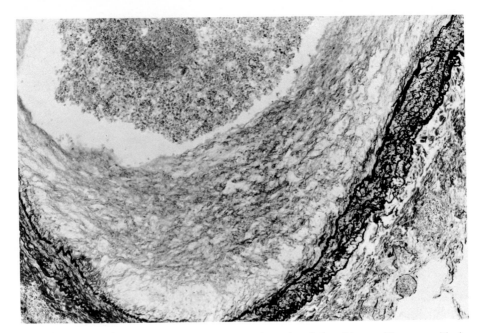

Figure 9-4. Elastic pulmonary artery with extensive atherosclerosis in a 34-year-old woman with rheumatic mitral stenosis (El.v.G., ×90).

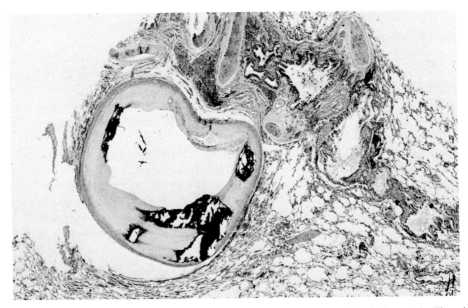

Figure 9-5. Elastic pulmonary artery in a 59-year-old woman with rheumatic mitral stenosis. There is marked intimal fibrosis and calcification of the arterial wall (H. and E., ×15).

disease is common. It was also one of the first cardiac conditions to be attacked by the cardiac surgeon, thus permitting study of lung biopsies taken during operation. In spite of that, the interpretation of the results is often difficult and controversial, especially with regard to the muscular pulmonary arteries and arterioles.

Often in cases of chronic pulmonary venous hypertension the intrapulmonary arteries are markedly or even severely affected. As we have seen, the changes are independent of the way obstruction to the pulmonary venous flow is brought about.

Correlation of the degree of the various lesions with the hemodynamic and clinical findings in the patients often presents serious problems as we will see later (p. 199).

Medial Hypertrophy

It is generally agreed that medial hypertrophy of muscular pulmonary arteries (Figure 9-6) is a common feature of chronic pulmonary venous hypertension, although various authors are less unanimous with regard to its incidence. According to some reports it is an almost constant finding (Heath and Whitaker, 1955; Harrison, 1960; Fichera and Hägerstrand, 1962). Others found it in only half of the cases or less (Henry, 1952).

In our own experience medial hypertrophy is present in the great majority of the cases (Wagenvoort, 1975). In a series of 20 autopsies of patients with chronic pulmonary venous hypertension due to mitral valve disease, the average thickness of the media, expressed as a percentage of the external vascular diameter, was 9.2 percent. It was within normal limits, that is below 7 percent in 3. In 12 patients it was between 7 and 12 percent, while 5 patients had a media of over 12 percent with 15.9 percent as a maximum.

In 300 lung biopsies from such patients, medial hypertrophy was judged absent or minimal in 45, mild to moderate in 218, and severe in 37 cases.

Medial hypertrophy is generally more severe in pulmonary venous hypertension than in pulmonary hypertension due to congenital cardiac shunts. This is the more remarkable because the latter group has a much higher average age and is consequently less influenced by the excessive medial hypertrophy so often observed in infants and young children.

As in other forms of pulmonary hypertension, medial hypertrophy is the first recognizable alteration in the arteries. This becomes particularly clear in young children with congenital mitral valve disease (Figure 9-7) and also in adults with early grades of pulmonary venous hypertension.

An increase in arterial smooth muscle, although most striking by the increased thickness of the media, also may be brought about by muscularization of arterioles (Heath and Edwards, 1959; Wagenvoort, 1975). This implies that small arteriolar branches, normally devoid of muscle cells, develop a muscular coat (Figure 9-8). While in normal lungs the arterioles loose their media when the diameter of these vessels becomes less than approximately 70 μ, in a case of chronic pulmonary venous hypertension arterioles of 50 to 30 μ, sometimes even of 20 μ or less, often possess a distinct muscular media. This indicates that there has been proliferation of muscle cells in a peripheral direction, or, more likely, that smooth muscle cells in these small vessels have developed from fibroblasts, endothelial cells, or more generally, from multifunctional mesenchymal cells (Wissler, 1967). The presence of

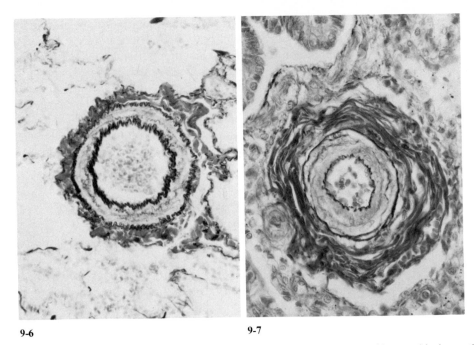

9-6   9-7

Figure 9-6. Muscular pulmonary artery with medial hypertrophy in a 45-year-old man with rheumatic mitral stenosis (El.v.G., ×230).

Figure 9-7. Marked medial hypertrophy of muscular pulmonary artery in a one-day-old male infant with congenital aortic atresia and mitral stenosis. On the average the media was considerably thicker than in normal newborn infants (El.v.G., ×350).

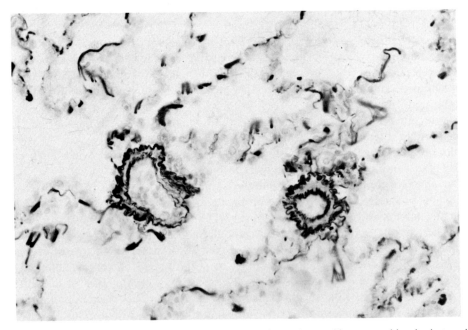

Figure 9-8. Pulmonary arterioles with muscularization in a 46-year-old woman with mitral stenosis. These arterioles measuring approximately 30 and 40 μ developed a distinct muscular coat between two elastic laminae (El.v.G., ×350).

186

a tone, and the eventual capacity to constriction in arterioles of such small caliber, obviously has marked consequences for the pulmonary vascular resistance.

Another form of muscular hyperplasia is the development of longitudinal smooth muscle cells. Bundles of these cells may be observed in close apposition to the media. They may be located in the intima (Hatt and Rouiller, 1958), often within duplications of the internal or external elastic lamina, (Figure 9-9) or in the adventitia (Figure 9-10) or both. Uncommonly a layer of longitudinal cells is seen within the media, thus between two layers of circularly arranged muscle (Figure 9-11).

The significance of these longitudinal muscle bundles is obscure. Their development, particularly at the intimal side, in cases of chronic bronchitis and in individuals living at high altitude is believed to be related to alveolar hypoxia (p. 239). In these cases, the bundles are virtually limited to small arteries and arterioles. In pulmonary venous hypertension, generally muscular arteries of larger caliber are involved. It is likely that the smooth muscle fibers are derived from multifunctional mesenchymal cells in the arterial wall (Wissler, 1967).

In the intima of systemic, notably of bronchial arteries, longitudinal muscle bundles are common, even in normal individuals. Weibel (1958) explained these as an adaptation to the stretch of these vessels during respiratory movements.

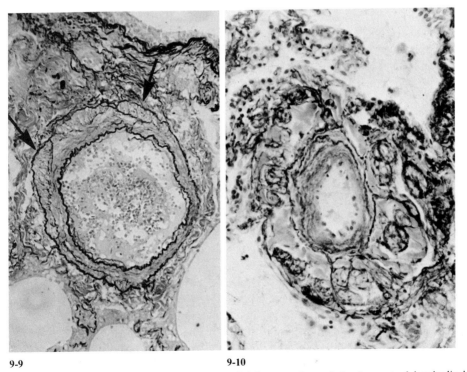

9-9   9-10

Figure 9-9. Muscular pulmonary artery with medial hypertrophy and development of longitudinal smooth muscle cells (arrows) in reduplications of the external elastic lamina. Woman aged 27 years with rheumatic mitral stenosis (El.v.G., ×140).

Figure 9-10. Muscular pulmonary artery with bundles of longitudinal smooth muscle cells in the adventitia in a 32-year-old woman with rheumatic mitral stenosis and incompetence (El.v.G., ×140).

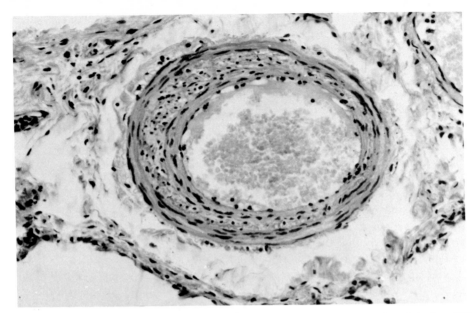

Figure 9-11.   Muscular pulmonary artery with a layer of longitudinal smooth muscle cells in the middle of the media. Man aged 58 years with rheumatic mitral stenosis (H. and E., ×230).

Wagenaar (1975), however, has thrown serious doubt on the validity of this concept by demonstrating that reparative processes of the arterial wall in the absence of stretch produce the same arterial lesions in experimental animals. He suggested that the longitudinal smooth muscle cells develop as a reparative process in response to stress and injury.

Burton (1954) showed on theoretical grounds that longitudinal muscle fibers, added to a circularly arranged muscular coat, would have a considerable mechanical advantage in withstanding the intraluminal pressure. Muscle fibers, even in the contracted state, are fairly easily distensible. A longitudinal fiber, if attached to a circumferential skeleton of collagen fibers, would be less affected by this distension.

If this hypothesis would appear to be correct, the development of the longitudinal muscle bundles, which in some instances may become very thick, could be considered as an additional muscular hypertrophy even though the bundles are not confined to the media.

Medial Fibrosis

Increase of collagen in the media of muscular pulmonary arteries is pronounced in cases of chronic pulmonary venous hypertension (Figure 9-12). Possibly, this medial fibrosis results from reparative processes as reaction to damage to the vascular wall.

It is likely that medial fibrosis will increase the rigidity of the walls of the muscular pulmonary arteries. This may have an effect on their ability to react to vaso-constrictive or vasodilator drugs (Harris and Heath, 1962).

Medial Atrophy

Thinning of the media to normal or subnormal dimensions, frequently found in individual arteries in pulmonary hypertension due to congenital cardiac shunts, is uncommon in chronic pulmonary venous hypertension. Marked dilatation of muscular pulmonary arteries and dilatation lesions with concomitant thinning of the media are not features of this type of pulmonary vascular disease.

Atrophy secondary to the development of severe intimal fibrosis is equally uncommon. It is striking that in these patients the media is so often hypertrophied even in the presence of subtotal obliteration of the lumen by intimal fibrosis (Figure 9-13).

Intimal Fibrosis

In the early stages of pulmonary vascular disease due to elevated pulmonary venous pressure, the intima is normal. In young children with congenital mitral stenosis, medial hypertrophy is usually very severe, as we have seen. When arterioles are constricted, the endothelial cells often bulge into the lumen but intimal fibrosis, as a rule, is absent. In most adult patients with pulmonary venous hypertension, however, intimal fibrosis is present (Figure 9-14), involving many muscular pulmonary arteries and arterioles (Parker and Weiss, 1936).

In a series of 20 autopsies, we (Wagenvoort, 1975) found intimal thickening, expressed as percentage of the internal vascular diameter—that is, in between opposite sides of the internal elastic lamina—of less than 12 percent in 3 cases. In 11 patients the average intimal thickness was between 12 and 20 percent and in 6 patients over 20 percent.

In our series of over 300 lung biopsies from patients with pulmonary venous hypertension, intimal fibrosis was within normal range in 37, mild to moderate in 236, and severe in 27 cases.

In evaluating these results, one may not overlook the fact that in normal individuals, intimal fibrosis of pulmonary arteries is common with increasing age (p.

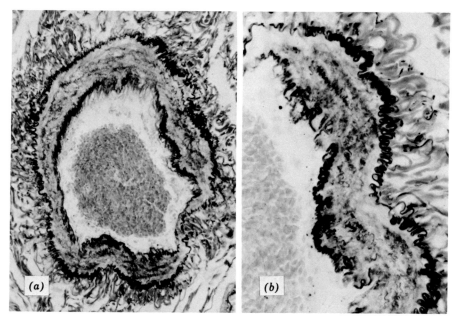

Figure 9-12. Muscular pulmonary artery (a) with hypertrophy and fibrosis of the media. In some areas (b) there is pronounced deposition of collagen with some elastic fibers. Woman aged 47 years with rheumatic mitral stenosis El.v.G., (a: ×140; b: ×350).

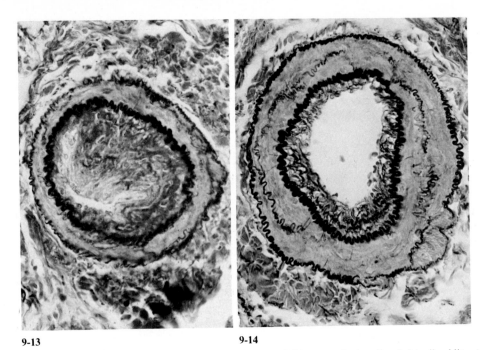

9-13   9-14

Figure 9-13. Muscular pulmonary artery with marked medial hypertrophy in spite of virtually obliterating intimal fibrosis. Woman aged 30 years with rheumatic mitral stenosis (El.v.G., ×250).

Figure 9-14. Muscular pulmonary artery with pronounced medial hypertrophy and moderate intimal fibrosis in a 23-year-old woman with rheumatic mitral stenosis (El.v.G., ×350).

36). But even if the age of the patients is taken into account, increased intimal fibrosis must be considered to be present in the majority of patients with pulmonary venous hypertension.

The type of intimal fibrosis, without being really characteristic for pulmonary venous hypertension, differs nonetheless from that observed in congenital cardiac shunts or in chronic thromboembolism. When the arteries are traced in serial sections, it appears that the length of the area with intimal fibrosis is much greater than that in thromboembolism. On cross section the fibrotic patch is either irregular, cushion-like and eccentric (Figure 9-15), crescent-shaped, (Figure 9-16) or concentric (Figure 9-17). It does not, or only rarely, show the laminar, onionskin-like arrangement that is so characteristic in cases of ventricular septal defect or patent ductus arteriosus.

Active cellular intimal proliferation is much more uncommon than in congenital heart disease, possibly because the disease runs a more protracted course with diminished chance for the early lesions to be caught in the histologic sections.

In the majority of the cases with marked intimal fibrosis, longitudinal smooth muscle cells can be found within the intimal thickening in at least some arteries (p. 187). Often there are only occasional muscle fibers that are easily overlooked but sometimes the thick intimal layer consists largely of smooth muscle cells (Figure 9-18).

Generally, however, the intimal thickening is brought about by paucicellular connective tissue with varying amounts of collagenous and elastic fibers. In some cases

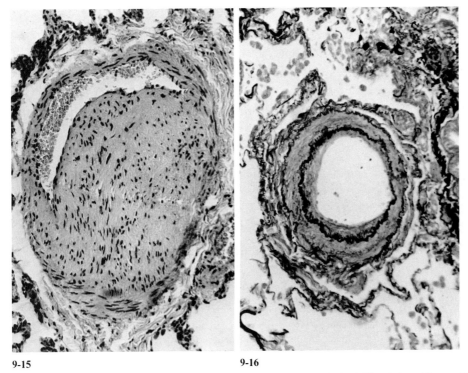

9-15   9-16

Figure 9-15. Muscular pulmonary artery with cushion-like eccentric intimal fibrosis in a 36-year-old woman with rheumatic mitral stenosis (H. and E., ×140).

Figure 9-16. Muscular pulmonary artery with crescent-shaped intimal fibrosis in a 43-year-old man with rheumatic mitral stenosis (El.v.G., ×140).

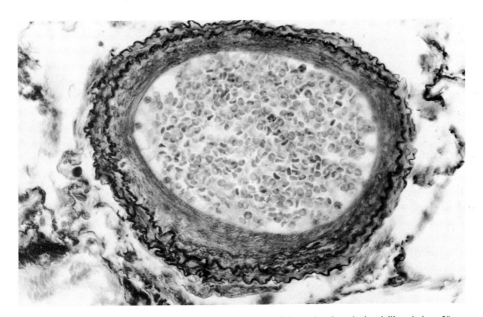

Figure 9-17. Muscular pulmonary artery with circumferential, nonlaminar intimal fibrosis in a 58-year-old man with rheumatic mitral stenosis (El.v.G., ×350).

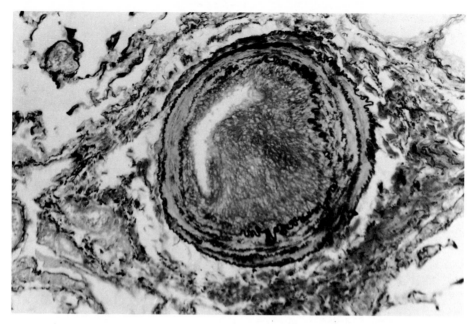

Figure 9-18. Muscular pulmonary artery with pronounced intimal thickening consisting of bundles of smooth muscle cells in a 52-year-old woman with rheumatic mitral stenosis (El.v.G., ×140).

there is marked elastosis of the thickened intima; in others, accumulation of acid mucopolysaccharides that stain positively with the alcian blue and result in pools of mucoid material. Incrustation with iron and calcium of intima and internal elastic lamina occasionally is observed (Walton and Heath, 1960).

The cause of the intimal fibrosis is not clear. In mitral valve disease thromboembolism to the pulmonary arteries is common (Thomas et al., 1956), particularly when atrial fibrillation and thrombosis of the right atrial appendage are present. In these instances the intimal fibrotic patches might well be due to organization of emboli. It is unlikely, however, that this should be responsible for the extensive intimal fibrosis in most cases of mitral valve disease and other conditions with elevated pulmonary venous hypertension. It does not explain the very long stretches of luminal obstruction by the intimal fibrosis and the virtual absence of recanalization with formation of intraluminal septa, so common in embolic pulmonary hypertension.

The possibility remains that intimal fibrosis results from organization of nonembolic thrombosis due to stasis or slow flow of the bloodstream in these cases (Inkley and Abbott, 1961; Wagenvoort, 1975).

Adventitia

The arterial adventitia is thick in patients with pulmonary venous hypertension (Figure 9-19). Its collagen content is increased. The thickness of the adventitia of injected arteries has been reported as averaging 10.5 percent of the arterial diameter against 4.6 percent in normal controls (Olsen, 1966).

Perivascular edema has been suggested by West et al. (1965) as a factor in raising the pulmonary vascular resistance by compressing the arteries and arterioles. They demonstrated this perivascular edema in experimental animals with raised pulmonary venous pressure by instant deep freezing of lung tissue. With ordinary morphologic techniques adventitial edema usually is not very conspicuous although it possibly induces the fibrosis of this layer (Olsen, 1966).

Pulmonary Arteritis

As in cases of congenital cardiac disease with a shunt, pulmonary hypertension in mitral valve disease may be complicated by fibrinous vasculosis which may proceed to necrotizing arteritis (Figure 9-20). In these instances fibrin probably is forced by the elevated pressure through the endothelium (Lendrum, 1955). It is deposited in the intima before passing through the media and finally into the adventitia (Figure 9-21). It may be accompanied by formation of a fibrin clot in the lumen.

In an early stage, an inflammatory reaction can be absent but pronounced accumulation of polymorphonuclear cells or lymphocytes throughout the wall and in the adjacent tissue may follow. Necrosis of the wall with loss of medial muscle tissue and disruption of elastic laminae often is present in these instances (Figure 9-22).

Single cases of pulmonary arteritis in mitral stenosis have been described by Symmers (1952), Hicks (1953), and Johnstone and Smith (1956). The particularly large number of 28 cases, reported by Spain (1956) included examples of supposedly healed arteritis. In our own experience pulmonary necrotizing arteritis is unusual in mitral valve disease and much rarer than in congenital cardiac shunts or in primary pulmonary hypertension, presumably because severe spastic contraction is uncommon in pulmonary venous hypertension.

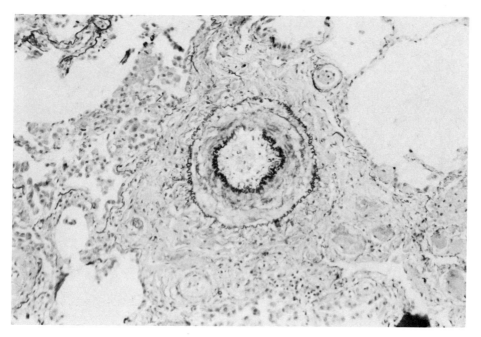

Figure 9-19. Muscular pulmonary artery with medial hypertrophy and fibrous thickening of the adventitia in a 46-year-old woman with rheumatic mitral stenosis (El.v.G., ×140).

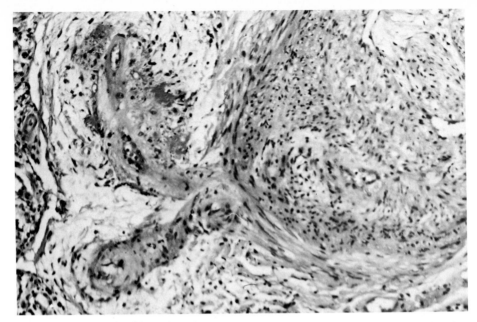

Figure 9-20. Muscular pulmonary artery with arteritis. There is fibrinoid necrosis in two branches (left). Woman aged 39 years with rheumatic mitral stenosis and incompetence (H. and E., ×140).

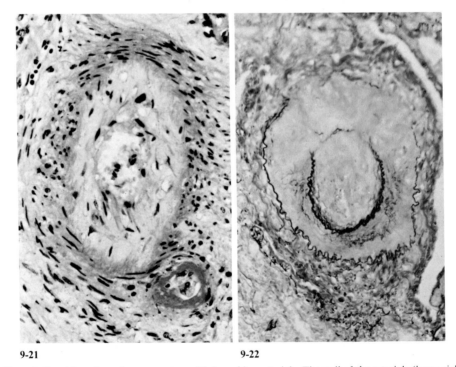

9-21   9-22

Figure 9-21. Muscular pulmonary artery with branching arteriole. The wall of the arteriole (lower right) is completely destroyed by fibrinoid necrosis. Woman aged 27 years with rheumatic mitral stenosis (H. and E., ×230).

Figure 9-22. Muscular pulmonary artery with a media swollen by fibrinoid necrosis and arteritis and with destruction of elastic laminae. Same case as Figure 9-21 (El.v.G., ×140).

194

The pulmonary arteritis has been misjudged as rheumatic vasculitis (Parker and Weiss, 1936; Elkeles and Glynn, 1946). It should not be confused with pulmonary arteritis resulting from embolism. After intravenous injections, cardiac catheterization, or intracardiac surgical procedures, particles of cotton-wool or gauze may be swept into the pulmonary circulation and become impacted in small arterial branches. There they often puncture the intima and internal elastic lamina, in this way causing a marked inflammatory reaction. Foreign body giant cells may be present in these instances. The particles appear to be birefringent when polarized light is used. Infected thromboemboli form another cause of pulmonary arteritis in mitral valve disease. It does not give rise to fibrinous vasculosis.

Dilatation Lesions and Plexiform Lesions

It is remarkable that dilatation lesions and plexiform lesions do not occur in chronic pulmonary venous hypertension (Wagenvoort, 1959) (p. 77). Since plexiform lesions are preceded by necrotizing pulmonary arteritis, which is uncommon in mitral valve disease, one might expect that these lesions are equally rare. Their total absence, however, requires a further explanation. Possibly the thick fibrous adventitia of the arteries in pulmonary venous hypertension prevents the dilatation of the affected segments and thus of the development of plexiform lesions.

Tandon and Kasturi (1975) claimed to have observed dilatation lesions in four patients, particularly in younger age groups. It is possible that in young patients with mitral stenosis, in whom there is less fibrosis of the muscular media, vaso-constriction is particularly severe and may occasionally proceed to dilatation lesions or plexiform lesions, but their illustrations are not convincing.

Obstruction to the pulmonary venous flow does not prevent the development of these structures, if it complicates arterial pulmonary hypertension resulting from cardiac malformations with a shunt. In patients with a common atrioventricular canal, and also when there is coexistent mitral incompetence, plexiform lesions are commonly found.

In patients with mitral atresia, plexiform lesions have been observed occasionally, but only when it was combined with large congenital shunts such as a common ventricle or a widely patent ductus arteriosus (Heath and Edwards, 1959; Kanjuh et al., 1964).

Pulmonary Veins and Venules

In chronic pulmonary venous hypertension, as a rule, there are changes in the pulmonary veins and venules. Such changes occasionally may be found in patients with pulmonary arterial hypertension, due to ventricular septal defect, chronic thromboembolism, or primary pulmonary hypertension (Wagenvoort and Wagenvoort, 1970). Almost certainly, however, this implies that in such a patient there is an additional hemodynamic disturbance, for instance as a result of left heart failure by which the pressure in the pulmonary veins is elevated.

In pulmonary venous hypertension, alterations in the walls of the pulmonary veins are common, although occasionally mild or even absent. If, however, the lesions are pronounced, as they often are in patients with mitral valve disease, for instance, the picture is characteristic. Sometimes, it may even demonstrate the presence of elevated pulmonary venous pressure in cases in which this was clinically unsuspected.

Medial Hypertrophy

Generally, in normal individuals, the pulmonary veins and venules have an irregular contour in histologic sections, in contrast to the arteries which, in cross section, tend to have a circular circumference. This, and the lack of a sharp demarcation between media and adventitia, make morphometric assessment of the veins more difficult and unreliable than of the arteries. Therefore, there is a danger of either overlooking or of overestimating the thickness of the venous wall, particularly of the media. Only in infants and young children is the contour of the pulmonary veins sufficiently regular to apply morphometry with confidence (Samuelson et al., 1970).

Medial hypertrophy of the veins in many cases of chronic pulmonary venous hypertension is so conspicuous, that it can be recognized without difficulty (Figure 9-23). In a series of 300 lung biopsies from such patients, this feature was absent or minimal in 162, moderate in 89, and severe in 49 cases. In autopsy material, however, it is present in the majority of the patients with mitral valve disease (Wagenvoort, 1970).

The hypertrophy of the media, with its increased content of smooth muscle fibers, suggests an adaptation to the elevated pressure and a capability for increasing the vascular tone and for contraction (p. 65). On the other hand, usually there is also marked fibrosis, often accompanied by elastosis, of the venous wall and this contributes to its thickness.

In congenital heart disease with obstructed pulmonary flow as in aortic atresia and anomalous pulmonary venous connection, the media of pulmonary veins may be

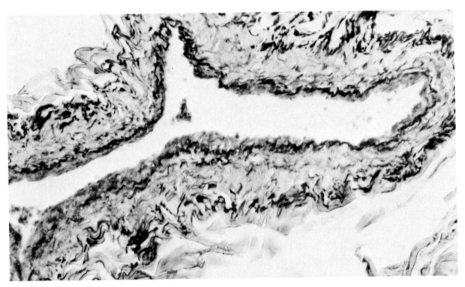

Figure 9-23. Pulmonary vein with pronounced medial hypertrophy in a 35-year-old woman with rheumatic mitral stenosis (El.v.G., ×200).

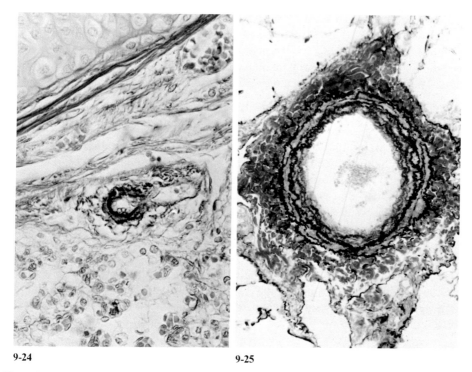

9-24   9-25

Figure 9-24. Pulmonary venule with medial hypertrophy and arterialization in a stillborn male infant with aortic atresia and prematurely closed foramen ovale (El.v.G., ×350).
Figure 9-25. Pulmonary vein with arterialization in a 35-year-old man with rheumatic mitral incompetence (El.v.G., ×140).

hypertrophied already in young infants and even during gestational age (Figure 9-24) (Samuelson et al., 1970; Wagenvoort, 1970).

In experimental stenosis of pulmonary venous trunks pronounced medial hypertrophy of the intrapulmonary veins has been produced in calves (Silove et al., 1972).

Arterialization

Within the normal pulmonary venous wall normally the elastic fibers are irregularly distributed. In chronic pulmonary venous hypertension the arrangement of the elastic fibers changes in such a way that there is a condensation into internal and external elastic laminae (Figure 9-25) with hardly any fibers in between (Heath and Edwards, 1959). This, in fact, is the same configuration as exists in pulmonary arteries. By this so-called arterialization (Wagenvoort, 1970), the veins may mimick arteries to such an extent that even the experienced worker may be fooled. If the localization of the vessel within the lung gives no clue to its identity, it sometimes is necessary to use serial sections in order to establish the nature of the vessel.

Smiley and coworkers (1966) showed that both medial hypertrophy and arterialization could be produced in dogs by reversing the bloodstream through a lobe of the lung in such a way that the veins had to withstand arterial pressures. An arrangement of the elastic tissue into two laminae apparently produces a better adaptation to pressure than the haphazard distribution of the fibers.

Arterialization is usually, although not always, accompanied by medial hypertrophy. It is often a more reliable indication of elevated pulmonary venous pressure, particularly when the venous wall is not markedly thickened.

Intimal Fibrosis

Intimal fibrosis, particularly of the hyalin, acellular type, in veins and venules of the lung of normal adult individuals is so common, that its presence in cases of chronic pulmonary venous hypertension must be judged with reservation.

It has been stated that it is not appreciably increased in these patients (Brenner, 1935; Heath and Whitaker, 1955). In our experience, however, venous intimal fibrosis in these instances is more widespread and more pronounced than in controls from similar age groups (Figure 9-26), even though severe obstruction is uncommon (Figure 9-27).

It is likely that the veins are very gradually silting up by a process of thrombosis with subsequent organization, in the same way as has been suggested for the pulmonary arteries. If this should happen very slowly, it would explain that a layer of recent thrombus rarely is observed.

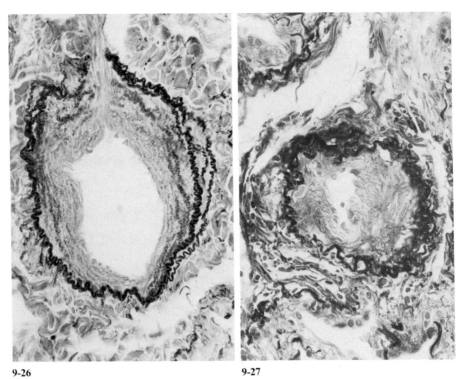

9-26   9-27

Figure 9-26. Pulmonary vein with intimal fibrosis. Woman aged 23 years with rheumatic mitral stenosis (El.v.G., ×350).

Figure 9-27. Pulmonary vein, almost obliterated by intimal fibrosis in a 39-year-old woman with rheumatic mitral stenosis (El.v.G., ×350).

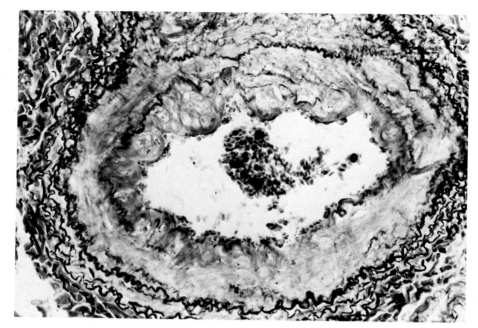

Figure 9-28. Pulmonary vein with medial hypertrophy and arterialization and severe intimal fibrosis, containing bundles of longitudinal smooth muscle cells. Man aged 52 years with rheumatic mitral stenosis (El.v.G., ×230).

As in the intima of pulmonary arteries, longitudinal smooth muscle cells may develop within the intimal fibrotic patches, although usually not to the same extent as in the arteries (Figure 9-28).

Pulmonary Varices

Varicosity of intrapulmonary veins occasionally has been described in chronic pulmonary venous hypertension (Castello et al., 1972; Kelvin et al., 1972). Sometimes a tumor-like mass is formed by a cluster of dilated veins (Eisenman et al., 1974).

The pulmonary venous trunks also have walls that are thicker than normal. Particularly the layer or cardiac muscle in continuity with hypertrophic left atrial myocardium is regularly increased in thickness.

Correlation of Pulmonary Vascular Lesions With Hemodynamic Data

Generally speaking, one would expect that the more severe the mitral stenosis, the higher the pulmonary arterial pressure and the more pronounced the vascular alterations will be. However, even when there is a tight stenosis of the mitral valve, development of severe pulmonary hypertension is not always predictable, and a high pulmonary vascular resistance develops only in a minority of the patients (Wood, 1958). Grover et al. (1963) suggested that this may be explained by individual hyper-reactivity of the pulmonary arteries, which are prone to constrict more in one individual than in the other.

In the presence of pulmonary hypertension some observers found a fairly close correlation between the degree of pulmonary arterial or venous pressures and the degree of medial hypertrophy and intimal fibrosis of the arteries and arterioles in individual patients with mitral stenosis (Heath and Whitaker, 1955; Bayer et al., 1957; Evans and Short, 1957). Roentgenologic narrowing of the arteries appeared to correlate with the elevation of pressure according to Davies et al. (1953) and Aber et al. (1963). Others, however, found only a superficial or hardly any connection between vascular changes and hemodynamic data (Henry, 1952; Goodale et al., 1955; Thomas et al., 1956; Jordan et al., 1966; Jorge, 1971).

In our own experience such a correlation, which is distinct in patients with congenital heart disease with a shunt, is poor in patients with mitral valve disease. This applies to pulmonary arterial medial hypertrophy as well as to intimal fibrosis and even to pulmonary venous lesions.

Pronounced vascular alterations were observed both in patients with high pulmonary arterial pressures or wedge pressures and in patients in whom these pressures were only mild. Conversely very mild vascular changes are sometimes observed in patients with severe pulmonary hypertension.

It is unlikely that this discrepancy is due to inadequacy of material or to errors in measuring or judgment. Lung biopsies were usually larger in patients with mitral valve disease than in those with congenital heart disease so that there is no reason why they should be less representative for the lung as a whole. Also the same results were obtained in cases in which autopsy material was available and whole lungs could be studied. From the latter studies it appeared that lack of correlation is due not merely to the site from where the biopsy was obtained, as suggested by Gough (1960).

In most of our patients and in those studied by others, pressures were recorded at rest. It is possible that if hemodynamic data would have been available during exercise, there would have been a closer relationship between the pressure recorded under these circumstances and the vascular alterations.

It also appears that increase of collagen and intercellular substance is to a large extent responsible for the marked increase in thickness of the media. This is shown by calculation of the number of smooth muscle cell nuclei per unit of medial cross-sectional area. In adult patients this number is only half of that in children with mitral stenosis and in patients with ventricular septal defect (Wagenvoort and Wagenvoort, unpublished data). Therefore the muscularity of the media is not so marked as its thickness might suggest.

Patients with mitral incompetence or with a combination of mitral stenosis and mitral incompetence generally exhibited more pronounced pulmonary arterial and venous lesions than those with mitral stenosis alone.

Bronchial Circulation and Anastomoses

In the intima of bronchial arteries, bundles of longitudinal smooth muscle cells occur in normal individuals (p. 45). In mitral valve disease these bundles are increased in number and in thickness (Figure 9-29) (Wagenaar, 1975).

The number of bronchopulmonary arteries, pulmobronchial arteries, and anastomoses between bronchial and pulmonary arteries is increased in infants with aortic

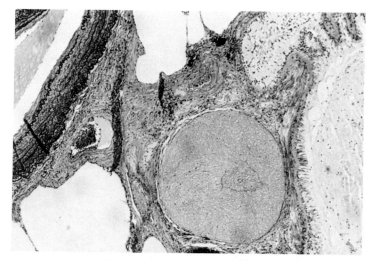

Figure 9-29. Bronchial artery, completely occluded by longitudinally arranged smooth muscle, in a 49-year-old woman with rheumatic mitral stenosis (El.v.G., ×50).

atresia when there is an additional premature closure of the foramen ovale (Wagenvoort et al., 1972). In these instances there is maximal obstruction to the pulmonary venous flow.

The flow through the bronchial veins probably is increased in mitral valve disease as a result of the presence of anastomotic connections with the pulmonary veins. Its morphologic counterpart is the striking dilatation of these veins around the bronchi (Figure 9-30) (Schoenmackers, 1960). In its extreme form varices may develop that may lead to hemoptysis (Ferguson et al., 1944). Extreme dilatation of the bronchial veins in congenital obstruction of the pulmonary venous flow has been reported in children (Becker et al., 1971).

The anastomoses between pulmonary veins and bronchial veins also are dilated, suggesting that blood is shunted away from the pulmonary veins to the pleurohilar bronchial veins and from there to the right atrium (Marchand et al., 1950). An increase in size and also in number of venous anastomoses was demonstrated in aortic atresia (Wagenvoort et al., 1972; Beckman et al., 1975).

Lymphatics

Since lymph flow in congested lungs is increased (p. 178), consequently the pulmonary lymphatics dilate and increase in number when elevated pulmonary venous pressure is produced (Uhley et al., 1962).

In the lungs of patients with obstructed pulmonary venous flow, the lymphatics are wide (Figure 9-31) and easily recognizable in the pleura, in the septa of the lung, and around vessels and bronchi (Gough, 1960; Heath and Hicken, 1960). They also can be demonstrated by injection of contrast medium in the lymphatic system (Servelle et al., 1968). The walls of the lymphatics are increased in thickness (Fi-

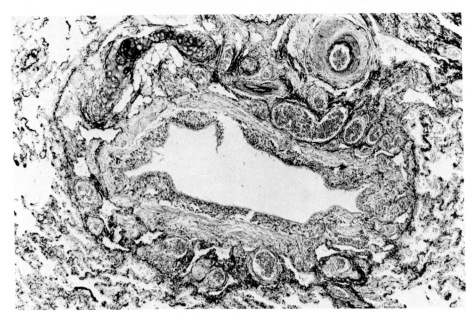

Figure 9-30. Bronchus surrounded by markedly dilated bronchial veins in a 56-year-old woman with rheumatic mitral stenosis (El.v.G., ×50).

chera and Hägerstrand, 1963) and usually contain more than normal smooth muscle cells (Figure 9-31).

Marked distension of the lymphatics together with edema of the connective tissue septa of the lung are responsible for the transient horizontal lines to be seen on the roentgenograms of patients with mitral valve disease. These so-called Kerley-B lines (p. 178) (Kerley, 1951) are found particularly in the lower parts of the lung.

Uncommonly, focal lymphangiectasis producing circumscript areas of dilated lymphatics is observed (Figure 9-32).

Lung Tissue and Alveolar Capillaries

While diffuse lung disease often has a marked effect on the pulmonary circulation (Chapter Twelve), alterations in the hemodynamics of the lung also may affect the pulmonary parenchyma. This is seen particularly in patients with chronic pulmonary venous hypertension. The lungs in cases of chronic congestion tend to be firm and can be cut easily (p. 181). This is due to increase of exudate and fibrous tissue. Moreover, the lung tissue is often brown due to congestion, scattered small hemorrhages, and particularly the deposition of iron pigment. The resulting brown induration is a late change and in many cases the fibrotic component is absent or inconspicuous.

Congestion, Edema, and Hemorrhage

In acute congestion, the pulmonary veins and the alveolar capillaries are engorged with blood. The alveolar walls are increased in thickness by the distension of the

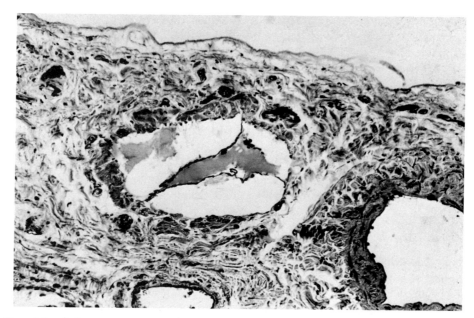

Figure 9-31. Dilated pleural lymphatics, one with a valve, in a 40-year-old woman with rheumatic mitral stenosis (H. and E., ×140).

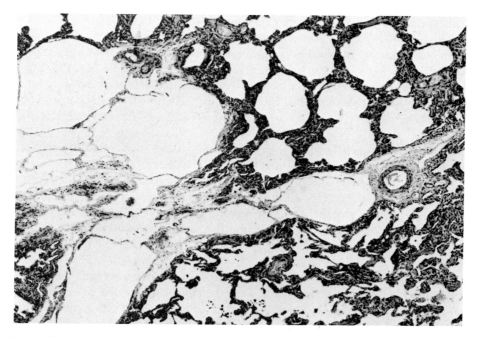

Figure 9-32. Focal lymphangiectasis involving intralobular connective tissue septa. Woman aged 18 years with rheumatic mitral stenosis (H. and E., ×50).

capillaries. Pulmonary edema can be recognized by its protein content as an eosinophilic granular precipitate within the alveolar spaces. Usually there is an admixture of erythrocytes that have escaped from the capillaries.

In chronic congestion, engorgement of alveolar capillaries and pulmonary edema often are absent or confined to small areas. This is particularly so when lung biopsies, taken during surgical procedures for mitral valve disease, are studied. In autopsy material, congestion and edema may be more marked. Apart from diapedesis of erythrocytes, distinct hemorrhages often are present, although it is uncommon that these become very large.

Hemorrhage is likely to occur on the basis of excessive dilatation of pulmonary venules and capillaries. In some instances dilated bronchial veins and their anastomoses with pulmonary veins may be the site of the bleeding.

Hemosiderosis

Red blood cells, having entered the alveolar spaces either by diapedesis or following rupture of venules or capillaries, are ingested by macrophages and broken down. Hemosiderin, deposited in these macrophages, is responsible for their brown granular pigmentation. If these cells are expectorated in the sputum they are known as "heart failure cells."

The hemosiderin-containing macrophages can be scattered over large areas of lung tissue (Figure 9-33) but they often form dense clusters of up to 2 or 3 mm in diameter (Figure 9-34) (Taylor and Strong, 1955). Hemosiderosis in chronic pulmonary venous congestion, therefore, may be diffuse as well as focal.

Iron pigment also is found outside macrophages in alveolar walls and particularly in the connective tissue of septa (Figure 9-35), pleura, and around bronchi. Vascular walls of arteries and veins also may be impregnated with iron. Uncommonly incrustation of elastic laminae of blood vessels becomes severe (Walton and Heath, 1960).

On chest radiograms basal horizontal lines, not to be confused with the transient Kerley B-lines (p. 178) have been ascribed by Fleischner and Reiner (1954) to the deposition of hemosiderin in the connective tissue septa between secondary lobules of the lung tissue. These so-called Fleischner lines also have been attributed to plate-like areas of atelectasis, edema of the septa (Gough, 1960), and to old embolic events.

Lendrum (1955) believed that the degree of hemosiderosis is related to the elevation of pulmonary arterial pressure. Heath and Whitaker (1956) in their study of lung biopsies from patients with mitral stenosis found no direct correlation with the degree of either pulmonary arterial or pulmonary venous pressures, although hemosiderosis was present only when there was associated pulmonary venous hypertension. Gough (1960) suggested that this lack of correlation might be due to these biopsies, taken from the lingula, not being representative for the lung as a whole.

We ourselves, however, could not find a distinct correlation between the degree of hemosiderosis on the one hand and hemodynamic data on the other, neither in patients from whom lung biopsies were available nor in those who came to autopsy and in whom whole lungs were studied. There is no doubt that, although pulmonary hemosiderosis may occur in other forms of pulmonary hypertension, it is by far most common in chronic pulmonary venous hypertension.

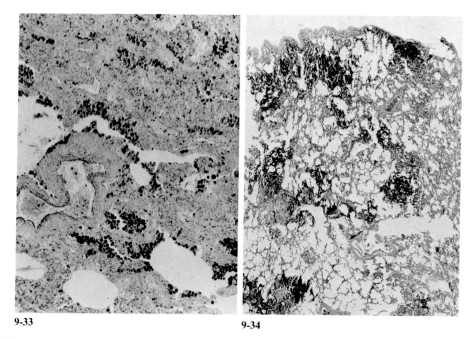

9-33

9-34

Figure 9-33. Diffuse hemosiderosis in alveolar macrophages in a 66-year-old man with left ventricular failure following myocardial infarction (H. and E., ×50).

Figure 9-34. Focal hemosiderosis with large clusters of hemosiderin-containing alveolar macrophages in a 52-year-old man with rheumatic mitral stenosis (Perl's iron stain, ×25).

Interstitial Fibrosis

Fibrosis of lung tissue in chronic congestion is due partly to organization of fibrinous exudate from pulmonary edema or superimposed infection. This form of fibrosis is intra-alveolar, and Heard et al. (1968) have stressed its importance in patients with left ventricular failure.

More characteristic is interstitial fibrosis with thickening of alveolar walls (Figure 9-36). Interstitial fibrosis may be diffuse or localized and often subpleural.

Parker and Weiss (1936) commented on the thickening of the capillary basement membrane, the interstitial edema, the increase of collagen within the alveolar walls, and the lining of these walls by cuboidal epithelium. O'Neal et al. (1955, 1957) in contrast, never found generalized and only occasionally localized interstitial fibrosis in mitral stenosis. This is contrary to the experience of others. Evans and Short (1957) believed that a marked degree of interstitial fibrosis together with marked pulmonary vascular lesions would impair a lasting benefit of valvotomy, but this was denied by Goodale et al. (1955). Bayer et al. (1957) described the process of interstitial fibrosis in lung biopsies from 92 patients with mitral stenosis. Edema of the alveolar wall was followed by an increase in reticulin fibers around the alveolar capillaries and eventually by the deposition of collagen. In progressive sclerosis of the alveolar walls the number of capillaries was reduced. Marked or severe degrees of interstitial fibrosis were observed in half of their cases. They also found a positive correlation with pulmonary arterial pressures. In our own material such a correlation with pressures was rather vague.

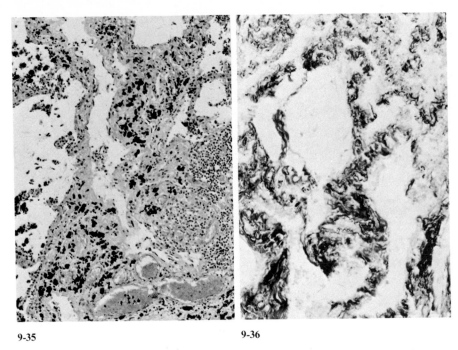

9-35   9-36

Figure 9-35. Hemosiderosis in interlobular fibrous septa and in thickened alveolar walls. Same case as Figure 9-34 (H. and E., ×50).
Figure 9-36. Interstitial fibrosis with deposition of collagen in alveolar walls. Same case as Figure 9-34 (El.v.G., ×90).

Electron-microscopy also showed that the alveolar wall and the capillaries of the lung often are affected in mitral stenosis with swelling of endothelial cells, thickening of the capillary basement membrane (Coalson et al., 1967), and proliferation of cells with increase of collagen (Figure 9-37) (Hatt and Rouiller, 1958). Payan et al. (1970) stressed that, even when the alveolar septa appear normal in light-microscopic studies, electron-microscopic studies often reveal edema of these septa and some cellular hyperplasia. The term interstitial pneumonia, used by these authors, to indicate these alterations, is confusing.

Electron-microscopic studies by Kay and Edwards (1973) revealed that the endothelial cells of the alveolar capillaries in mitral stenosis were swollen and edematous with vacuolated cytoplasm. The capillary basement membrane was thickened and sometimes split, while there was an increase in collagen and elastic fibers. In areas of cuboidal cell metaplasia, thin membranous pneumocytes were replaced by thick granular pneumocytes. These contained lamellar bodies and microvilli on their surface.

It is likely that interstitial edema is basic to the thickening and fibrosis of the alveolar walls (Figure 9-37), rather than incorporation of organized intra-alveolar edema into the walls as suggested by Heath and Edwards (1959).

Alveolar wall fibrosis is more likely to develop when pulmonary venous pressure is high. It is independent of the way in which the chronic elevation of pressure is brought about, so that it is also observed in conditions like mediastinal fibrosis with

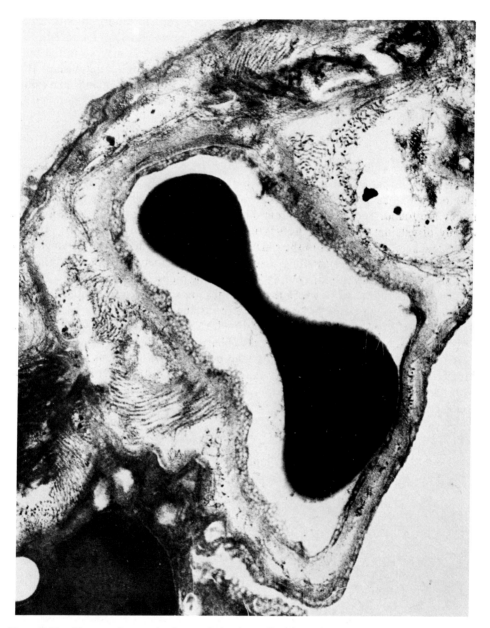

Figure 9-37. Electronmicrograph of part of alveolar wall with capillary in a 37-year-old woman with rheumatic mitral stenosis. There is a marked increase in the thickness of the air-blood barrier due to the deposition of collagen and reticulin fibers. The endothelial layer is swollen. The lumen contains an erythrocyte (×17,800).

occlusion of pulmonary veins (Andrews, 1957), left cardiac failure due to diffuse myocardial fibrosis (Heath et al., 1957), or left atrial myxoma (Solomon, 1960).

In many instances interstitial fibrosis and hemosiderosis are marked in the same lungs or even in the same circumscript areas, suggesting some relationship. It is unlikely, however, that the iron pigment induced fibrosis of alveolar walls and examples of cases in which either of these lesions occur in the absence of the other are plentiful.

Microlithiasis

In the lungs of patients with mitral valve disease or other conditions with elevated pulmonary venous pressure, small round concrements with concentric layering commonly are found. These so-called microliths or calcospherites (Figure 9-38) consist mainly of calcium phosphate, have a fairly uniform appearance, and are lying in alveolar spaces. Their size is in the range of 100 to 600 μ in diameter. Although they are usually scattered over the lung tissue and although their number in a histologic section is limited, they are fairly often found in lung biopsies.

Cases of microlithiasis in which the microliths are so numerous that they lie close together in the lung tissue are rare. In these instances the lung may become very heavy and firm or stone-hard, may be difficult to remove from the thorax, and has to be dissected by saw rather than by knife (Sharp and Danino, 1953).

It is likely that microliths develop in the presence of a fibrinous exudate in the alveolar spaces, but it is not known exactly how these little concrements develop. They are much more common in pulmonary venous hypertension than in other

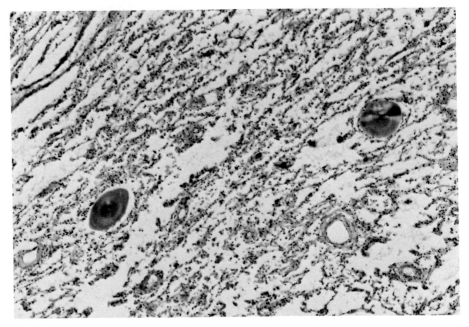

Figure 9-38.   Two microliths in lung tissue of a 47-year-old woman with rheumatic mitral stenosis (H. and E., ×90).

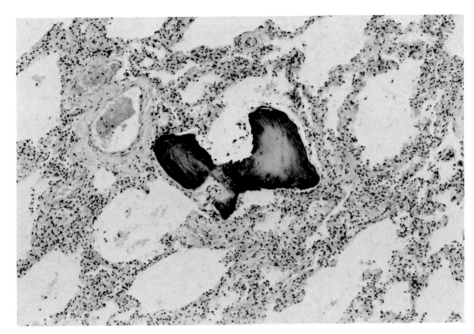

Figure 9-39. Osseous nodule with tuberous form and smooth outline in lung tissue of a 56-year-old woman with rheumatic mitral stenosis (H. and E., ×90).

forms of pulmonary hypertension. Occasionally they may be found in the absence of hemodynamic disturbances, and then even in large numbers (Abdel-Hakim et al., 1959).

If microlithiasis is marked, the condition may be recognized on a chest radiogram, since it produces numerous small opacities (Sharp and Danino, 1953).

Ossification

Formation of bone in lung tissue is related to chronic pulmonary congestion. Just as in the case of microlithiasis, bone formation may occur in the absence of pulmonary hypertension (Daust, 1929; Reingold and Mizunoue, 1961) and in cases of pulmonary hypertension without elevation of pulmonary venous pressure (Davidson and Heath, 1960; Lendrum, 1960), but it is far more common in pulmonary venous hypertension (Hicks, 1953; Johnstone and Smith, 1956; Heath and Edwards, 1959; Galloway et al., 1961).

In these instances osseous nodules are found in alveolar spaces (Figure 9-39) probably on the basis of fibrinous precipitate (Lendrum, 1960), although actual organization of this exudate with transition to bone, is not proven.

The bony nodules have a tuberous form and usually a smooth outline. Their size varies from half a millimeter or less to several millimeters. The larger ones may contain bone marrow.

Osseous nodules are usually fairly scarce in the lungs and never reach the great density, sometimes although rarely, observed in microlithiasis. On the other hand, by the size of the nodules, the condition is usually even more striking and more readily recognizable on chest radiograms than microlithiasis (Whitaker et al., 1955).

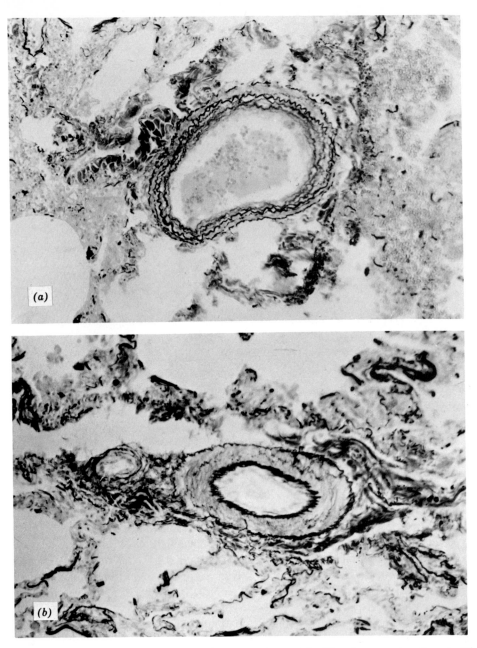

Figure 9-40. (*a*) Muscular pulmonary artery from apex of upper lobe. There is a normal media and mild intimal fibrosis. (*b*) Muscular pulmonary artery from basis of lower lobe. There is marked medial hypertrophy and no intimal fibrosis. Both arteries are from a 27-year-old woman with rheumatic mitral stenosis (*Both*: El.v.G., ×140).

Regional Distribution of Lesions

In most forms of pulmonary hypertension, the pulmonary vascular lesions are distributed equally over both lungs. In chronic pulmonary venous hypertension there are distinct differences between the alterations in upper and lower parts of the lungs.

Medial hypertrophy of muscular pulmonary arteries is more severe in the lower lobes than in the apex of the lungs (Figure 9-40) (Doyle et al., 1957, Ferencz and Dammann, 1957; Harrison, 1958; Heath and Edwards, 1959; Gough, 1960). In the tip of the lingula these alterations resemble those at the basis of the lungs. The average medial thickness of muscular pulmonary arteries in 20 autopsy cases of patients with mitral valve disease was 9.2 and 8.4 percent for apex upper lobe and apex lower lobe respectively and 11.0 and 9.7 percent for tip of lingula and basis of lower lobe respectively (Wagenvoort, 1975). These differences may be related to the effect of hydrostatic pressure in the lower parts of the lungs and also to the low flow in these areas.

It is not always clear from the various reports whether intimal fibrosis of pulmonary arteries also is considered more severe in the lower parts of the lungs. In our experience, however, it is rather the other way round (Figure 9-40). The mean intimal thickness in a group of 20 patients with mitral valve disease, was 17.9 percent in the apex of the upper lobe, 19.9 percent in the lingula, 9.8 percent in the apex of the lower lobe, and 13.8 percent at its basis (Wagenvoort, 1975).

In the pulmonary veins, medial hypertrophy and arterialization were more marked in the lower parts of the lungs than in the upper parts, while intimal fibrosis was more pronounced in the upper lobes.

It seems likely that the development of smooth muscle cells in both arteries and veins is related to the higher pressure, whereas intimal fibrosis in either type of vessel is thrombotic in origin and unrelated to the pressure.

Dilated lymphatics in our experience are more common and more conspicuous in the upper than in the lower lobes of lungs from most patients with mitral valve disease who come to autopsy. This may be related to the observation of Doyle et al. (1957) and Gough (1960) that congestion in the final stages is usually more severe in the upper than in the lower parts of the lungs.

According to Gough (1960), hemosiderosis is more severe in the upper than in the lower lobes. Generally, this is also borne out by our own autopsy material, although such a distribution was not constant. The lingula, which in Gough's opinion contains much less iron pigment than the remainder of the lungs, was in our material intermediate between apex and basis.

Also interstitial fibrosis of the lungs has been reported by Gough to be more severe at the basis of the lungs. We found so many exceptions to this rule that we consider this relationship unreliable.

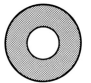 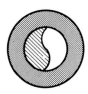 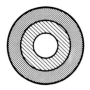

Congestive hypertensive vascular lesions: Severe medial hypertrophy and eccentric or concentric (non-laminar) intimal fibrosis of arteries (*left*). Medial hypertrophy, arterialization and intimal fibrosis of veins (*right*).

REFERENCES

Abdel-Hakim, M., El-Mallah, S., Hashem, M., and Abdel-Halim, S.: Pulmonary alveolar microlithiasis. *Thorax.* **14:** 263, 1959.

Aber, C. P., Campbell, J. A., and Meecham, J.: Arterial patterns in mitral stenosis. *Brit. Heart J.* **25:** 109, 1963.

Andrews, E. C.: Five cases of an undescribed form of pulmonary interstitial fibrosis caused by obstruction of the pulmonary veins. *Bull. J. Hopk. Hosp.* **100:** 28, 1957.

Arnott, M. W.: The lungs in mitral stenosis. *Brit. Med. J.* **ii:** 765, 823, 1963.

Bader, M. E., Bader, R. A., and Dack, S.: Alterations in lung function and anatomy in heart failure with particular reference to mitral stenosis. *Dis. Chest* **28:** 141, 1955.

Bayer, O., Grosse-Brockhoff, F., Loogen, F. and Meessen, H.: Vergleichende klinische pathophysiologische und pathologisch-anatomische Untersuchungen bei Mitralstenose. *Arch. Kreislaufforsch.* **26:** 238, 1957.

Becker, A. E., Becker, M. J., and Edwards, J. E.: Dilated bronchial veins within pulmonary parenchyma. Observations in congenital pulmonary venous obstruction. *Arch. Path.* **91:** 256, 1971.

Beckman, C. B., Moller, J. H., and Edwards, J. E.: Alternate pathways to pulmonary venous flow in left-sided obstructed anomalies. *Circulation* **52:** 509, 1975.

Botticelli, J. T., Schlueter, D. F., and Lange, R. I.: Pulmonary venous and arterial hypertension due to chronic fibrous mediastinitis. Hemodynamics and pulmonary function. *Circulation* **33:** 862, 1966.

Braun, K., and Stern, S.: Functional significance of the pulmonary venous system. *Amer. J. Cardiol.* **20:** 56, 1967.

Brenner, O.: Pathology of the vessels of the pulmonary circulation. *Arch. Int. Med.* **56:** 724, 1935.

Burton, A. C.: Relation of structure to function of the tissues of the wall of blood vessels. *Physiol. Review* **34:** 619, 1954.

Carlill, S. D., Duke, H. N., and Jones, M.: Some observations on pulmonary hemodynamics in the cat. *J. Physiol.* **136:** 112, 1957.

Castello, J., Perez Gomez, F., and Marazuela, A.: Varicosidad pulmonar. *Rev. Esp. Cardiol.* **25:** 175, 1972.

Charms, B. L., Brofman, B. L., and Kohn, P. M.: Pulmonary resistance in acquired heart disease. *Circulation* **20:** 850, 1959.

Coalson, J. J., Jacques, W. E., Campbell, G. S., and Thompson, W. M.: Ultrastructure of the alveolar-capillary membrane in congenital and acquired heart disease. *Arch. Path.* **83:** 377, 1967.

Daust, W.: Über verästete Knochenspangenbildung in der Lunge. *Frankf. Z. Path.* **37:** 313, 1929.

Davidson, L., and Heath, D.: Gonadal dysgenesis with cor pulmonale. *Circulation* **21:** 419, 1960.

Davies, L. G., Goodwin, J. F., Steiner, R. E., and Van Leuven, B. D.: The clinical and radiological assessment of the pulmonary arterial pressure in mitral stenosis. *Brit. Heart J.* **15:** 393, 1953.

Davies, L. G., Goodwin, J. F., and Van Leuven, B. D.: The nature of pulmonary hypertension in mitral stenosis. *Brit. Heart J.* **16:** 440, 1954.

Dexter, L.: Pathologic physiology of mitral stenosis and its surgical implications. *Bull. N. Y. Acad. Med.* **28:** 90, 1952.

Dexter, L.: Physiologic changes in mitral stenosis. *New Engl. J. Med.* **254:** 829, 1956.

Dexter, L., Dow, J. W., Haynes, F. W., Whittenberger, J. L., Ferris, B. G., Goodale, W. T., and Hellems, H. K.: Studies of pulmonary circulation in man at rest. Normal variations and interrelations between increased pulmonary blood flow, elevated pulmonary arterial pressure, and high pulmonary "capillary" pressures. *J. Clin. Invest.* **29:** 602, 1950.

Dollery, C. T., and West, J. B.: Regional uptake of radioactive oxygen, carbon monoxide and carbon dioxide in the lungs of patients with mitral stenosis. *Circ. Res.* **8:** 765, 1960.

Donald, K. W.: Pulmonary vascular resistance in mitral valvular disease. In Adams, W. A., and Veith, I., *Pulmonary Circulation*. Grune and Stratton, New York, London, 1959.

Doyle, A. E., Goodwin, J. F., Harrison, C. V., and Steiner, R. E.: Pulmonary vascular patterns in pulmonary hypertension. *Brit. Heart J.* **19:** 353, 1957.

Edwards, J. E.: Congenital stenosis of pulmonary veins. Pathologic and developmental considerations. *Lab. Invest.* **9**: 46, 1960.

Edwards, J. E., and Burchell, H. B.: Multilobar pulmonary venous obstruction with pulmonary hypertension. *Arch. Int. Med.* **87**: 372, 1951.

Edwards, J. E., and Burchell, H. B.: Effects of pulmonary hypertension of the tracheobronchial tree. *Dis. Chest* **38**: 272, 1960.

Eisenman, B., Durand, M., Soyer, R., Menasche, P., and Dubost, C.: Dilatation anévrysmale des veines pulmonaires par insuffisance mitrale. *Nouv. Presse Méd.* **45**: 2729, 1974.

Elkeles, A., and Glynn, L. E.: Disseminated parenchymatous ossification in the lungs associated with mitral stenosis. *J. Path. Bact.* **58**: 518, 1946.

Evans, W., and Short, D. S.: Pulmonary hypertension in mitral stenosis. *Brit. Heart J.* **19**: 457, 1957.

Ferencz, C., and Dammann, J. F.: Significance of the pulmonary vascular bed in congenital heart disease. V. Lesions of the left side of the heart causing obstruction of the pulmonary venous return. *Circulation* **16**: 1046, 1957.

Ferguson, F. C., Kobilak, R. E., and Deitrick, J. E.: Varices of the bronchial veins as a source of hemoptysis in mitral stenosis. *Amer. Heart J.* **28**: 445, 1944.

Fichera, G., and Hägerstrand, I.: Studies on vascular changes in chronic lung congestion. *Acta Path. Microbiol. Scand.* **56**: 377, 1962.

Fichera, G., and Hägerstrand, I.: Studies of vascular changes in chronic lung congestion. 2. Lymphatic vessels. *Acta Path. Microbiol. Scand.* **57**: 31, 1963.

Fleischner, F. G., and Reiner, L.: Linear X-ray shadows in acquired pulmonary hemosiderosis and congestion. *New Engl. J. Med.* **250**: 900, 1954.

Friedman, W. F., and Braunwald, E.: Alterations in regional pulmonary blood flow in mitral valve disease studied by radioisotope scanning. *Circulation* **34**: 363, 1966.

Galloway, B. W., Epstein, E. J., and Coulshed, N.: Pulmonary ossific nodules in mitral valve disease. *Brit. Heart J.* **23**: 297, 1961.

Goodale, F., Sanchez, G., Friedlich, A. L., Scannel, J. G., and Myers, G. S.: Correlation of pulmonary arteriolar resistance with pulmonary vascular changes in patients with mitral stenosis before and after valvulotomy. *New Engl. J. Med.* **252**: 979, 1955.

Gough, J.: The lungs in mitral stenosis. In Harrison, C. V., *Recent Advances in Pathology.* J. & A. Churchill, Ltd., London, 1960.

Grover, R. F., Vogel, J. H. K., Averill, K. H., and Blount, S. G.: Pulmonary hypertension. Individual and species variability relative to vascular reactivity. *Amer. Heart J.* **66**: 1, 1963.

Harris, P.: Patent ductus arteriosus with pulmonary hypertension. *Brit. Heart J.* **17**: 85, 1955.

Harris, P., and Heath, D.: *The Human Pulmonary Circulation. Its Form and Function in Health and Disease.* E. & S. Livingstone, Ltd., Edinburgh, London, 1962.

Harrison, C. V.: The pathology of the pulmonary vessels in pulmonary hypertension. *Brit. J. Radiol.* (*n.s.*) **31**: 217, 1958.

Harrison, C. V.: Diseases of arteries. In *Recent Advances in Pathology.* J. & A. Churchill, Ltd., London, 1960.

Hatt, P. Y., and Rouiller, C.: Les ultrastructures pulmonaires et le régime de la petite circulation. I. Au cours du rétrécissement mitral serré. *Sem. Hôp.* **17**: 1371, 1958.

Heard, B. E., Steiner, R. E., Herdan, A., and Gleason, D.: Oedema and fibrosis of the lungs in left ventricular failure. *Brit. J. Radiol.* **41**: 161, 1968.

Heath, D., and Whitaker, W.: The pulmonary vessels in mitral stenosis. *J. Path. Bact.* **70**: 291, 1955.

Heath, D., and Whitaker, W.: The relation of pulmonary hemosiderosis to hypertension in the pulmonary arteries and veins in mitral stenosis and congenital heart disease. *J. Path. Bact.* **72**: 531, 1956.

Heath, D., Cox, E. V., and Harris-Jones, J. N.: The clinico-pathological syndrome produced by co-existing pulmonary arterial and venous hypertension. *Thorax* **12**: 321, 1957.

Heath, D., and Edwards, J. E.: Histological changes in the lung in diseases associated with pulmonary venous hypertension. *Brit. J. Dis. Chest* **53**: 8, 1959.

Heath, D., and Hicken, P.: The relation between left atrial hypertension and lymphatic distension in lung biopsies. *Thorax* **15**: 54, 1960.

Henry, E. W.: The small pulmonary vessels in mitral stenosis. *Brit. Heart J.* **14:** 406, 1952.

Hicks, J. D.: Acute arterial necrosis in the lungs. *J. Path. Bact.* **65:** 333, 1953.

Inkley, S. R., and Abbott, G. R.: Unilateral pulmonary arteriosclerosis. *Arch. Int. Med.* **108:** 903, 1961.

Isemein, L., Payan, H., Gerard, R., and Clement, J. P.: Un cas d'anévrisme de la branche droite de l'artère pulmonaire. *Presse Méd.* **70:** 1865, 1962.

Jebavý, P., Runczik, I., Oppelt, A., Tilsch, J., Stanék, V., and Widimský, J.: Regional pulmonary function in patients with mitral stenosis in relation to hemodynamic data. *Brit. Heart J.* **32:** 330, 1970.

Johnstone, J. M., and Smith, G.: Pulmonary arteritis. *Scott. Med. J.* **1:** 396, 1956.

Jordan, S. C.: Development of pulmonary hypertension in mitral stenosis. *Lancet* ii: 322, 1965.

Jordan, S. C., Hicken, P., Watson, D. A., Heath, D., and Whitaker, W.: Pathology of the lungs in mitral stenosis in relation to respiratory function and pulmonary hemodynamics. *Brit. Heart J.* **28:** 101, 1966.

Jorge, P. A. R.: Correlacao clinico-anatomo patologica em casos di hypertensao pulmonar por doenca valvular mitral. *Arq. Bras. Cardiol.* **24:** 49, 1971.

Kanjuh, V. I., Sellers, R. D., and Edwards, J. E.: Pulmonary vascular plexiform lesion. *Arch. Path.* **78:** 513, 1964.

Kay, J. M., and Edwards, F. R.: Ultrastructure of the alveolar-capillary wall in mitral stenosis. *J. Path.* **111:** 239, 1973.

Kelvin, F. M., Boone, J. A., and Peretz, D.: Pulmonary varix. *J. Canad. Ass. Radiol.* **23:** 227, 1972.

Kerley, P.: In Shanks, S. C., and Kerley, P., *A Textbook of X-ray Diagnosis,* vol. 2, ed. 2, Lewis, London, 1951.

Klos, I.: Spontanruptur der Arteria pulmonalis bei Mitralstenose. *Z. Kreislaufforsch.* **58:** 860, 1969.

Lendrum, A. C.: Fibrinous vasculosis. *J. Clin. Path.* **8:** 180, 1955.

Lendrum, A. C.: Pulmonary hemosiderosis: pathological aspects. *Proc. Roy. Soc. Med.* **53:** 338, 1960.

Levy, H.: Partial rupture of pulmonary artery with lesions of medionecrosis in a case of mitral stenosis. *Amer. Heart J.* **62:** 31, 1961.

Lucas, R. V.: Congenital causes of pulmonary venous obstruction. *Cardiovasc. Clinics* **4:** 19, 1972.

Madeloff, S. M., and Rushton, D. G.: Rupture of the pulmonary artery associated with mitral stenosis and systemic hypertension. *Guy's Hosp. Rep.* **105:** 320, 1956.

Marchand, P., Gilroy, J. C., and Wilson, V. H.: An anatomical study of the bronchial vascular system and its variations in disease. *Thorax* **5:** 207, 1950.

Meszaros, W. T.: Lung changes in left heart failure. *Circulation* **47:** 859, 1973.

Meyer, W. M., and Richter, H.: Das Gewicht der Lungenschlagader als Gradmesser der Pulmonalarteriensklerose und als morphologisches Kriterium der pulmonalen Hypertonie. *Virch. Arch. Path. Anat.* **328:** 121, 1956.

Olsen, E. G. J.: Perivascular fibrosis in lungs in mitral valve disease. A possible mechanism of production. *Brit. J. Dis. Chest* **60:** 129, 1966.

O'Neal, R. M., Thomas, W. A., and Hartroft, P. M.: The media of small muscular pulmonary arteries in mitral stenosis. *Arch. Path.* **60:** 267, 1955.

O'Neal, R. M., Thomas, W. A., Kyn Taik Lee, and Rabin, E. R.: Alveolar walls in mitral stenosis. *Circulation* **15:** 64, 1957.

Parker, F., and Weiss, S.: The nature and significance of the structural changes in the lungs in mitral stenosis. *Amer. J. Path.* **12:** 573, 1936.

Payan, H., Chomette, G., Lebreuil, G., Auriol, M., Garbe, L., Durand, M., Césarini, J. P., and Sudan, N.: Modifications de la paroi alvéolaire en rapport avec les cardiopathies. *Arch. Anat. Path.* **18:** 59, 1970.

Rabin, E. R., and Meyer, E. C.: Cardiopulmonary effects of pulmonary venous hypertension with special reference to pulmonary lymphatic flow. *Circ. Res.* **8:** 324, 1960.

Reingold, I. M., and Mizunoue, G. S.: Idiopathic disseminated pulmonary ossification. *Dis. Chest* **40:** 543, 1961.

Ritchie, B. C., Schauberger, G., and Staub, N. C.: Inadequacy of perivascular edema hypothesis to account for distribution of pulmonary blood flow in lung edema. *Circ. Res.* **24:** 807, 1969.

Rudolph, A. M.: Pulmonary venomotor activity. *Med. Thorac.* **19:** 184, 1962.

Samuelson, A., Becker, A. E., and Wagenvoort, C. A.: A morphometric study of pulmonary veins in normal infants and infants with congenital heart disease. *Arch. Path.* **90:** 112, 1970.

Sanger, P. W., Robicsek, F., Taylor, F. H., Magistro, R., and Foti, E.: Observations on pulmonary vasomotor reflexes. *J. Thorac. Surg.* **17:** 774, 1959.

Schoenmackers, J.: Über Bronchialvenen und ihre Stellung zwischen groszem und kleinem Kreislauf. *Arch. Kreislaufforsch.* **32:** 1, 1960.

Seidenberg, B., Bloomberg, A. E., and Hurwitt, E. S.: Delayed rupture of the pulmonary artery following mitral commissurotomy. *J. Thorac. Cardiovasc. Surg.* **44:** 813, 1962.

Selzer, A.: Hemodynamic sequelae of sustained elevation of left atrial pressure. *Circulation* **20:** 243, 1959.

Servelle, M., Soulié, J., Andrieux, J., Poncey, J. J., Daloche, A., and Nussaume, O.: Les lymphatiques du poumon cardiaque. *Arch. Mal. Coeur* **61:** 620, 1968.

Sharp, M. E., and Danino, E. A.: An unusual form of pulmonary calcification: "microlithiasis alveolaris pulmonum." *J. Path. Bact.* **65:** 389, 1953.

Silove, E. D., Tavernor, W. D., and Berry, C. L.: Reactive pulmonary arterial hypertension after pulmonary venous constriction in the calf. *Cardiovasc. Res.* **6:** 36, 1972.

Smiley, R. H., Jaques, W. E., and Campbell, G. S.: Pulmonary vascular changes in lung lobes with reversed pulmonary blood flow. *Surgery* **59:** 529, 1966.

Solomon, M.: Interstitial pulmonary fibrosis secondary to pulmonary venous hypertension. Report of a case due to myxoma of the left atrium. *J.A.M.A.* **174:** 464, 1960.

Spain, D. M.: Necrotizing and healing pulmonary arteritis with advanced mitral stenosis. *Arch. Path.* **62:** 489, 1956.

Stanek, V., Oppelt, A., Jebavý, P., and Widimský, J.: A contribution to the mechanism of the distribution of pulmonary blood flow in patients with mitral stenosis. *Bull. Physio-path. Resp.* **7:** 913, 1971.

Symmers, W. S. C.: Necrotizing pulmonary arteriopathy associated with pulmonary hypertension. *J. Clin. Path.* **5:** 36, 1952.

Tandon, H. D., and Kasturi, J.: Pulmonary vascular changes associated with isolated mitral stenosis in India. *Brit. Heart J.* **37:** 26, 1975.

Taylor, H. E., and Strong, G. F.: Pulmonary hemosiderosis in mitral stenosis. *Ann. Int. Med.* **42:** 26, 1955.

Thomas, A. J., James, W. R. L., and Owen, G. M.: Abnormalities in the pulmonary arterioles in some cases of coronary artery disease. *Brit. Heart J.* **24:** 110, 1962.

Thomas, G. C., Whitelaw, D. M., and Taylor, H. E.: Rupture of the pulmonary artery complicating rheumatic mitral stenosis. *Arch. Path.* **60:** 99, 1955.

Thomas, W. A., Kyo Taik Lee, Rabin, E. R., and O'Neal, R. M.: Mitral stenosis and pulmonary arteriosclerosis. Correlation of pulmonary arteriosclerosis, right ventricular hypertrophy, and thrombo-embolism in autopsied patients who died with mitral stenosis. *Arch. Path.* **62:** 257, 1956.

Tredal, S. M., Carter, J. B., and Edwards, J. E.: Cystic medial necrosis of the pulmonary artery. *Arch. Path.* **97:** 183, 1974.

Uhley, H. N., Leeds, S. E., Sampson, J. J., and Friedman, M.: Role of pulmonary lymphatics in chronic edema. *Circ. Res.* **11:** 966, 1962.

Urbanek, K.: Zur Kenntnis der mykotischen und rheumatischen Aneurysmen der Lungenschlagader. *Z. Kreislaufforsch.* **37:** 419, 1945.

Wagenaar, S. S.: Histologie en histopathologie van bronchiale arterien. Thesis, Amsterdam, 1975.

Wagenvoort, C. A.: The morphology of certain vascular lesions in pulmonary hypertension. *J. Path. Bact.* **78:** 503, 1959.

Wagenvoort, C. A.: Morphologic changes in intrapulmonary veins. *Human Path.* **1:** 205, 1970.

Wagenvoort, C. A.: Pathology of congestive pulmonary hypertension. *Progr. Resp. Res.* **9:** 195, 1975.

Wagenvoort, C. A., Heath, D., and Edwards, J. E.: *The Pathology of the Pulmonary Vasculature.* Charles C Thomas, Springfield, Ill., 1964.

Wagenvoort, C. A., and Wagenvoort, N.: Primary pulmonary hypertension. A pathologic study of the lung vessels in 156 clinically diagnosed cases. *Circulation* **42**: 1163, 1970.

Wagenvoort, C. A., Wagenvoort, N., and Becker, A. E.: The effect of obstructed pulmonary venous blood flow on the development of alternative pathways in the lung. *J. Path.* **107**: 21, 1972.

Walton, K. W., and Heath, D.: Iron incrustation of the pulmonary vessels in patent ductus arteriosus with congenital mitral disease. *Brit. Heart J.* **22**: 440, 1960.

Weibel, E. R.: Die Entstehung der Längsmuskulatur in den Ästen der A. bronchiales. *Z. Zellforsch.* **47**: 440, 1958.

West, J. B., and Dollery, C. T.: Distribution of blood flow and ventilation-perfusion ratio in the lung, measured with radioactive CO_2. *J. Appl. Physiol.* **15**: 405, 1960.

West, J. B., Dollery, C. T., and Heard, B. E.: Increased vascular resistance in the lower zone of the lung caused by perivascular edema. *Lancet* **ii**: 181, 1964.

West, J. B., Dollery, C. T., and Heard, B. E.: Increased pulmonary vascular resistance in the dependent zone of the isolated dog lung caused by perivascular edema. *Circ. Res.* **17**: 191, 1965.

Whitaker, W., Black, A., and Warrack, A. J. N.: Pulmonary ossification in patients with mitral stenosis. *J. Fac. Radiol.* **7**: 29, 1955.

Wissler, R. W.: The arterial medial cell, smooth muscle or multifunctional mesenchyme? *Circulation* **36**: 1, 1967.

Wood, P.: Pulmonary hypertension with special reference to the vasoconstrictive factor. *Brit. Heart J.* **20**: 557, 1958.

Wood, P., Besterman, E. M., Towers, M. K., and McIlroy, M. B.: The effect of acetylcholine on pulmonary vascular resistance and left atrial pressure in mitral stenosis. *Brit. Heart J.* **19**: 279, 1957.

Yacoub, M. H., and Thompson, V. C.: Chronic idiopathic pulmonary hilar fibrosis. *Thorax* **26**: 365, 1971.

Yoshida, Y.: Studies on the pathologic physiology of pulmonary hypertension in mitral valvular disease. I. The role of sympathetic nervous system on the increment of pulmonary vascular resistance. *Jap. Circ. J.* **33**: 359, 1969.

Yu, P. N., Beatty, D. C., Lovejoy, F. W., Nye, R. E., and Joos, W. A.: Studies of pulmonary hypertension. VII. Hemodynamic effects of acute hypoxia in patients with mitral stenosis. *Amer. Heart J.* **52**: 683, 1956.

CHAPTER TEN

Pulmonary Veno-occlusive Disease

Among the patients with pulmonary hypertension of unknown origin, there is a small group in whom the pattern of the pulmonary vascular lesions is distinctive and different from that in patients with the plexogenic form of primary pulmonary hypertension or with thromboembolism. Progressive obstruction of pulmonary veins and particularly of pulmonary venules is characteristic for this group of patients. The pulmonary arteries and arterioles may be involved but to a lesser extent and in part probably secondary to alterations in the pulmonary venous system.

The case described by Höra in 1934 usually is considered the first acceptable report on this condition. Although he used the term "Primäre Pulmonalsklerose," the brunt of the vascular lesions was in the veins and venules of the lung rather than in the arteries.

In deciding whether a case belongs in this category, distal obstruction to the pulmonary venous flow, such as mitral valve disease, left atrial myxoma, or processes narrowing the pulmonary venous trunks, must be excluded. In all these instances, the intrapulmonary veins and venules, as we have seen in Chapter Nine, may become involved with narrowing by intimal fibrosis, even though this rarely results in generalized severe obstruction (Wagenvoort, 1970). Nasrallah et al. (1975) warned about confusing this condition with congenital atresia of pulmonary veins. Also cases with coexisting generalized thrombosis and phlebitis of both systemic and pulmonary veins (Manzini, 1947) should be excluded. What remains is a small group of patients.

Pulmonary veno-occlusive disease, as it was termed by Heath and coworkers (1966), is undoubtedly an uncommon condition and until recently very few pathologists had experience with its morphologic picture. From the records, however, it seems that in the last years either its frequency has increased or the condition is better recognized than before. In 1971, we could only collect 11 acceptable cases from the literature (Wagenvoort et al., 1971). Not included were 16 cases, briefly mentioned by Liebow et al. (1967) and Carrington and Liebow (1970), without detailed information. Since that time, the number of case reports has been rising steadily so that in 1975 the number of cases that have been published, or were submitted to us, came to 31 (Wagenvoort, 1976).

SEX AND AGE

Pulmonary veno-occlusive disease affects predominantly children and young adults. Of the 31 patients just mentioned, 14 were 16 years or older and 17 below that age. Four were younger than 2 years and an 8-week old infant is the youngest patient on record (Wagenvoort et al., 1971). In this case and in that described by Le Tan Vinh and coworkers (1974) an intrauterine origin has been assumed. The oldest patient was 48 years (Höra, 1934).

There is no sex difference as in primary pulmonary hypertension, where there is a pronounced preponderance of the female sex, at least in adult patients. In pulmonary veno-occlusive disease, of the 31 patients, 17 were male and 14 female.

FAMILY HISTORY

In one instance two siblings were affected by the disease (Wagenvoort, 1972). The patient of Heath and coworkers (1966) was the mother of three children with congenital cyanotic heart disease. Another patient had a brother who died from an Eisenmenger syndrome (Rosenthal et al., 1963).

CLINICAL AND HEMODYNAMIC FINDINGS

The clinical picture of pulmonary veno-occlusive disease, as it evolves from the description of mostly single cases, resembles in many respects that of primary pulmonary hypertension. The duration of the illness may be a few weeks in infants but averages between one and 2 years. Seven years in the cases of Heath et al. (1966) and Braun et al. (1973) was the maximum.

Fatigue and dyspnea on exertion are usually the first symptoms, which become gradually progressive. Eventually clinical signs of pulmonary hypertension and of congestion and edema of the lungs may develop. Cyanosis, syncope, hemoptysis, and finger clubbing have been present in some patients.

In several patients, although not in all, the chest roentgenogram is helpful (Scheibel et al., 1972). There is often a vague patchy or reticulate pattern, associated with Kerley B-lines and increased vascular markings, while the large pulmonary veins are not prominent as they are in mitral valve disease. A roentgenologic indication of postcapillary pulmonary hypertension in a patient without signs of increased left atrial pressure may suggest the correct diagnosis.

Cardiac catheterization will reveal that the pulmonary arterial pressure is elevated. The wedge pressure may be increased but usually only mildly, while it is often within normal limits. Therefore the wedge pressure is of little value in differentiating pulmonary veno-occlusive disease from the plexogenic form of primary pulmonary hypertension.

Carrington and Liebow (1970) explained the low wedge pressure in these instances as a result of the partial blockage of pulmonary and collateral bronchial venules, leading to a gradual fall of capillary pressure, after the inflow through the pulmonary artery has been interrupted by the wedged catheter. When the obstruction of the pulmonary venous outflow is located more distally as in mitral stenosis, the wedge pressure is high because the pulmonary veins will receive a flow from adjacent areas supplied by arteries not blocked by the catheter.

Slow drainage through the few remaining patent vessels, eventually resulting in a low wedge pressure, also was suggested by Brown and Harrison (1966) who found that flushing the wedged catheter with saline solution resulted in a disproportionally large rise in pressure, falling slowly to a low base level.

On the whole, the clinical diagnosis presents grave problems. Lung biopsies have permitted the diagnosis during life (Brown and Harrison, 1966; Wagenvoort and Wagenvoort, 1974), but the clinical diagnosis also may be established without morphologic criteria when the possibility of this rare condition is considered (Clinicopathological Conference, 1972; Liebow et al., 1973).

The prognosis of pulmonary veno-occlusive disease is bleak, since almost all cases have been fatal. Anticoagulant therapy has only been temporarily effective if at all. Only in one case were the results considered encouraging (Liu and Sackler, 1972). The poor effect in most cases is not surprising since the majority of the venules are irreversibly obstructed.

MORPHOLOGIC FINDINGS

In all patients the heart is enlarged with marked right ventricular hypertrophy. Congenital malformations are not part of the picture. Pleural effusions are common. The lungs are large, firm and congested, moist and dark, or have dark spots on cut surface.

The most striking histologic findings are in the smaller pulmonary veins and venules. Many veins and venules exhibit narrowing or even complete occlusion by fibrous tissue. This is almost always paucicellular and usually loose and edematous with only scarce collagenous fibers (Figure 10-1). In some instances there is a larger content of collagenous fibers with some admixture of elastin, resulting in a dense occlusive mass (Figure 10-2). On the whole, the intimal alterations strongly suggest a thrombotic origin (Liebow et al., 1967; Wagenvoort and Wagenvoort, 1974). A single narrow lumen in the center may represent the remainder of the original lumen (Figure 10-2) but multiple channels, suggestive of recanalization (Figure 10-3) and even leading to intravascular fibrous septa (Figure 10-4), do occur.

In most cases up to 95 percent of veins and venules are affected (Heath et al., 1966). The percentage of totally or subtotally occluded vessels also may be high. On the other hand, in some cases (Rosenthal et al., 1972; Wagenvoort, 1972) although many venules were narrowed (Figure 10-5), complete occlusion was uncommon.

The media of the small pulmonary veins is often unremarkable but may show arterialization (Figure 10-6) with the formation of internal and external elastic

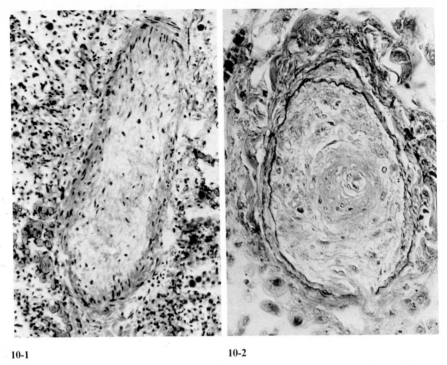

10-1   10-2

Figure 10-1. Pulmonary vein completely obstructed by loose, edematous connective tissue in a 4-year-old girl with pulmonary veno-occlusive disease (H. and E., ×120).

Figure 10-2. Pulmonary vein with subtotal occlusion by collagen-rich fibrous tissue in a 9-year-old girl with pulmonary veno-occlusive disease (El.v.G., ×350).

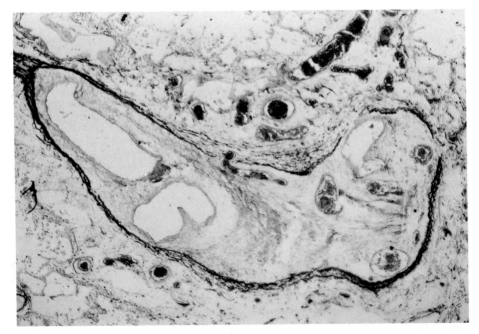

Figure 10-3. Pulmonary vein obstructed by connective tissue with multiple recanalization channels. Man aged 33 years with pulmonary veno-occlusive disease (El.v.G., ×35).

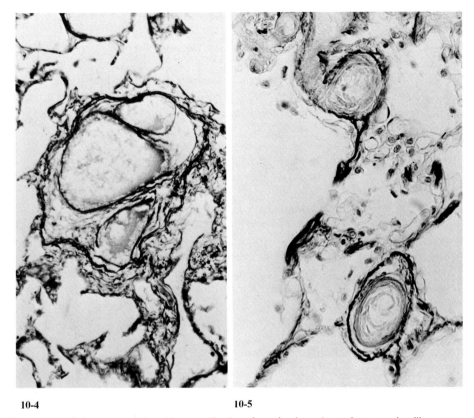

10-4   10-5

Figure 10-4. Pulmonary venule with recanalization channels given rise to intravascular fibrous septa. Woman aged 45 years with pulmonary veno-occlusive disease (El.v.G., ×140).

Figure 10-5. Pulmonary venules with narrowing by intimal fibrosis. There is still a patent lumen. Girl aged 13 years with pulmonary veno-occlusive disease (El.v.G., ×350).

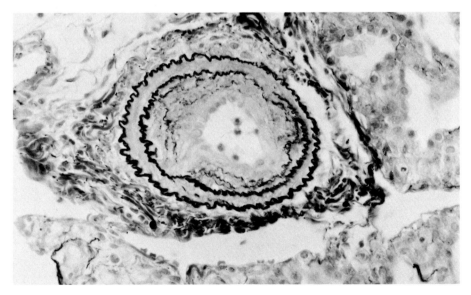

Figure 10-6. Pulmonary vein with pronounced medial hypertrophy and arterialization and narrowing by intimal fibrosis in a 3-month-old male infant with pulmonary veno-occlusive disease (El.v.G., ×350).

221

laminae on either side of the thickened media (Wagenvoort, 1972). This, as we have discussed before (p. 197), indicates an adaptation to an increased pressure which in turn will be due to obstruction further downstream. Larger pulmonary veins indeed often are involved. Organized and recanalized masses with the formation of intraluminal fibrous septa often are observed in large veins (Figure 10-7) even close to the hilar region (Crane and Grimes, 1960; Stovin and Mitchison, 1965; Heath et al., 1966; Braun et al., 1973; Wagenvoort and Wagenvoort, 1974).

Also bronchopulmonary venous anastomoses and bronchial veins sometimes were affected and partly or completely obstructed (Figure 10-8) (Wagenvoort et al., 1971).

As compared to the veins, the changes in the pulmonary arteries are much more limited (Bürki, 1963). Medial hypertrophy is often not severe and may be mild or even absent. In 2 of 13 cases in which we studied the pulmonary arteries morphometrically, the mean medial thickness expressed as percentage of the external diameter, was within normal limits, that is, below 7 percent (Wagenvoort and Wagenvoort, 1974). In 5 cases it varied from 7 to 10 percent, and in 3 it was between 12 and 16 percent. Only in 2 infants was there very severe medial hypertrophy, that is, over 20 percent, but in infants the media is usually very thick in the presence of pulmonary hypertension.

In the majority of the patients, some or even many pulmonary arteries contain thrombi (Figure 10-9) with transitions to crescent-shaped or patchy intimal fibrosis (Figure 10-10) (Wagenvoort and Wagenvoort, 1974; Thadani et al., 1975). In 3 patients (Stovin and Mitchison, 1965; Weisser, 1967; Heath et al., 1971) fibrinoid necrosis was observed in some arteries but other changes characteristic of primary

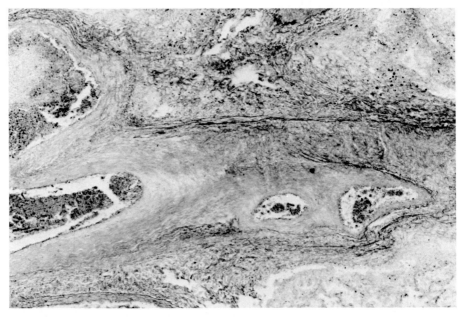

Figure 10-7.   Large pulmonary veins close to the hilar region, largely obstructed by intimal fibrosis in an 8-week-old male infant with pulmonary veno-occlusive disease (El.v.G., ×50).

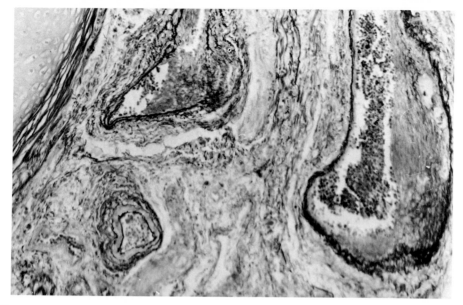

Figure 10-8. Bronchial vein (top) and bronchopulmonary venous anastomosis (right), both severely narrowed by intimal fibrosis. Same case as Figure 10-7 (El.v.G., ×140).

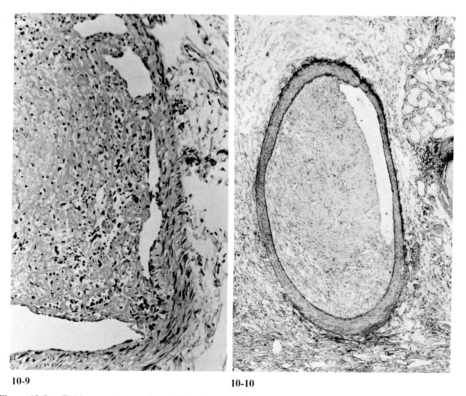

10-9   10-10

Figure 10-9. Fairly recent thrombus with early organization in muscular pulmonary artery in a 13-year-old girl with pulmonary veno-occlusive disease (H. and E., ×300).

Figure 10-10. Large muscular pulmonary artery subtotally obstructed by intimal fibrosis based on organized thrombus. Girl aged 13 years with pulmonary veno-occlusive disease (El.v.G., ×35).

pulmonary hypertension, such as concentric-laminar intimal fibrosis, arteritis, and plexiform lesions, are always absent.

In the lung tissue there is pulmonary edema. Congestion is usually limited to small areas which also show interstitial fibrosis (Figure 10-11) and often interstitial pneumonia with polymorphonuclear leucocytes (Braun et al., 1973) or plasma cells and lymphocytes (Wagenvoort, 1972) in the thickened alveolar walls (Figure 10-12). Marked hemosiderosis also prevails in these areas (Figure 10-13). Hemosiderosis may be so pronounced that the condition may simulate idiopathic pulmonary hemosiderosis (Carrington and Liebow, 1970). There are, however, also cases in which hemosiderin deposits are mild (Mallory, 1937). Microlithiasis is observed occasionally.

The focal interstitial fibrosis and pneumonia is sometimes so extensive as to become confluent (Figure 10-14) so that whole lobes are affected (Figure 10-15). Bronchopneumonia and the formation of hyaline membranes (Figures 10-16 and 10-17) occasionally is added to the picture (Wagenvoort and Wagenvoort, 1974).

In several cases there is an increase of bronchial mucous glands or of mucus-secreting goblet cells in the bronchial epithelial lining or both (Figure 10-18). Pulmonary lymphatics were almost always dilated.

The pathologic lesions of the lung tissue and of the vessels are sometimes equally distributed over both lungs and over the lobes of one lung. Höra (1934) had the impression that the right lower lobe was less affected than the remainder of the lungs. Brown and Harrison (1966) reported that the lesions in a biopsy from the left lower lobe were more severe than in that from the lingula but later, when the same case was published as a clinicopathological conference (1968), after the autopsy results were known, an equal distribution over both lungs was established. In the

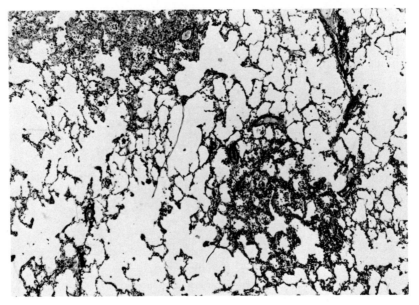

Figure 10-11. Focal areas of congestion and interstitial fibrosis of the lung in a 16-year-old boy with pulmonary veno-occlusive disease (H. and E., ×35).

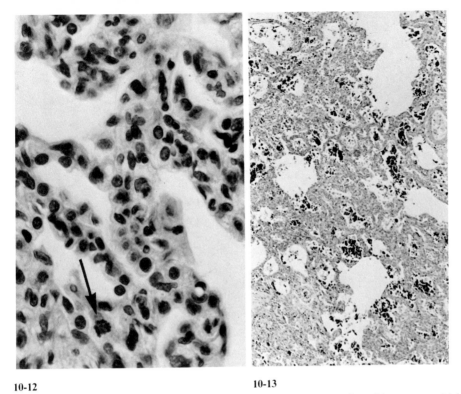

10-12   **10-13**

Figure 10-12. Lung tissue with interstitial pneumonia. A mitotic figure is indicated by an arrow. Male infant aged 3 months with pulmonary veno-occlusive disease (H. and E., ×560).

Figure 10-13. Pulmonary hemosiderosis with focal accumulations of hemosiderin-laden macrophages in a 12-year-old girl with pulmonary veno-occlusive disease (Perl's iron stain, ×50).

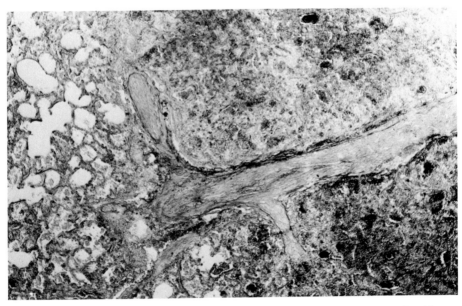

Figure 10-14. Lung tissue with confluent area of interstitial pneumonia (right). A totally obliterated pulmonary vein is cut longitudinally. Same case as Figure 10-13 (El.v.G., ×35).

225

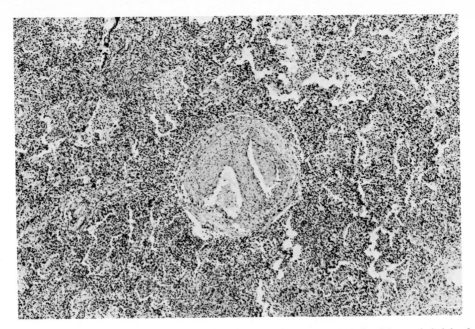

Figure 10-15. Lung tissue with extensive and confluent interstitial pneumonia involving a whole lobe. In the center there is a partially obstructed pulmonary vein. Male infant aged 8 weeks with pulmonary veno-occlusive disease (H. and E., ×35).

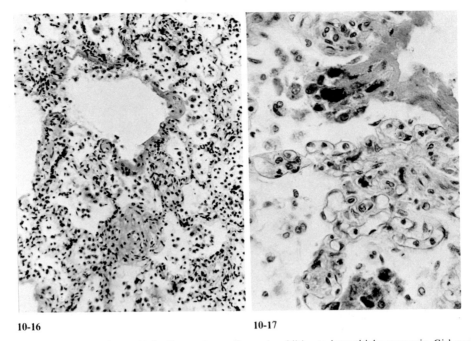

10-16   10-17

Figure 10-16. Lung tissue with hyalin membrane disease in addition to interstitial pneumonia. Girl aged 13 years with pulmonary veno-occlusive disease (H. and E., ×120).

Figure 10-17. Lung tissue with hyalin membranes, congested alveolar capillaries, and hemosiderin-containing macrophages. Same case as Figure 10-16 (H. and E. ×350).

226

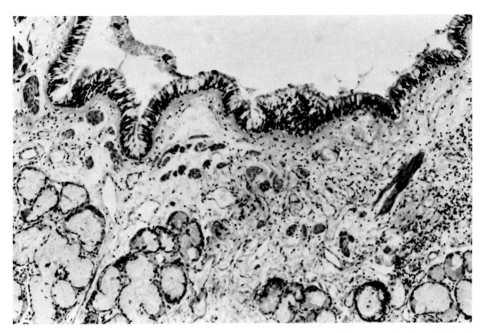

Figure 10-18. Bronchial wall with hyperplastic active mucous glands and increase of goblet cells in the bronchial epithelial lining. Girl aged 12 years with pulmonary veno-occlusive disease (H. and E., ×90).

case of Calderon and Burdine (1974), asymmetrical involvement of major pulmonary veins was responsible for absence of unilateral pulmonary perfusion.

In our own experience, there are cases in which the lungs are totally involved with an equal distribution of the various lesions over the lung tissue. In other cases the pulmonary vascular and parenchymal changes are much more severe in some parts of the lungs than in others and this distribution is not a constant one. In two cases there were extensive and severe alterations in the lower lobes, while the upper lobes, including the lingula, were virtually without any lesions. In another case it was just the other way round and the alterations were practically limited to the upper lobes.

As a matter of fact, such an unequal distribution may have consequences when lung biopsies are taken for diagnostic purposes.

Outside the lungs, the blood vessels of other organs are reportedly normal.

ETIOLOGY

The cause of pulmonary veno-occlusive disease is unknown. As to the pathogenesis of the obstructive changes, in the pulmonary veins, however, most authors agree that these are caused by thrombosis (Stovin and Mitchison, 1965; Brown and Harrison, 1966; Heath et al., 1966, 1971; Tingelstad et al., 1969; Carrington and Liebow, 1970; Dainauskas et al., 1971; Wagenvoort et al., 1971; Liu and Sackler, 1972; Braun et al., 1973; Wagenvoort, 1976). The common presence of recognizable thrombi, either recent or in the early stages of organization, and the regular occurrence of intraluminal septa as late stages of recanalization indicate this. Thrombi also were found fairly often in pulmonary arteries (Höra, 1934; Wagenvoort, 1972).

In 1967, Liebow and his coworkers were the first to comment on a possible connection between pulmonary veno-occlusive disease and a preceding febrile influenza-like illness. There is indeed a fairly large number of cases in which such a relation with a preceding infection of the respiratory tract is mentioned (Brewer and Humphreys, 1960; Crane and Grimes, 1960; Tingelstad et al., 1969; Wagenvoort et al., 1971; Wagenvoort, 1972). The serologic reactions in the patient described by Stovin and Mitchison (1965) suggested a toxoplasmosis infection, but the overall evidence for toxoplasmosis as a cause for the condition is weak.

A viral origin of the disease could explain the frequent occurrence of interstitial pneumonia, which in turn may lead to interstitial fibrosis. The hemosiderosis in the affected areas was held by Carrington and Liebow (1970) as an argument against such an origin of interstitial fibrosis and in favor of a congestive origin. This is not necessarily true since the occlusion of pulmonary veins will cause congestion anyway in the affected areas, so that hemosiderosis will develop irrespective of the way in which the interstitial fibrosis was brought about.

The one case with development of hyaline membranes and the regularly occurring hyperplasia of bronchial mucous glands and goblet cells may indicate an infective and possibly viral origin. Simultaneous occurrence of subacute myocarditis (Figure 10-19) in an infant, 8 weeks old, who probably acquired the disease in utero following an infectious respiratory illness of the mother in the thirty-fourth week of pregnancy, may point in the same direction.

It could then be asummed that a virus is responsible for the thrombus formation in the lung vessels. In an Annotation in the *British Medical Journal* (1972) the possibility is put forward that in pulmonary veno-occlusive disease, an infective agent might selectively attack the pulmonary venous endothelium and deplete its plasminogen activator. As the activator content is low anyway in the endothelium of pulmonary veins, inhibited lysis and thrombus formation might result.

In one case (Corrin et al., 1974) the presence of irregular deposits of IgG and complement was established in alveolar walls within a lung biopsy. It was suggested that immune complexes, possibly stemming from a viral infection, may have initiated thrombosis by activation of "contact" clotting factors or platelets.

Proof for the viral hypothesis, however, is lacking since so far all attempts to identify an infectious agent have failed.

Whether genetic factors contribute to the chances of acquiring the disease, remains undecided in view of the limited number of known cases.

There are other etiologic possibilities such as inhalation or ingestion of toxic substances but most case histories do not support such an origin. Only one case history, that of a 14-year-old boy, suggested sniffing of powdered household cleanser as a possible cause of pulmonary veno-occlusion (Liu and Sackler, 1972).

Veno-occlusive disease of the liver in the West Indies has been demonstrated to result from ingestion of Crotalaria alkaloids in the form of bush tea (Bras et al., 1957). In rats, fulvine, one of the alkaloids from the Crotalaria group, produces obstructive lesions not only in pulmonary arteries but also in pulmonary veins (Wagenvoort et al., 1974). However, patients with veno-occlusive disease of the liver reportedly have a normal pulmonary vasculature, and there is no distinct indication

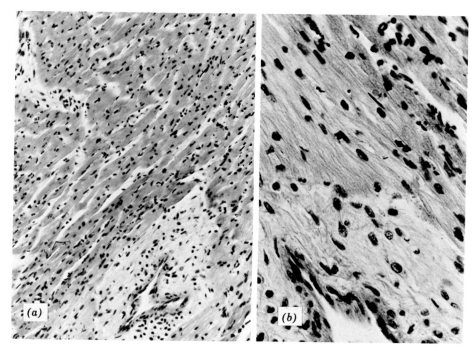

Figure 10-19. (*a*) Left ventricular myocardium of a 8-week-old male infant with pulmonary veno-occlusive disease. There is subacute myocarditis with an inflammatory exudate of polymorphonuclear and mononuclear cells and with occasional necrosis of individual muscle fibers. (*b*) Detail of *a* (H. and E., *a*: ×100, *b*: ×250).

that herbs or drugs were involved in any of the patients with veno-occlusive disease of the lungs.

Since several patients with pulmonary veno-occlusive disease had neither a history of infectious upper respiratory disease nor signs of an inflammatory reaction in the lungs, it is possible that in this condition thrombosis of pulmonary veins is elicited by various agents. This would mean that pulmonary veno-occlusive disease is a syndrome, rather than an etiologic entity (Wagenvoort, 1976).

Pulmonary veno-occlusive disease: Arteries (*left*) with some medial hypertrophy and eccentric intimal fibrosis. Veins, particularly small ones (*right*), with obliterating intimal fibrosis and intravascular fibrous septa.

REFERENCES

Annotation: Pulmonary veno-occlusive disease. *Brit. Med. J.* **3**: 369, 1972.

Bras, G., Berry, D. M., and György, P.: Plants as aetiological factors in veno-occlusive disease of the liver. *Lancet* **i**: 960, 1957.

Braun, A., Greenberg, S. D., Malik, S., and Jenkins, D. E.: Pulmonary veno-occlusive disease associated with pulmonary phlebitis. *Arch. Path.* **95**: 67, 1973.

Brewer, D. B., and Humphreys, D. R.: Primary pulmonary hypertension with obstructive venous lesions. *Brit. Heart J.* **22**: 445, 1960.

Brown, C. H., and Harrison, C. V.: Pulmonary veno-occlusive disease. *Lancet* **ii**: 61, 1966.

Bürki, K.: Eine primäre isolierte obliterierende Pulmonalvenenveränderung als Ursache eines chronischen Cor pulmonale. *Arch. Kreislaufforsch.* **40**: 35, 1963.

Calderon, M., and Burdine, J. A.: Pulmonary veno-occlusive disease. *J. Nucl. Med.* **15**: 455, 1974.

Carrington, C. B., and Liebow, A. A.: Pulmonary veno-occlusive disease. *Human Path.* **1**: 322, 1970.

Clinicopathological conference: A case of veno-occlusive disease. *Brit. Med. J.* **i**: 816, 1968.

Clinicopathological conference: Heart failure in a middle-aged woman. *Brit. Med. J.* **ii**: 773, 1972.

Corrin, B., Spencer, H., Turner-Warwick, M., Beales, S. J., and Hamblin, J. J.: Pulmonary veno-occlusion—An immune complex disease? *Virch. Arch. A Path. Anat. Histol.* **364**: 81, 1974.

Crane, J. T., and Grimes, O. F.: Isolated pulmonary venous sclerosis: a cause of cor pulmonale. *J. Thorac. Cardiovasc. Surg.* **40**: 410, 1960.

Dainauskas, J. R., Hughes, R. L., and English, J. T.: Clinical pathologic conference. *Amer. Heart J.* **82**: 817, 1971.

Heath, D., Segel, N., and Bishop, J.: Pulmonary veno-occlusive disease. *Circulation* **34**: 242, 1966.

Heath, D., Scott, O., and Lynch, J.: Pulmonary veno-occlusive disease. *Thorax* **26**: 663, 1971.

Höra, J.: Zur Histologie der klinischen "Primären Pulmonalsklerose." *Frankf. Z. Path.* **47**: 100, 1934.

Le Tan Vinh, Tran Van Duc, Huault, G., Gallet, J.-P., Joly, C., Aussannaire, M., and Thieffry, S.: La maladie veino-occlusive du poumon. *Arch. Franc. Pédiatr.* **31**: 187, 1974.

Liebow, A. A., McAdams, A. J., Carrington, C. B., and Viamonte, M.: Intrapulmonary veno-obstructive disease. *Circulation* (suppl. II) **35, 36**: 172, 1967.

Liebow, A. A., Moser, K. M., and Southgate, M. T.: Rapidly progressive dyspnea in a teenage boy. *J.A.M.A.* **223**: 1243, 1973.

Liu, L., and Sackler, J. P.: A case of pulmonary veno-occlusive disease. *Angiology* **23**: 299, 1972.

Mallory, T. B.: Case records of the Massachusetts General Hospital: Case 23511. *New Engl. J. Med.* **217**: 1045, 1937.

Manzini, C.: Endophlebitis obliterans universalis, vorwiegend der Lungenvenen, mit konsekutivem Cor pulmonale. *Path. Bacteriol.* **10**: 309, 1947.

Nasrallah, A. T., Mullins, C. E., Singer, D., Harrison, G., and McNamara, D. G.: Unilateral pulmonary vein atresia: diagnosis and treatment. *Amer. J. Cardiol.* **36**: 969, 1975.

Rosenthal, A., Vawter, G., and Wagenvoort, C. A.: Intrapulmonary veno-occlusive disease. *Amer. J. Cardiol.* **31**: 78, 1973.

Scheibel, R. L., Dedeker, K. L., Gleason, D. F., Pliego, M., and Kieffer, S. A.: Radiographic and angiographic characteristics of pulmonary veno-occlusive disease. *Radiology* **103**: 47, 1972.

Stovin, P. G. I., and Mitchinson, M. J.: Pulmonary hypertension due to obstruction of the intrapulmonary veins. *Thorax* **20**: 106, 1965.

Thadani, U., Burrow, C., Whitaker, W., and Heath, D.: Pulmonary veno-occlusive disease. *Quart. J. Med.* **44** (n.s.): 173, 1975.

Tingelstad, J. B., Aterman, K., and Lambert, E. C.: Pulmonary venous obstruction. Report of a case mimicking primary pulmonary artery hypertension, with a review of the literature. *Amer. J. Dis. Child.* **117**: 219, 1969.

Wagenvoort, C. A.: Morphologic changes in intrapulmonary veins. *Human Path.* **1**: 205, 1970.

Wagenvoort, C. A.: Vasoconstrictive primary pulmonary hypertension and pulmonary veno-occlusive disease. *Cardiovasc. Clinics* **4:** 97, 1972.

Wagenvoort, C. A.: Pulmonary veno-occlusive disease. Entity or syndrome? *Chest* **69:** 82, 1976.

Wagenvoort, C. A., Losekoot, G., and Mulder, E.: Pulmonary veno-occlusive disease of presumably intrauterine origin. *Thorax* **26:** 429, 1971.

Wagenvoort, C. A., and Wagenvoort, N.: The pathology of pulmonary veno-occlusive disease. *Virch. Arch. A Path. Anat. Histol.* **364:** 69, 1974.

Wagenvoort, C. A., Wagenvoort, N., and Dijk, H. J.: Effect of fulvine on pulmonary arteries and veins of the rat. *Thorax* **29:** 522, 1974.

Weisser, K., Wyler, F., and Gloor, F.: Pulmonary veno-occlusive disease. *Arch. Dis. Childh.* **42:** 322, 1967.

CHAPTER ELEVEN

Hypoxic Pulmonary Hypertension

Hypoxia may be a cause of elevated pulmonary arterial pressure and right ventricular hypertrophy, irrespective of the way the hypoxia is brought about. Widely differing conditions, such as lung diseases, kyphoscoliosis, muscular dystrophy, Pickwickian syndrome, and high altitude residence, therefore, may give rise to this form of pulmonary hypertension.

HEMODYNAMICS

It has long been known that alveolar hypoxia causes a rise in pulmonary arterial pressure, as becomes apparent on breathing low oxygen mixtures (Von Euler and Liljestrand, 1946; Motley et al., 1947; Westcott et al., 1951; Fishman et al., 1952). Unilateral breathing of such mixtures increases the vascular resistance of the hypoxic lung (Dirken and Heemstra, 1948a; Fishman et al., 1955). Von Euler and Liljestrand (1946) pointed out that a localized effect of hypoxia might thus influence the distribution of the blood flow within the lung, by shunting away the blood from hypoxic areas to better aerated parts.

Up to now, there is still some uncertainty as to the exact site of increased resistance within the pulmonary vasculature, and particularly, there is no unanimity as to how the pressor response to hypoxia is mediated (Fishman, 1976).

Hypercapnia and acidosis are also likely to influence pulmonary vascular resistance, although this does not mean that the site of action and the mechanisms involved are the same.

It is possible that in part the increased pulmonary arterial pressure is caused by a shift of blood from systemic to pulmonary circulation coupled with an increased cardiac output. This would mean that the rise in pressure should be passive rather than active (Fishman et al., 1955; Wilcox et al., 1964). On the other hand, although this effect may contribute to hypoxic pulmonary hypertension, an increased blood flow can account only to a limited extent for the increased pressure (Lewis et al., 1952; Stroud and Conn, 1954; Fishman et al., 1960; Wilcox et al., 1964).

Increased blood viscosity due to a rise in hematocrit, as may become apparent in chronic hypoxic pulmonary hypertension, and increased alveolar capillary and left atrial pressures have been considered as factors involved in the development of pulmonary hypertension in hypoxia. But among other considerations these factors would not explain the instantaneous rise in pressure in acute hypoxia and, therefore, could be only contributing factors in the more chronic forms of the disease (Aviado, 1965; Bergofsky, 1974).

Constriction of lung vessels is almost certainly the most important factor in elevating the resistance in hypoxia (Cournand, 1958) and the available evidence points to vasoconstriction at precapillary level (Bergofsky, 1974). Acetylcholine, a known vasodilator for the pulmonary circulation, can relieve the vascular resistance induced by hypoxia (Harris, 1957; Fritts et al., 1958).

Additional vasomotor activity in the postcapillary vessels has been suggested (Kuida et al., 1963; Naeye, 1965). It has been shown that, while the pulmonary arterial pressure rises gradually with increasing alveolar hypoxia and arterial undersaturation (Fritts et al., 1960; Harris and Heath, 1962), the wedge pressure remains unaffected (Westcott et al., 1951; Doyle et al., 1952; Sieker et al., 1955; Estes et al., 1957). Even so the morphologic evidence, as we will see (p. 240), suggests that the pulmonary veins are also influenced by hypoxia and/or hypercapnic acidosis, even if their effect on the pulmonary circulation is much more limited than the arterial response.

Vasoconstriction at pulmonary arterial or arteriolar level, in principle, could be induced by alveolar hypoxia, as well as by hypoxemia of the mixed venous blood. The latter possibility has been stressed by Bergofsky and coworkers (1963). They found that a diminished oxygen tension of mixed venous blood caused increase of pressure and resistance in pulmonary arteries. Other studies, however, did not sustain such an effect of the mixed venous blood (Aviado, 1960; Duke et al., 1960). Hauge (1970) suggested, that while pulmonary arterial hypoxemia alone, in the absence of air way hypoxia, does not produce a pressor response, it is still possible that a low oxygen content of the blood determines the vasoconstrictive response to ventilation hypoxia. This, however, does not explain unilateral increase of vascular resistance when one lung is ventilated with a hypoxic gas mixture. Therefore, it seems more likely that alveolar hypoxia is responsible for the increased resistance.

There is no clear-cut understanding of the underlying mechanisms of hypoxic pulmonary vasoconstriction. The central nervous system apparently is not involved, as was demonstrated by Reeves and Leathers (1964). The sympathetic nervous system has long been thought to play a part in the mediation of the hypoxic stimulus. The various results of experimental work, however, have been contradictory. Valenca et al. (1971) concluded from lung reimplantation studies in dogs, that the response to hypoxia should be a reflex, mediated through the sympathetic system. Kalemi et al. (1972) demonstrated that sympathectomy in animals caused depression or even blockade of the vascular response to hypoxia.

On the other hand, much evidence has accumulated indicating that the importance of sympathetic pathways is very limited (Duke, 1957; Fishman, 1961;

Lloyd, 1966). Blockade of adrenergic receptors does not alter significantly the pressor response to hypoxia (Silove and Grover, 1968; Badder et al., 1973).

The possibility that vasoconstriction is induced by various humoral agents, which may occur naturally in the pulmonary circulation, has been extensively studied (Dirken and Heemstra, 1948b; Harris, 1970). However, it appears very difficult to assess the action of substances like catecholamines and serotonin on the pulmonary circulation, in view of simultaneous effects on the systemic circulation.

The lung is an active metabolizing organ with a capacity to synthetize various substances (Fishman and Pietra, 1974). Hauge (1970) showed that the hypoxic response in rat lungs is temperature dependent and suggested that reduction of available oxygen might cause a rapid change in the concentration of various metabolites.

The role of angiotensin in the production of hypoxic pulmonary hypertension was stressed by Zakheim et al. (1975). Prostaglandins, and particularly prostaglandin $F_{2\alpha}$, also have been considered (Tyler et al., 1975), but their role as a mediator for the hypoxic pressor response seems an additional rather than a primary one (Bergofsky, 1974).

Histamine is another substance suggested as mediator for hypoxic vasoconstriction (Aviado et al., 1966). There is a correlation between the amount of histamine in lung tissue in rats and the pressure response to hypoxia (Hauge, 1968), while this response can be completely, although temporarily, blocked by histamine-releasing agents (Hauge and Staub, 1969). Also the work of Susmano and Carleton (1973) lends support to this hypothesis, while Fishman (1976) concluded that of all humoral agents, histamine is the most likely to act as an intrinsic mediator of the pulmonary pressure response.

Kay et al. (1974) stressed the importance of perivascular lung mast cells in this connection, since inhibition of mast cell degranulation also inhibited the expected rise in pulmonary arterial resistance. The mast cells, therefore, were supposed to act as chemoreceptors, thus monitoring the alveolar oxygen tension. Mast cells are increased in numbers at high altitude in various species of animals. Their numbers show a correlation with the degree of right ventricular hypertrophy (Reeves et al., 1974), although in hypoxic rats mast cell hyperplasia may lag behind hypertrophy of the right ventricle (Mungall, 1976).

Reflex vasoconstriction of the pulmonary vessels due to stimulation of carotid or aortic bodies also has been considered (Aviado et al., 1957). In this respect it is important to note that the carotid bodies undergo enlargement in various states of hypoxia and even may become the site of tumors (p. 242).

Bergofsky and Holtzman (1967) suggested that hypoxia may induce depolarization of the pulmonary arterial smooth muscle cells since it caused a reversible loss of potassium and gain of sodium in samples of vascular smooth muscle tissue. Such a depolarization could bring the muscle cell closer to its excitatory threshold, thus providing an important factor in initiating vasoconstriction. Although these investigators studied both "large" and "small" arteries, it is not clear from their account whether any muscular pulmonary arteries, that is, of a diameter below 1000 μ, were involved in their studies. Older reports (Smith and Coxe, 1951) indicate that strips of media of elastic pulmonary arteries do not react to hypoxia.

The anatomic relation of the smallest muscular pulmonary arteries to the alveolar air spaces is such that changes in alveolar oxygen tension may have a direct effect through diffusion of gas, on these arteries. In this respect the small arteries are in a somewhat better position than the veins of similar caliber (Staub, 1961; Jamieson, 1964; Hasleton et al., 1968). Hauge (1970) has suggested that the effector area must be localized at a precapillary level. He believes that these segments of the pulmonary vascular bed are the ones most sensitive to hypoxia.

There is evidence that the action of hypercapnic acidosis on the other hand is not limited to the smallest arteries but that it acts over a much longer stretch of the muscular pulmonary arteries (Bergofsky, 1974).

The above review of physiologic principles underlying hypoxic pulmonary hypertension, even though far from complete, indicates that much is controversial and that little has been established beyond doubt. This is even more accentuated by the fact that the various data are only partly derived from studies in man but mostly from work done in animals and hypoxia may well act differently in various species.

It seems likely that multiple factors, although of course not necessarily to the same extent, are involved in mediating the hypoxic stimulus resulting in elevated pulmonary vascular pressure and that this may happen in multiple stages.

The contribution the pathologist may provide in solving these problems is limited, although not entirely profitless.

MORPHOLOGY

Right Ventricular Hypertrophy

Hypoxia causes right ventricular hypertrophy in a variety of animal species (Valdivia, 1957; Hultgren et al., 1963; Recavarren and Arias-Stella, 1964; Hultgren and Miller, 1965; James and Thomas, 1968; Kay and Smith, 1973). This hypertrophy develops within weeks and appears to be readily reversible after return to normal environment (Heath et al., 1973a).

Also in the human, hypoxia results in an increased weight of the right ventricle although with considerable variation (Hultgren and Miller, 1967). Children born and raised at the low barometric pressures of high altitude, fail to reduce their right ventricular weight after birth and may show prominent right ventricular hypertrophy, particularly after the age of 4 months (Arias-Stella and Recavarren, 1962).

In other states of chronic hypoxia, such as chronic bronchitis (Figure 11-1) and Pickwickian syndrome, the right ventricle is also usually hypertrophied. In pulmonary emphysema, in which hypoxia is supposed to be instrumental in bringing about pulmonary hypertension (Riley et al., 1948; Evans et al., 1963), right ventricular hypertrophy is variable, as will be discussed in Chapter Twelve.

Pulmonary Trunk, Main Arteries, and Elastic Arteries

The effect of hypoxia on the structure of the extrapulmonary arteries has been studied mainly with regard to residents of high altitudes. Saldana and Arias-Stella (1963a,b) demonstrated that in these individuals the thickness of the media of the pulmonary trunk is increased, while the aortic type of elastic configuration in the main pulmonary arteries is retained till the age of approximately 9 years and even

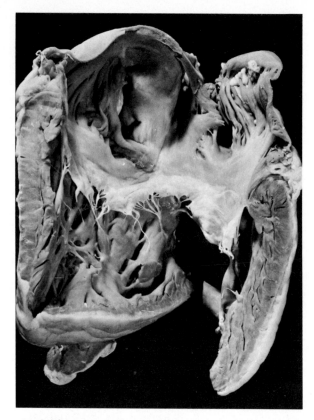

Figure 11-1. Pronounced right ventricular hypertrophy in a 61-year-old man with chronic bronchitis and emphysema. For a reliable assessment it is usually necessary to establish the weight of the right ventricular mass.

may persist much longer. Elevation of pulmonary arterial pressure is apparently basic to these findings.

Castillo et al. (1967) confirmed these results and assessed the extensibility of the pulmonary trunk for a given extensible force. It appeared that the extensibility of the vessel was inappropriately low in these individuals. Heath et al. (1968) reported similar findings in various animals living at high altitude although some animals (cattle, sheep, llama) have much more muscle in the media of the pulmonary trunk than is found in man or dog.

Chronic hypoxia in the rat results in an increased medial thickness of the pulmonary trunk and in similar changes in elastic configuration as in man (Heath, 1972). These changes are reversible upon return to normal atmospheric conditions (Heath et al., 1973a).

The intima of the pulmonary trunk may be thickened with atherosclerotic patches but apparently this is directly related to the elevation of pressure. In hypercholesterolemic rabbits, hypoxia was a distinct factor in producing atherosclerosis in the pulmonary trunk (Altland and Highman, 1960).

Muscular Pulmonary Arteries and Arterioles

In most forms of pulmonary hypertension in man, medial hypertrophy of muscular pulmonary arteries develops irrespective of the caliber of these vessels. It is present in arteries with a diameter of 300 to 400 μ just as well as in arterioles. As we have seen (p. 65) the muscular coat even may extend in a peripheral direction so that arterioles as small as 30 to 20 μ in diameter may become muscularized.

Hypoxic pulmonary hypertension is an exception because the response of the pulmonary arterioles to hypoxia is stronger than that of the muscular arteries. The small muscular pulmonary arteries, therefore, usually exhibit marked medial hypertrophy with muscularization of arterioles (Figure 11-2), while in the larger muscular arteries the media is normal (Figure 11-3) or only mildly hypertrophied. Such a differential effect on muscular pulmonary arteries of various sizes is independent of the way hypoxia is brought about. It has been observed in residents of high altitude areas (Arias-Stella and Saldana, 1963), as well as in patients suffering from chronic bronchitis and emphysema, kyphoscoliosis, and Pickwickian syndrome (Naeye, 1961a,b; Heath, 1963; Hicken et al., 1965; Hasleton et al., 1968). The medial hypertrophy is reversible when its cause has been removed (Hasleton et al., 1968; Heath et al., 1973a).

In some individuals who have always lived at high altitude not only the small arterioles but also larger muscular pulmonary arteries of an external diameter in the range of 100 to 200 μ show distinct medial hypertrophy (Figure 11-4), so that the

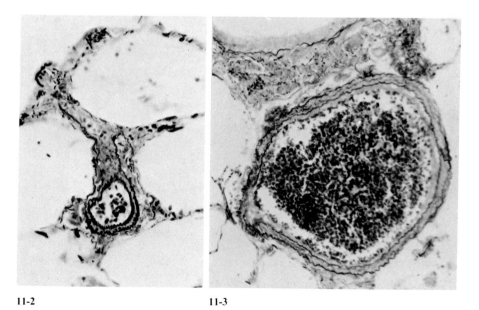

11-2   11-3

Figure 11-2. Pulmonary arteriole with muscularization of its wall in a 35-year-old man, native to an altitude of 3300 meters (El.v.G., ×230).

Figure 11-3. Muscular pulmonary artery with normal medial thickness from the same case as Figure 11-2 (El.v.G., ×230).

differential effect of hypoxia on the arteries has shifted to a larger caliber, but this is not the rule.

As a consequence of muscularization of arterioles, the number of muscular pulmonary arteries with a caliber below 70 μ is distinctly increased (Wagenvoort and Wagenvoort, 1973).

Similar changes, occurring predominantly in the smallest arteries, have been described in animals during chronic hypoxia (Alexander and Jensen, 1963a; Naeye, 1969; Abraham et al., 1971; Will and Kay, 1974). In our own experience this hypoxic effect on the small pulmonary arteries in rats may already be distinct after one to 2 weeks exposure (Figures 11-5 and 11-6), particularly after instillation of the lungs by fixative whereby constricted arteries tend to have a crenated and non-constricted vessels a smooth internal elastic lamina. Intermittent hypoxia produces the same effect (Urbanova et al., 1973). Female rats have been reported to show more severe medial hypertrophy of pulmonary arteries in response to hypoxia than male animals (Smith et al., 1974).

Intimal fibrosis generally is not a feature of hypoxic pulmonary hypertension. In inhabitants of high altitude regions, intimal fibrosis, if present at all, is only mild as an age change and not more striking than at sea level. In kyphoscoliosis and chronic bronchitis, it is often more marked (p. 266) but clearly secondary to thrombi or emboli or related to previous inflammation of lung tissue (Wagenvoort and Wagenvoort, 1973).

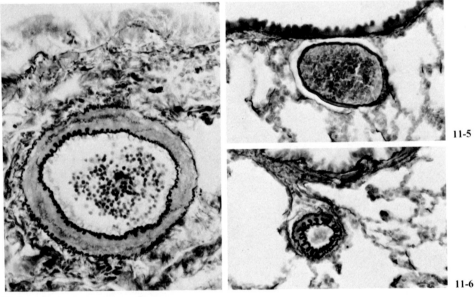

11-5

11-6

11-4

Figure 11-4. Muscular pulmonary artery with medial hypertrophy in a 21-year-old man, native to an altitude of 3300 meters (El.v.G., ×230).

Figure 11-5. Normal muscular pulmonary artery in a rat after instillation of the lungs with fixative. The artery is thin-walled with smooth elastic laminae (El.v.G., ×230).

Figure 11-6. Constricted muscular pulmonary artery in a rat exposed for 14 days to a hypoxic environment. The medial thickness is increased and the lumen is narrow. In spite of instillation with fixative, the elastic laminae are crenated (El.v.G., ×230).

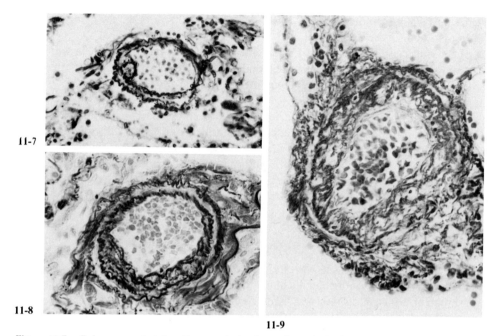

Figure 11-7. Pulmonary arteriole with muscularization and one intimal bundle of longitudinal smooth muscle cells in a 50-year-old man, native to an altitude of 4000 meters (El.v.G., ×230).

Figure 11-8. Small muscular pulmonary artery with crescent-shaped intimal layer of longitudinal smooth muscle cells in a 62-year-old man, native to an altitude of 3300 meters (El.v.G., ×350).

Figure 11-9. Muscular pulmonary artery with continuous and relatively thick intimal layer of longitudinal smooth muscle cells, from the same case as Figure 11-8 (El.v.G., ×350).

A rather characteristic pulmonary vascular lesion in chronic hypoxia, however, is the development of longitudinal smooth muscle cells in the intima of muscular pulmonary arteries (Hicken et al., 1965; Hasleton et al., 1968, Heath, 1970; Wagenvoort and Wagenvoort, 1973). In cross section these muscle bundles sometimes form small patches (Figure 11-7), but more often they form crescent-shaped (Figure 11-8) or continuous concentric layers, which uncommonly cause pronounced narrowing of the lumen (Figure 11-9). The smooth muscle cells usually are embedded in collagen and elastic fibers. The bundles may be present over long distances within the arteries.

Longitudinal muscle bundles in the intima are found most commonly in small muscular pulmonary arteries. Hasleton and coworkers (1968) described them in arteries in the range of 38 to 300 μ, particularly in those between 65 and 200 μ external diameter.

In our experience they are almost exclusively seen in arteries between 50 and 150 μ. The total number of arterial and arteriolar cross sections provided with longitudinal muscle bundles is fairly small. Often several histologic sections of lung tissue must be studied before their presence can be established.

These intimal muscle bundles are not pathognomonic for hypoxic pulmonary hypertension. Such bundles also are seen commonly in congestive pulmonary hypertension, as in mitral stenosis, but then usually in larger pulmonary arteries even up to 500 μ in diameter (p. 187), and occasionally in other forms of hypertensive pulmonary vascular disease.

The combination, however, of a normal media in the larger muscular pulmonary arteries, muscularization of arterioles, and the occurrence of intimal smooth muscle bundles strongly suggests a hypoxic origin of the elevated pulmonary arterial pressure.

Fibrin thrombi in pulmonary arteries have been reported in chronic mountain sickness (p. 247) and in high altitude pulmonary edema (p. 249). Fibrinoid necrosis of pulmonary arteries and arteritis are very rare in hypoxic pulmonary hypertension. Dunnill (1960) described these lesions in a patient who died from chronic bronchitis with right cardiac insufficiency. Plexiform lesions and dilatation lesions never have been reported.

Lung Tissue and Alveolar Capillaries

Even though the lung tissue with its alveolar capillaries depends heavily on aerobic metabolism, it can withstand local hypoxia remarkably well (Fisher et al., 1972; Fishman and Pietra, 1974). In individuals exposed to the low barometric pressure of high altitude, generally the lung tissue and the capillary network are morphologically normal, suggesting that their structure is not appreciably influenced by the hypoxia. In some instances, however, endothelial damage has been reported in both man and experimental animals (p. 249). Alterations of lung tissue in other conditions in which hypoxia prevails, such as chronic bronchitis, are clearly secondary to episodes of inflammation.

Pulmonary Venules and Veins

The veins and venules of the lung in chronic hypoxia have received little attention and are generally believed to be normal. However, in a series of 14 individuals from altitudes over 3000 meters we noticed prominent thickening of the venous media along with arterialization (Figure 11-10) in 5. More than average intimal fibrosis of veins and venules (Figure 11-11) was observed in 7 and the development of longitudinally arranged smooth muscle cells in the venous intima (Figure 11-12) in 2 individuals. Generally these changes were present in those patients who also had pulmonary arterial manifestations of hypoxia (Wagenvoort and Wagenvoort, 1976).

The venous alterations were even more marked in patients with chronic bronchitis. Smooth muscle cell development in the intima of pulmonary veins was encountered in the majority of these cases.

These observations could lend support to the opinion expressed by others (Kuida et al., 1963; Naeye, 1965) that to some extent hypoxia acts on pulmonary veins and venules as well as on pulmonary arteries and arterioles.

Carotid and Aortic Bodies

The function of the carotid and aortic bodies is generally supposed to be that of chemoreceptor organs, sensitive to P_{O_2}, P_{CO_2}, and pH (De Castro, 1928; Heymans et

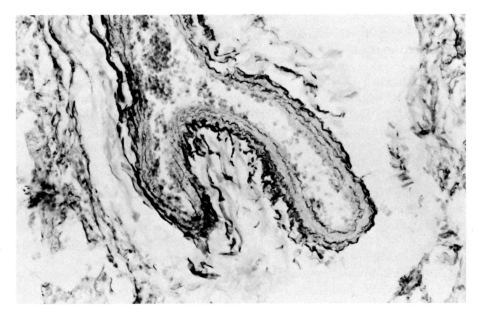

Figure 11-10. Pulmonary vein with medial hypertrophy and arterialization in a 42-year-old woman, native to an altitude of 4000 meters (El.v.G., ×230).

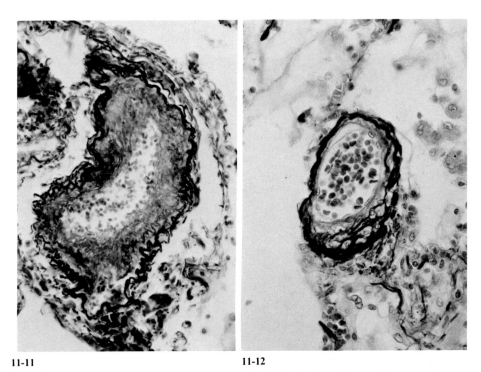

11-11   11-12

Figure 11-11. Pulmonary vein with pronounced intimal fibrosis in a 40-year-old man, native to an altitude of 4000 meters (El.v.G., ×230).
Figure 11-12. Pulmonary venule with a crescent-shaped layer of longitudinal smooth muscle cells in a 48-year-old woman, native to an altitude of 4000 meters (El.v.G., ×350).

al., 1930; Comroe, 1964), but the physiologic and morphologic implications of this concept are not easily reconciled (Becker, 1973).

The interest in these small organs recently received a new impetus by the finding that they are increased in size in states of hypoxia. This was found in individuals living at high altitudes (Arias-Stella, 1969; Arias-Stella and Valcarcel, 1973), as well as in some patients with Pickwickian syndrome or chronic bronchitis and emphysema (Figure 11-13). In the latter group there was no relation between total carotid body weight and type and severity of the emphysema (Heath et al., 1970; Edwards et al., 1971a). On the other hand, it seems that there is a correlation with the degree of right ventricular hypertrophy and thus possibly with hypoxic pulmonary hypertension (Heath, 1973).

Also in animals, hypoxia leads to an increased weight of the carotid bodies as could be demonstrated in animals collected at high altitude (Edwards et al., 1971b) as well as in animals kept in low-pressure chambers or exposed to hypoxic gas mixtures (Figure 11-14). The changes appear to be reversible after return to normal atmospheric conditions (Blessing and Wolff, 1973; Heath et al., 1973a).

The enlargement of the carotid body is caused by increase in size and possibly in number of the type I glomus cells, which show a clear cytoplasm with vacuolization, suggesting that these cells are mainly responding to the hypoxia (Edwards et al., 1971b; Blessing and Wolff, 1973; Laidler and Kay, 1975).

Recent reports have demonstrated that chronic stimulation of glomus tissue by hypoxia may eventually lead to development of carotid body tumors and

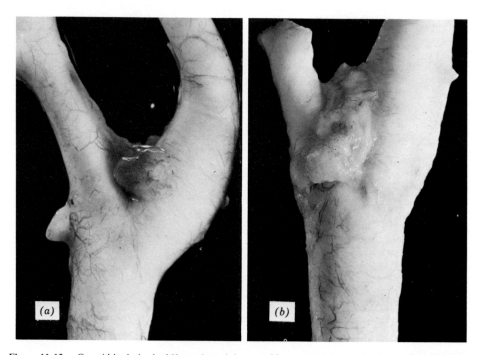

Figure 11-13.   Carotid body in the bifurcation of the carotid artery. (*a*) Normal individual, man aged 52 years. (*b*) Man, aged 71 years with chronic bronchitis and emphysema. In the latter patient the carotid body is markedly enlarged.

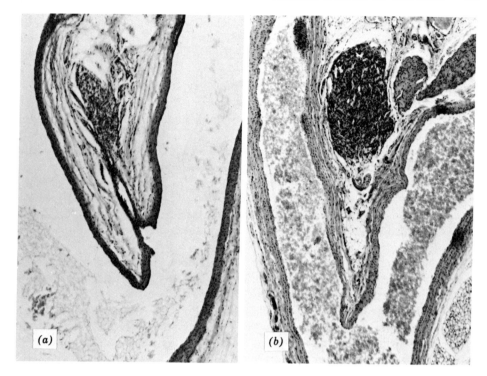

Figure 11-14. Carotid body in the bifurcation of the carotid artery of the rat. (*a*) Normal rat. (*b*) Rat exposed to hypoxia for 2 weeks. In both instances, sections are through the middle of the carotid body, which is enlarged in the hypoxic animal (H. and E., ×50).

chemodectomas. Among six patients with such tumors described by Chidid and Jao (1974), four had lung disease with chronic hypoxia. Saldana et al. (1973) reported chemodectomas in a series of 30 patients living at high altitudes in the Andes. An interesting but unexplained note to these findings was that they occurred six to seven times more often in females than in males.

VARIOUS STATES OF HYPOXIA

The mode of action of hypoxia in producing pulmonary hypertension is likely to be independent of the cause of the hypoxia. Also the effect with regard to the pulmonary vasculature is in principle the same in various situations in which hypoxia prevails. Even so it may be advantageous to review briefly the various states in which hypoxia occurs.

High Altitude

On the average, the pulmonary arterial pressure in residents of altitudes above 3000 meters is increased as compared to that of individuals living at sea level. This increase is more or less proportional to the level of altitude (Cruz-Jibaba et al.,

1964). The differences are moderate at rest. The mean pulmonary arterial pressure in young healthy individuals averaged 15 mmHg in Denver (Colorado), altitude 1600 meters, as compared to 25 mmHg in Leadville (Colorado), altitude 3100 meters (Blount and Vogel, 1967). During exercise, however, the difference becomes considerably greater. In Denver it rose from 12 to 16 mmHg at rest to 18 to 25 mmHg after exercise, but in Leadville it rose from 25 to 54 mmHg (Vogel et al., 1962). In Mexico City (altitude 2200 meters) similar mean pressures were obtained as in Denver (DeMicheli et al., 1960).

In Morococha in the Peruvian Andes at an altitude of 4500 meters, Peñaloza et al. (1962) studied a group of native residents and found mean pulmonary arterial pressures of 28 mmHg as compared to 12 mmHg in sea level subjects. These pressures rose to respectively 60 and 18 mmHg during exercise and could be reduced by administering oxygen. When natives from the Andean mountains are brought to sea level, their pressures drop but rise again upon their return to high altitude (Sime et al., 1971).

It is interesting to see that, while there is apparently a critical altitude in the range of 3000 meters at which pulmonary arterial pressures begins to rise significantly, the pressure increase at 4500 meters is not so great as would be expected. This has led to the interesting speculation that the inhabitants of the high Andes, who have lived at these altitudes for many generations, possibly have some inherited adaptation to their environment, absent in the population of Leadville, which generally lived there for only one generation (Vogel et al., 1962).

On the other hand, there are also reports that natives to the high mountain regions have higher pressures than temporary residents (Rotta et al., 1956; Peñaloza et al., 1963), although the latter group consisted of persons living for approximately one year at high altitude.

The response to high altitude hypoxia is not the same in all individuals. The usual pattern of hypoxic pulmonary hypertensive changes in the lung vessels, including medial hypertrophy of small arterioles, in contrast to the larger muscular arteries which are normal, and the presence of longitudinal muscle bundles, certainly is not always present, not even in natives who always have lived at high altitudes. In a number of cases the pulmonary vasculature in these individuals is perfectly normal, while in others medial hypertrophy of pulmonary arterioles may be very marked. There is an indication that with increasing altitudes the number of individuals with medial hypertrophy of the pulmonary arteries increases (Wagenvoort and Wagenvoort, 1973).

In newborn infants and during the first weeks of life, there are no differences in pulmonary arterial pressure between those born at high altitudes and those born at sea level. But while at sea level, pressures drop rapidly to the same levels as in adults, the high altitude infants have a much slower decrease of pulmonary arterial pressure, while their electrocardiograms show definite development of right ventricular hypertrophy (Peñaloza et al., 1960, 1963; Vogel et al., 1964).

The weight of the right ventricle in the high altitude infant at birth, is similar to that in the sea level newborn, but right ventricular hypertrophy is a regular finding in the older infants and children from high altitudes (Arias-Stella and Recavarren, 1962; Hultgren and Miller, 1965). Similarly, the pulmonary arteries and arterioles in the newborn are normal but fail to decrease their medial thickness at the same rate as sea level infants do. Therefore, there is medial hypertrophy of these arteries from the age of one month onward (Naeye, 1965; Arias-Stella and Castillo, 1966).

Individual Variability

Grover and his coworkers (1963a) have stressed that there is both a species and an individual variability in the response to high altitude hypoxia. In cattle there is a strong tendency to develop hypoxic pulmonary hypertension with vascular altera- tions (Alexander et al., 1960; Will et al., 1962; Alexander and Jensen, 1963; Grover et al., 1963b), while this is absent or minimal in sheep, cats, and rabbits (Reeves et al., 1963a,b). Individual hyper-reactivity of the pulmonary vasculature was demonstrated in cattle. One third of the animals developed pulmonary hypertension at an altitude of 3000 meters, while the others preserved pressures within normal range. At 3900 meters, however, pulmonary hypertension was present in all.

When in cattle one pulmonary artery is ligated, the mild hypoxia of an altitude of 1600 meters, may be enough for the development of progressive pulmonary hypertension (Vogel et al., 1967). Moreover, the contralateral lung may exhibit pronounced medial thickening of pulmonary arteries (Figure 11-15) (Wagenvoort et al., 1969) as compared to those in normal sea level animals (Figure 11-16) (Wagenvoort and Wagenvoort, 1969). Also these studies suggested a marked varia- tion in individual reactivity to hypoxia.

Probably there are different populations in cattle each with their own ability to adapt to high altitude environment (Cueva and Will, 1968). Weir et al. (1974) raised two stocks of cattle, one from "hyper-reactive" and one from "hyporeactive" ani- mals, for three generations. The results strongly suggested that hyper-reactivity as well as hyporeactivity in these animals was hereditarily determined. It also appeared that the influence of hypoxia on pulmonary arterial pressure was less in cattle native to high altitudes than in newcomers (Will et al., 1975).

The llama, which lives naturally on very high Andean slopes, shows complete adaptation since there is no right ventricular hypertrophy nor medial hypertrophy of large or small pulmonary arteries (Heath et al., 1974).

The significance of pulmonary vascular reaction and of pulmonary hypertension in response to hypoxia, is not well understood. Grover et al. (1963b) have suggested that the elevated pressure might have a beneficial effect in that it may result in more effective perfusion of all the areas of lung tissue, thus improving oxygen saturation of the arterial blood. This mechanism, however, would apply particularly to deep- chested animals with large hydrostatic pressures. Natural acclimatization to high altitude apparently is an extremely complex mechanism and far from being solved.

Mountain Sickness

Adaptation to high altitude hypoxia may be congenital or acquired. The presence of arterial oxygen desaturation, polycythemia, and mild pulmonary arterial hyperten- sion does not necessarily prevent an individual to pursue his physical and mental activities in the same way as others do at sea level. Such an acclimatization may be attained by people born at low altitudes, who have lived in the high mountains for a period of time, as well as by natives of high altitude areas.

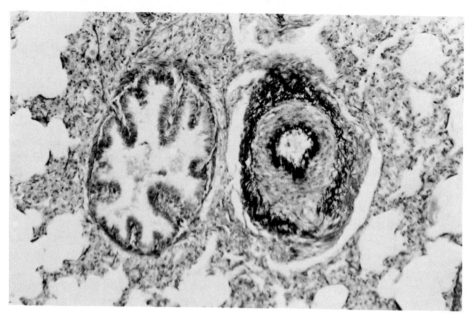

Figure 11-15. Muscular pulmonary artery with pronounced medial hypertrophy from the right lung of a young cow that was exposed to mild high altitude hypoxia after left pulmonary artery ligation (El.v.G., ×140).

The process of acclimatization, which may last from months to years, may evolve without clinical symptoms, but often produces usually mild symptoms such as shortness of breath, cyanosis, nausea, vomiting, muscular cramps, and general decrease of physical and mental fitness. This acute mountain sickness is cured by oxygen or return to sea level but may disappear spontaneously as a result of acclimatization to life at high altitude.

More severe symptoms may be present when there is maladaptation, which is not uncommon. The clinical picture varies widely and for the resulting condition, the terms chronic mountain sickness, high altitude disease, Andes disease, soroche and Monge's disease have been used. Although this disease was known, and its relation to high altitude appreciated in the Inca period, the first description of it as a clinical entity was by Monge (1928).

Chronic mountain disease, which is not uncommon above 3500 meters, may be either due to impaired acclimatization or to loss of natural adaptation, as observed in some natives of the high Andean plateaux. Good descriptions of the clinical picture have been given by Monge (1937, 1942), Hurtado (1942, 1960), Rotta et al. (1956), Peñaloza et al. (1963), and Monge and Monge (1966). The symptoms include congestion, cyanosis, headache, nausea, insomnia, paraesthesia, and impaired vision. Pulmonary arterial pressures are twice as high as in adapted high altitude residents (Saldana, 1968). Polycythemia and increased blood volume and hematocrit almost always are present.

At high altitudes hyperventilation is normal. It is an important mechanism in the adaptation, since it keeps alveolar P_{O_2} at a level of approximately 50 mmHg. In chronic mountain disease, however, there is no hyperventilation, or there may be hypoventilation, apparently due to a decreased response of the respiratory center to carbon dioxide stimulation (Hurtado, 1942, 1960).

Chronic mountain disease may abate or even be cured when the sufferer descends to sea level. This explains why very little is known about the cardiopulmonary histopathology of the entity. Arias-Stella et al. (1973a), impressed by the variety in signs and symptoms, proposed a classification of chronic mountain disease into three types. Type I, or "chronic soroche," is the process as found in individuals born at sea level who come to live in the mountains but fail to adapt. Type II, or Monge's syndrome, may occur both in native and in relatively recent residents of high altitudes but only in the presence of other organic disorders that aggravate hypoxia, such as kyphoscoliosis or obesity. Type III is designated by Arias-Stella et al. as Monge's disease. It is seen both in acclimatized and native residents of high altitude, who lost their adaptation probably by a gradual insensitivity of the respiratory center to carbon dioxide, leading to hypoventilation and further alveolar hypoxia.

There are no autopsy records of any patient falling into this last category, and Heath (cited by Arias-Stella et al., 1973a) has challenged the existence of Monge's disease as a clinicopathologic entity, although from the clinical point of view such cases are well documented.

The autopsy findings in one patient, suffering from chronic mountain disease, were described by Arias-Stella et al. (1973b), but this patient had pronounced kyphoscoliosis and, therefore, belonged to type II in their classification. The pulmonary arteries in this case showed prominent medial hypertrophy, intimal fibrosis, and multiple thrombi. Formation of thrombi with subsequent occlusion of vessels as a cause of high altitude pulmonary hypertension has been suggested by Singh and coworkers (1965, 1972). One of their arguments was that sufferers from this disease ameliorated little or not at all on descent to sea level. Peñaloza et al.

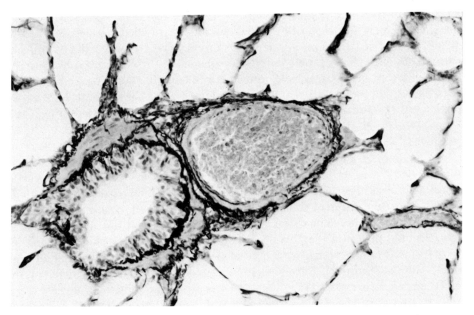

Figure 11-16. Muscular pulmonary artery with thin media from a normal sea-level cow of the same age as the animal in Figure 11-15 (El.v.G., ×140).

(1962), however, had exactly the opposite experience and, therefore, concluded that there must be an important functional factor in the elevation of pulmonary arterial pressure. Autopsy data are clearly necessary to decide this issue and the controversy over Monge's disease.

Brisket Disease

Cattle, when brought to mountainous regions over 3000 meters during the summer months, may develop a subacute illness which has been compared to chronic mountain sickness in man. This disease, first described in 1917 by Glover and Newsom (cited by Hecht et al., 1959), was shown by Hecht et al. (1959, 1962) to be related to high altitude hypoxia. While patients with chronic mountain disease rarely develop right heart failure, this is the most characteristic feature in these animals. In the late stages fluid collects in the subcutaneous tissue, particularly in the skin fold between the forelegs, the brisket. Also the lower jaw may be involved causing a characteristic and grotesque appearance. Edema often is associated with pleural effusions and ascites. The disease does not affect all herds or all animals within one herd equally. Also younger animals are particularly susceptible. The condition is often fatal unless the animals are brought to lower altitudes.

Pulmonary hypertension in the animals is reflected by marked right ventricular hypertrophy and by often severe medial hypertrophy of pulmonary arteries and arterioles along with some intimal fibrosis, particularly in the larger arteries (Alexander and Jensen, 1963b). Astrup et al. (1968) have suggested that decreased fibrinolytic activity, resulting in delayed resolution of fibrin, may be a factor in determining susceptibility of cattle to brisket disease.

High Altitude Pulmonary Edema

Sometimes at high altitudes a form of acute pulmonary edema, clearly related to hypoxia, is observed in man, although the mechanisms by which this is brought about are obscure. High altitude pulmonary edema was first described by Hurtado (1937). Since then many cases have been described from the Peruvian Andes and the United States, but particularly from the Himalaya region. These reports have drawn attention to the clinical features and hemodynamic implications (Houston, 1960; Alzamora-Castro et al., 1961; Hultgren et al., 1961, 1964, 1971; Fred et al., 1962; Wyss, 1963; Singh, 1965; Singh et al., 1965; Roy et al., 1968) and to the morphologic findings at autopsy in fatal cases (Hultgren et al., 1962; Arias-Stella and Kruger, 1963; Nayak et al., 1964). High altitude pulmonary edema may occur at any age. It is observed particularly in natives or other acclimatized residents of high altitudes, who after a stay of some days or weeks at sea level, return to their homes in the mountains. The chances for developing the condition are much greater in these categories than in sea level residents who have just arrived at high altitudes for the first time. Permanent residents and acclimatized plainsmen remaining at high altitudes are not susceptible. The higher the altitude an individual is arriving at, the greater the risk he is exposed to, although it seems that the vulnerable altitude varies in different parts of the world (Singh, 1965). Other important factors in bringing about an attack of pulmonary edema, apart from individual susceptibility (Hultgren et al., 1961), are the rapidity of ascent and particularly physical exertion and exposure to cold. Usually oxygen gives immediate relief of symptoms.

The clinical picture does not differ essentially from that observed in other cases of acute pulmonary edema. There is pronounced elevation of pulmonary arterial pressure—much higher than in normal individuals at these altitudes—while it has been shown that pulmonary venous and left atrial pressures are normal (Fred et al., 1962; Hultgren et al., 1964). Therefore, pulmonary edema is not based on left ventricular failure.

Although the mechanism by which fluid seeps out of the pulmonary vascular bed is unexplained, it has been suggested that constriction of pulmonary veins and venules results in increased capillary pressure and pulmonary edema (Fred et al., 1962). Wedge pressures, however, are normal (Hultgren et al., 1964; Roy et al., 1969). This would appear to rule out obstruction at a venous level, although Recavarren (1966) and Saldana (1968) pointed out that measurements always have been made after lung edema became manifest so that the capillary hydrostatic pressure could have decreased subsequently.

Recavarren (1966) suggested that by elevation of pulmonary arterial pressure, preterminal arterioles are opened, thus permitting this pressure to be transmitted to the capillary bed.

If pulmonary edema develops, there is usually a delay of several hours to a few days after arrival at high altitude. This fact has led to the speculation that hypoxia does not act directly on the pulmonary vasculature but that its effect is mediated via the hypothalamus, resulting in constriction of venous reservoirs in the body and in excess blood volume within the pulmonary circulation (Singh, 1965). An increased pulmonary blood volume also has been noted by Roy et al. (1968).

The role of the pulmonary capillary endothelium which may be damaged directly by hypoxia, resulting in an increased permeability, has also been stressed (Recavarren, 1966; Roy et al., 1969). Heath et al. (1973b) described changes in the endothelium of alveolar capillaries in rats, with the formation of vesicles in the cytoplasm of these cells, when the animals were kept at simulated high altitude for 12 hours.

Possibly endothelial damage is one of the factors inducing sludging of erythrocytes in alveolar capillaries and the formation of thrombi in arterioles. The latter changes have been regarded as one of the causes of pulmonary hypertension, particularly when the pressure does not come down upon removal of the patient to sea level (Singh, 1965).

The number of autopsies performed on patients who died from high altitude pulmonary edema is fairly limited. Arias-Stella and Kruger (1963) found alveolar and bronchiolar edema in two patients. In addition there were recent thrombi in capillaries and sometimes in pulmonary arterioles and arteries along with hyalin membranes in respiratory bronchioles. The histochemical composition of these membranes was the same as of those observed in newborn infants. Moreover, they described medial hypertrophy of muscular pulmonary arteries, muscularization of arterioles, and even intimal fibrosis.

Similar findings, particularly with regard to the presence of fibrin thrombi in arteries and hyalin membranes in lung tissue in these instances, have been made by Hultgren et al. (1962). Also Nayak et al. (1964) stressed the occurrence of intra-alveolar fibrin, hemorrhage, and the formation of hyalin membranes in the lungs in most of the 13 cases from which they studied material. Moreover, hyalin thrombi occurred regularly in alveolar capillaries.

Chronic Bronchitis and Emphysema

Pulmonary hypertension and heart failure may complicate severe chronic lung disease. There are several factors that cause or contribute to the elevation of pulmonary arterial pressure in various diseases of the lung. One of the factors, however, is likely to be chronic hypoxia. Particularly in some cases of chronic bronchitis and emphysema, hypoxic pulmonary hypertension may develop in a manner similar to that observed at high altitude (Evans et al., 1963; Abraham et al., 1968, 1969).

The morphologic findings in the vasculature of the lung in some of these cases are also identical to those found in patients with hypoxic pulmonary hypertension from other causes. This means that medial hypertrophy of small caliber pulmonary arteries and the development of longitudinal intimal muscle cells are the characteristic features (Hicken et al., 1965; Hasleton et al., 1968; Heath, 1970; Wagenvoort and Wagenvoort, 1973). This lends support to the view that similar mechanisms are involved in producing pulmonary hypertension in chronic hypoxia and pulmonary emphysema. The subject, however, will be discussed more extensively in connection with other forms of chronic lung disease associated with pulmonary hypertension, in Chapter Twelve.

Pickwickian Syndrome

The association of obesity, excessive appetite, somnolence, polycythemia, and cardiopulmonary disease has long been known, but the first systematic description of this syndrome was given by Sieker et al. in 1955. They reported on four patients with these symptoms. Several other cases were described within the next two years (Auchincloss et al., 1955; Burwell et al., 1956; Carroll, 1956; Counihan, 1956; Estes et al., 1957; Seide, 1957).

Burwell and his associates (1956) coined the term "Pickwickian syndrome" in reference to Charles Dickens' description of an extremely fat and somnolent youth, named Joe, who figures in *The Pickwick Papers* as Mr. Wardle's boy. The term has been criticized on the basis that it was not Mr. Pickwick who suffered from this syndrome, but it is obvious that Burwell, in proposing the term, had *The Pickwick Papers* in mind, rather than the main character of the book.

Although the term Pickwickian syndrome is well established, the syndrome itself is not always clearly defined. Burwell and associates considered shallow breathing with alveolar hypoventilation induced by extreme obesity to result in chronic hypoxia and hypercapnia. The hypercapnia would be responsible for the somnolence, although this view has been challenged (Escande et al., 1967). Somnolence was not always a symptom in patients described as suffering from the syndrome (Naeye, 1961b). Escande et al. (1967) feel that such cases should be excluded from it.

Hypoxic pulmonary hypertension which eventually may lead to cardiac failure is one of the most severe components of the Pickwickian syndrome. The condition may be reversible following weight loss (Burwell et al., 1956). Sudden death has been repeatedly reported in these patients (Counihan, 1956; Estes et al., 1957; Jenab et al., 1959; MacGregor et al., 1970; James et al., 1973).

While intrinsic cardiac or pulmonary disease is absent, right ventricular hypertrophy usually is pronounced. The muscular pulmonary arteries exhibit the same features as those in patients with other forms of chronic hypoxia. Medial hypertrophy is particularly severe in the smallest arteries and arterioles and absent or slight in the larger ones (Heath, 1963; Naeye, 1969). Longitudinal smooth muscle bundles in the intima are commonly observed (Heath, 1963; Hasleton et al., 1968). Intimal fibrosis of the pulmonary arteries is not an outstanding feature, but multiple thrombi or thromboemboli may be found in some cases (Seide, 1957; James et al., 1973).

Hypoxia Due to Muscular and Skeletal Disorders

Shallow breathing and impaired ventilation with subsequent alveolar hypoxia, in the long course, may give rise to pulmonary hypertension in patients with muscular disease involving the respiratory musculature or with deformities of the thoracic cage.

Paralysis of the respiratory musculature, which sometimes results in hypoxic pulmonary hypertension, may be related to direct damage of the respiratory center (Naeye, 1961c), to generalized muscle disease like progressive muscular dystrophy (De Fraiture, 1957; Davies and Reid, 1971), or to poliomyelitis (Lukas and Plum, 1952).

Kyphoscoliosis by whatever cause, influences the size of the lungs and their capacity to increase alveolar ventilation during exercise. The resulting hypoxia may lead to pulmonary hypertension and heart failure (Hanley et al., 1958). Davies and Reid (1971) pointed out that in children with scoliosis the limitation and distortion of the space available to the lungs in the thoracic cavity affects the growth of the lungs with decreased numbers of alveoli. Even so, in two of their four cases there was right ventricular hypertrophy and medial hypertrophy of muscular pulmonary arteries and this was attributed by them to the existing hypoxemia. Also Naeye (1961a) suggested that the combination of reduction of the pulmonary vascular bed in these small lungs and chronic hypoxemia is responsible for the changes in the pulmonary arteries and in the right ventricle. Medial hypertrophy of these arteries was mild in the case described by Davidson and Heath (1960). Later, Heath (1970) stated that in kyphoscoliosis the same features can be observed in the pulmonary vasculature as in other states of hypoxia. The occurrence of pulmonary hypertension in thoracic ankylosing spondylitis (Talbot, 1971), in which ventilation rather than the available thoracic space is restricted, suggests that hypoxia is a prominent factor in the production of pulmonary hypertension and heart failure.

Chronic Upper Airway Obstruction

Chronic upper airway obstruction due to enlarged tonsils or adenoids is common in children. The clinical syndrome in which this is combined with alveolar hypoventilation, somnolence, hypoxic pulmonary hypertension, and heart failure has been described only fairly recently (Cox et al., 1965; Menashe et al., 1965; Luke et al., 1966; Levy et al., 1967; Ainger, 1968; Gerald and Duncan, 1968). Pulmonary hypertension is reversible when tonsillectomy and adenoidectomy are performed (Menashe et al., 1965; Macartney et al., 1969). Apparently there is some racial predilection since most patients described were negroes (Bland et al., 1969). In the case described by Don and Siggers (1971), the facial deformities as part of Crouzon's disease were suggested to have contributed to the upper airway obstruction, although adenotonsillectomy resulted in improvement. Also the syndrome of Pierre-Robin, due to its cranial deformities with narrowing of the upper airways, may be associated with pulmonary hypertension (Cogswell and Easton, 1974).

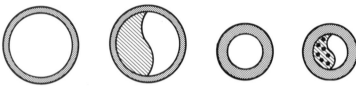

Hypoxic hypertensive vascular lesions: Muscular arteries with normal media and sometimes (in chronic lung disease) eccentric intimal fibrosis. Arterioles with medial hypertrophy and longitudinal muscle bundles in intima.

REFERENCES

Abraham, A. S., Cole, R. B., and Bishop, J. M.: Reversal of pulmonary hypertension by prolonged oxygen administration to patients with chronic bronchitis. *Circ. Res.* **23:** 147, 1968.

Abraham, A. S., Cole, R. B., Green, I. D., Hedworth-Whitty, R. B., Clarke, S. W., and Bishop, J. M.: Factors contributing to the reversible pulmonary hypertension of patients with acute respiratory failure studied by serial observations during recovery. *Circ. Res.* **24:** 51, 1969.

Abraham, A. S., Kay, J. M., Cole, R. B., and Pincock, A. C.: Haemodynamic and pathological study of the effect of chronic hypoxia and subsequent recovery of the heart and pulmonary vasculature of the rat. *Cardiovasc. Res.* **5:** 95, 1971.

Ainger, L. E.: Large tonsils and adenoids in small children with cor pulmonale. *Brit. Heart J.* **30:** 356, 1968.

Alexander, A. F., Will, D. H., Grover, R. F., and Reeves, J. T.: Pulmonary hypertension and right ventricular hypertrophy in cattle at high altitude. *Amer. J. Vet. Res.* **21:** 199, 1960.

Alexander, A. F., and Jensen, R.: Pulmonary vascular pathology of high altitude-induced pulmonary hypertension in cattle. *Amer. J. Vet. Res.* **24:** 1112, 1963a.

Alexander, A. F., and Jensen, R.: Pulmonary vascular pathology of bovine high mountain disease. *Amer. J. Vet. Res.* **24:** 1098, 1963b.

Altland, P. D., and Highman, B.: Effects of high altitude on cholesterol-fed rabbits. Production of severe pulmonary atherosclerosis with calcification. *Arch. Path.* **70:** 349, 1960.

Alzamora-Castro, V., Garrido-Lecca, G., and Battilana, G.: Pulmonary edema of high altitude. *Amer. J. Cardiol.* **7:** 769, 1961.

Arias-Stella, J.: Human carotid body at high altitude. Meet. Amer. Ass. Path. Bact., San Francisco, 1969, abstract 150.

Arias-Stella, J., and Recavarren, S.: Right ventricular hypertrophy in native children living at high altitude. *Amer. J. Path.* **41:** 55, 1962.

Arias-Stella, J., and Saldana, M.: The terminal portion of the pulmonary arterial tree in people native to high altitudes. *Circulation* **28:** 915, 1963.

Arias-Stella, J., and Kruger, H.: Pathology of high altitude pulmonary edema. *Arch. Path.* **76:** 147, 1963.

Arias-Stella, J., and Castillo, Y.: The muscular pulmonary arterial branches in stillborn natives of high altitude. *Lab. Invest.* **15:** 1951, 1966.

Arias-Stella, J., and Valcarcel, J.: The human carotid body at high altitudes. *Path. Microbiol.* **39:** 292, 1973.

Arias-Stella, J., Kruger, H., and Recavarren, S.: On the pathology of chronic mountain sickness. *Path. Microbiol.* **39:** 283, 1973a.

Arias-Stella, J., Kruger, H., and Recavarren, S.: Pathology of chronic mountain sickness. *Thorax* **28:** 701, 1973b.

Astrup, T., Glas, P., and Kok, P.: Lung fibrinolytic activity and bovine high mountain disease. *Proc. Soc. Exp. Biol. Med.* **127:** 273, 1968.

Auchincloss, J. H., Cook, E., and Renzetti, A. D.: Clinical and physiological aspects of a case of obesity, polycythemia and alveolar hypoventilation. *J. Clin. Invest.* **34:** 1537, 1955.

Aviado, D. M.: Pharmacology of the pulmonary circulation. *Pharmacol. Rev.* **12:** 159, 1960.

Aviado, D. M.: *The Lung Circulation,* vol. 1. Pergamon Press, 1965.

Aviado, D. M., Ling, J. S., and Schmidt, C. F.: Effects of anoxia on pulmonary circulation; reflex pulmonary vasoconstriction. *Amer. J. Physiol.* **189:** 253, 1957.

Aviado, D. M., Samanék, M., and Folle, L. E.: Cardiopulmonary effects of tobacco and related substances. I. Release of histamine during inhalation of cigarette smoke and anoxemia in the heart-lung and intact dog preparation. *Arch. Environ. Health* **12:** 705, 1966.

Badder, E., Magill, T., and Gump, F. E.: Regional alpha-adrenergic blockade and the pulmonary pressor response to hypoxia. *Surgery* **74:** 555, 1973.

Becker, A. E.: Normal structure, ultrastructure and enzyme content of glomic cells. *Path. Microbiol.* **39:** 287, 1973.

Bergofsky, E. H.: Mechanisms underlying vasomotor regulation of regional pulmonary blood flow in normal and disease states. *Amer. J. Med.* **57:** 378, 1974.

Bergofsky, E. H., Bass, B. G., Ferretti, R., and Fishman, A. P.: Pulmonary vasoconstriction in response to precapillary hypoxemia. *J. Clin. Invest.* **42:** 1201, 1963.

Bergofsky, E. H., and Holtzman, S.: A study of the mechanisms involved in the pulmonary arterial pressor response to hypoxia. *Circ. Res.* **20:** 506, 1967.

Bland, J. W., Edwards, F. K., and Brinsfield, D.: Pulmonary hypertension and congestive heart failure in children with chronic upper airway obstruction. New concepts of etiologic factors. *Amer. J. Cardiol.* **23:** 830, 1969.

Blessing, M. H., and Wolff, H.: The carotid bodies at simulated high altitude. *Path. Microbiol.* **39:** 310, 1973.

Blount, S. G., and Vogel, J. H. K.: Pulmonary hypertension. *Modern Conc. Cardiov. Dis.* **36:** 61, 1967.

Burwell, C. S., Robin, E. D., Whaley, R. D., and Bickelmann, A. G.: Extreme obesity associated with alveolar hypoventilation. A Pickwickian syndrome. *Amer. J. Med.* **21:** 811, 1956.

Carroll, D.: A peculiar type of cardiopulmonary failure associated with obesity. *Amer. J. Med.* **21:** 819, 1956.

Castillo, Y., Kruger, H., Arias-Stella, J., Hurtado, A., Harris, P., and Heath, D.: Histology, extensibility and chemical composition of pulmonary trunk in persons living at sea-level and at high altitude in Peru. *Brit. Heart J.* **29:** 120, 1967.

Chidid, A., and Jao, W.: Hereditary tumors of the carotid bodies and chronic obstructive pulmonary disease. *Cancer* **33:** 1635, 1974.

Cogswell, J. J., and Easton, D. M.: Cor pulmonale in the Pierre-Robin syndrome. *Arch. Dis. Childh.* **49:** 905, 1974.

Comroe, J. H.: The peripheral chemoreceptors. In *Handbook of Physiology,* section B, Respiration, vol. 1. Washington, 1964.

Counihan, T. B.: Heart failure due to extreme obesity. *Brit. Heart J.* **18:** 425, 1956.

Cournand, A.: Control of the pulmonary circulation in normal man. In J. McMichael, *Circulation.* Blackwell, Oxford, 1958.

Cox, M. A., Schiebler, G. L., Taylor, W. J., Wheat, M. W., and Krovetz, L. J.: Reversible pulmonary hypertension in a child with respiratory obstruction and cor pulmonale. *J. Pediatr.* **67:** 192, 1965.

Cruz-Jibaja, J., Banchero, N., Sime, F., Peñaloza, D., Gamboa, R., and Marticorena, E.: Correlation between pulmonary artery pressure and level of altitude. *Dis. Chest* **46**: 446, 1964.

Cueva, S., and Will, D. H.: Blood oxygen transport in cattle "susceptible" and "resistant" to high mountain disease. In *Current Research in Chronic Respiratory Disease*. Publ. Health Serv. Public. nr. 1879, 1968.

Davidson, L., and Heath, D.: Gonadal dysgenesis with cor pulmonale. *Circulation* **21**: 419, 1960.

Davies, G., and Reid, L.: Effect of scoliosis on growth of alveoli and pulmonary arteries and on right ventricle. *Arch. Dis. Childh.* **46**: 623, 1971.

De Castro, F.: Sur la structure et l'innervation du sinus carotidien de l'homme et des mammifères. Nouveaux faits sur l'innervation et la fonction du glomus caroticum. Etudes anatomiques et physiologiques. *Trab. Lab. Invest. Biol. Univ. Madrid* **25**: 331, 1928.

De Fraiture, W. H.: Een zeldzame oorzaak van chronisch cor pulmonale. *Ned. Tijdschr. Geneesk.* **101**: 399, 1957.

DeMicheli, A., Villacis, E., Guzzi, P., and Rubio, V.: Observaciones sobre los valores hemodinamicos y respiratorios obtenidos en sujetos normales. *Arch. Inst. Cardiol. Mexico* **30**: 507, 1960.

Dirken, M. N. J., and Heemstra, H.: The adaptation of the lung circulation to the ventilation. *Quart. J. Exp. Physiol.* **34**: 213, 1948a.

Dirken, M. N. J., and Heemstra, H.: Agents acting on the lung circulation. *Quart. J. Exp. Physiol.* **34**: 227, 1948b.

Don, N., and Siggers, D. C.: Cor pulmonale in Crouzon's disease. *Arch. Dis. Childh.* **46**: 394, 1971.

Doyle, J. T., Wilson, J. S., and Warren, J. V.: Pulmonary vascular responses to short-term hypoxia in human subjects. *Circulation* **5**: 263, 1952.

Duke, H. N.: Observations on the effects of hypoxia on the pulmonary vascular bed. *J. Physiol.* **135**: 45, 1957.

Duke, H. N., Killick, E. M., and Marchant, J. V.: Changes in pH of the perfusate during hypoxia in isolated perfused cat lungs. *J. Physiol.* **153**: 413, 1960.

Dunnill, M. S.: Fibrinoid necrosis in the branches of the pulmonary artery in chronic non-specific lung disease. *Brit. J. Dis. Chest* **54**: 355, 1960.

Edwards, C., Heath, D., and Harris, P.: The carotid body in emphysema and left ventricular hypertrophy. *J. Path.* **104**: 1, 1971a.

Edwards, C., Heath, D., Harris, P., Castillo, Y., Kruger, H., and Arias-Stella, J.: The carotid body in animals at high altitude. *J. Path.* **104**: 231, 1971b.

Escande, J.-P., Schwartz, B.-A., Gentilini, M., Hazard, J., Choubrac, P., and Domart, A.: Le syndrome Pickwickien. *Presse Méd.* **75**: 1607, 1967.

Estes, E. H., Sieker, H. O., McIntosh, H. D., and Kelser, G. A.: Reversible cardiopulmonary syndrome with extreme obesity. *Circulation* **16**: 179, 1957.

Evans, T. O., van der Reis, L. and Selzer, A.: Circulatory effects of chronic pulmonary emphysema. *Amer. Heart J.* **66**: 741, 1963.

Fisher, A. B., Hyde, R. W., and Reif, J. S.: Insensitivity of the alveolar septum to local hypoxia. *Amer. J. Physiol.* **223**: 770, 1972.

Fishman, A. P.: Respiratory gases in the regulation of the pulmonary circulation. *Physiol. Rev.* **41**: 214, 1961.

Fishman, A. P.: Hypoxia on the pulmonary circulation. How and where it acts. *Circ. Res.* **38**: 221, 1976.

Fishman, A. P., McClement, J., Himmelstein, A., and Cournand, A.: Effects of acute anoxia on the circulation and respiration in patients with chronic pulmonary disease studied during the "steady state." *J. Clin. Invest.* **31**: 770, 1952.

Fishman, A. P., Himmelstein, A., Fritts, H. W., and Cournand, A.: Blood flow through each lung in man during unilateral hypoxia. *J. Clin. Invest.* **34**: 637, 1955.

Fishman, A. P., Fritts, H. W., and Cournand, A.: Effects of breathing carbon dioxide upon the pulmonary circulation. *Circulation* **22**: 220, 1960.

Fishman, A. P., and Pietra, G. G.: Handling of bioactive materials by the lung. *New Engl. J. Med.* **291**: 884, 953, 1974.

Fred, H. L., Schmidt, A. M., Bates, T., and Hecht, H. H.: Acute pulmonary edema of altitude. Clinical and physiological observations. *Circulation* **25**: 929, 1962.

Fritts, H. W., Harris, P., Clauss, R. H., Odell, J. E., and Cournand, A.: The effect of acetylcholine on the human pulmonary circulation under normal and hypoxic conditions. *J. Clin. Invest.* **37**: 99, 1958.

Fritts, H. W., Odell, J. E., Harris, P., Braunwald, E. W., and Fishman, A. P.: Effects of acute hypoxia on the volume of blood in the thorax. *Circulation* **22**: 216, 1960.

Gerald, B., and Duncan, W. T.: Cor pulmonale and pulmonary edema in children secondary to chronic upper airway obstruction. *Radiology* **90**: 679, 1968.

Grover, R. F., Vogel, J. H. K., Averill, K. H., and Blount, S. G.: Pulmonary hypertension. Individual and species variability relative to vascular reactivity. *Amer. Heart J.* **66**: 1, 1963a.

Grover, R. F., Reeves, J. T., Will, D. H., and Blount, S. G.: Pulmonary vasoconstriction in steers at high altitude. *J. Appl. Physiol.* **18**: 567, 1963b.

Hanley, T., Platts, M. M., Clifton, M., and Morris, T. L.: Heart failure of the hunchback. *Quart. J. Med.* (n.s.) **27**: 155, 1958.

Harris, P.: Influence of acetylcholine on the pulmonary arterial pressure. *Brit. Heart J.* **29**: 272, 1957.

Harris, P.: The pharmacology of some naturally occurring substances in the human pulmonary circulation. *Progr. Resp. Res.* **5**: 100, 1970.

Harris, P., and Heath, D.: *The Human Pulmonary Circulation. Its Form and Function in Health and Disease.* E. & S. Livingstone, Ltd., Edinburgh, London, 1962.

Hasleton, P. S., Heath, D., and Brewer, D. B.: Hypertensive pulmonary vascular disease in states of chronic hypoxia. *J. Path. Bact.* **95**: 431, 1968.

Hauge, A.: Role of histamine in hypoxic pulmonary hypertension in the rat. I. Blockade or potentiation of endogenous amines, kinins and ATP. *Circ. Res.* **22**: 371, 1968.

Hauge, A.: The pulmonary vasoconstrictor response to acute hypoxia. Studies on mechanism and site of action. *Progr. Resp. Res.* **5**: 145, 1970.

Hauge, A., and Staub, N. C.: Prevention of hypoxic vasoconstriction in cat lung by histamine-releasing agent 48/80. *J. Appl. Physiol.* **26**: 693, 1969.

Heath, D.: Longitudinal muscle in pulmonary arteries. *J. Path. Bact.* **85**: 407, 1963.

Heath, D.: Hypoxic hypertensive pulmonary vascular disease. *Progr. Resp. Res.* **5**: 13, 1970.

Heath, D.: The histological features and physical characteristics of the pulmonary trunk at high altitude. *Path. Microbiol.* **38**: 266, 1972.

Heath, D.: The carotid body in human cardiopulmonary disease. *Path. Microbiol.* **39**: 305, 1973.

Heath, D., Harris, P., Castillo, Y., and Arias-Stella, J.: Histology, extensibility and chemical composition of the pulmonary trunk of dogs, sheep, cattle and llamas living at high altitude. *J. Path. Bact.* **96**: 161, 1968.

Heath, D., Edwards, C., and Harris, P.: Post-mortem size and structure of the human carotid body. Its relation to pulmonary disease and cardiac hypertrophy. *Thorax* **25**: 129, 1970.

Heath, D., Edwards, C., Winson, M., and Smith, P.: Effects on the right ventricle, pulmonary vasculature, and carotid bodies of the rat of exposure to, and recovery from, simulated high altitude. *Thorax* **28**: 24, 1973a.

Heath, D., Moosavi, H., and Smith, P.: Ultrastructure of high altitude pulmonary oedema. *Thorax* **28**: 694, 1973b.

Heath, D., Smith, P., Williams, D., Harris, P., Arias-Stella, J., and Kruger, H.: The heart and pulmonary vasculature of the llama (Lama glama). *Thorax* **29**: 463, 1974.

Hecht, H. H., Lange, R. L., Carnes, W. H., Kuida, H., and Blake, J. T.: Brisket disease. I. General aspects of pulmonary hypertensive heart disease in cattle. *Transact. Ass. Amer. Physic.* **72**: 157, 1959.

Hecht, H. H., Kuida, H., Lange, R. L., Thorne, J. L., and Brown, A. M.: Brisket disease. II. Clinical features and hemodynamic observations in altitude-dependent right heart failure of cattle. *Amer. J. Med.* **32**: 171, 1962.

Heymans, C., Bouckaert, J. J., and Dautrebande, L.: Sinus carotidien et réflexes respiratoires. II. Influences respiratoires réflexes de l'acidose, de l'alcalose, de l'anhydride carbonique, d l'ion hydrogène et de l'anoxémie. Sinus carotidien et échanges respiratoires dans les poumons et au-delà des poumons. *Arch. Int. Pharmacodyn.* **39**: 400, 1930.

Hicken, P., Heath, D., Brewer, D. B., and Whitaker, W.: The small pulmonary arteries in emphysema. *J. Path. Bact.* **90**: 107, 1965.

Houston, C. S.: Acute pulmonary edema of high altitude. *New Engl. J. Med.* **263**: 478, 1960.

Hultgren, H. N., Spickard, W. B., Hellriegel, K., and Houston, C. S.: High altitude pulmonary edema. *Medicine* **40**: 289, 1961.

Hultgren, H. N., Spickard, W. B., and Lopez, C. E.: Further studies of high altitude pulmonary oedema. *Brit. Heart J.* **24**: 95, 1962.

Hultgren, H. N., Marticorena, E., and Miller, H.: Right ventricular hypertrophy in animals at high altitude. *J. Appl. Physiol.* **18**: 913, 1963.

Hultgren, H. N., Lopez, C. E., Lundberg, E., and Miller, H.: Physiologic studies of pulmonary edema at high altitude. *Circulation* **29**: 393, 1964.

Hultgren, H. N., and Miller, H.: Right ventricular hypertrophy at high altitude. *Ann. N.Y. Acad. Sci.* **127**: 627, 1965.

Hultgren, H. N., and Miller, H.: Human heart weight at high altitude. *Circulation* **35**: 207, 1967.

Hultgren, H. N., Grover, R. F., and Hartley, L. H.: Abnormal circulatory responses to high altitude in subjects with a previous history of high-altitude pulmonary edema. *Circulation* **44**: 759, 1971.

Hurtado, A.: Aspectos fisiopatologicos y patologicos de la vida en la altura. Lima, 1937.

Hurtado, A.: Chronic mountain sickness. *J.A.M.A.* **120**: 1278, 1942.

Hurtado, A.: Some clinical aspects of life at high altitudes. *Ann. Int. Med.* **53**: 247, 1960.

James, W. R. L., and Thomas, A. J.: The effect of hypoxia on the heart and pulmonary arterioles of mice. *Cardiovasc. Res.* **2**: 278, 1968.

James. T. N., Frame, B., and Coates, E. O.: De subitaneis mortibus. III. Pickwickian syndrome. *Circulation* **48**: 1311, 1973.

Jamieson, A. G.: Gaseous diffusion from alveoli into pulmonary arteries. *J. Appl. Physiol.* **19**: 448, 1964.

Jenab, M., Lade, R. I., Chiga, M., and Diehl, A. M.: Cardio-respiratory syndrome of obesity in a child. *Pediatrics* **24**: 23, 1959.

Kalemi, A., Bruschke, P. E., and Parsons, E. F.: Role of the autonomic nervous system in hypoxic response of the pulmonary vascular bed. *Resp. Physiol.* **15**: 245, 1972.

Kay, J. M., and Smith, P.: The small pulmonary arteries in rats at simulated high altitude. *Path. Microbiol.* **39**: 270, 1973.

Kay, J. M., Waymire, J. C., and Grover, R. F.: Lung mast cell hyperplasia and pulmonary histamine-forming capacity in hypoxic rats. *Amer. J. Physiol.* **226**: 178, 1974.

Kuida, H., Tsagaris, T. J., and Hecht, H. H.: Evidence for pulmonary venoconstriction in brisket disease. *Circ. Res.* **12**: 182, 1963.

Laidler, P., and Kay, J. M.: The effect of chronic hypoxia on the number and nuclear diameter of type I cells in the carotid bodies of rats. *Amer. J. Path.* **79**: 311, 1975.

Levy, A. M., Tabakin, B. S., Hanson, J. S., and Nakewicz, R. M.: Hypertrophied adenoids causing pulmonary hypertension and severe congestive failure. *New Engl. J. Med.* **277**: 506, 1967.

Lewis, B. M., Gorlin, R., Houssay, H. E. J., Haynes, F. W., and Dexter, L.: Clinical and physiological correlations in patients with mitral stenosis. *Amer. Heart J.* **43**: 2, 1952.

Lloyd, T. C.: Role of nerve pathways in the hypoxic vasoconstriction of lung. *J. Appl. Physiol.* **21**: 1351, 1966.

Lukas, D. S., and Plum, F.: Pulmonary function in patients convalescing from acute poliomyelitis with respiratory paralysis. *Amer. J. Med.* **12**: 388, 1952.

Luke, M. J., Mehrizi, A., Folger, G. M., and Rowe, R. D.: Chronic nasopharyngeal obstruction as a cause of cardiomegaly, cor pulmonale, and pulmonary edema. *Pediatrics* **37**: 762, 1966.

Macartney, F. J., Panday, J., and Scott, O.: Cor pulmonale as a result of chronic nasopharyngeal obstruction due to hypertrophied tonsils and adenoids. *Arch. Dis. Childh.* **44**: 585, 1969.

MacGregor, M. I., Block, A. J., and Ball, W. C.: Serious complications and sudden death in the Pickwickian syndrome. *Johns Hopk. Med. J.* **126**: 279, 1970.

Menashe, V. D., Farrchi, C., and Miller, M.: Hypoventilation and cor pulmonale due to chronic upper airway obstruction. *J. Pediatr.* **57**: 198, 1965.

Monge, C.: Enfermedad de los Andes. Estudio fisiologico. *An. Fac. Med.* Lima **11**: 1, 1928.

Monge, C.: High altitude disease. *Arch. Int. Med.* **59**: 32, 1937.

Monge, C.: Life in the Andes and chronic moutain sickness. *Science* **95**: 79, 1942.

Monge, C., and Monge, C. C.: *High Altitude Diseases. Mechanism and Management.* Charles C Thomas, Springfield, Ill., 1966.

Motley, H. L., Cournand, A., Werko, L., Himmelstein, A., and Dresdale, D.: Influence of short periods of induced acute anoxia upon pulmonary artery pressures in man. *Amer. J. Physiol.* **150**: 315, 1947.

Mungall, I. P. F.: Hypoxia and lung mast cells: influence of disodium cromoglytate. *Thorax* **31**: 94, 1976.

Naeye, R. L.: Kyphoscoliosis and cor pulmonale. A study of the pulmonary vascular bed. *Amer. J. Path.* **38**: 561, 1961a.

Naeye, R. L.: Hypoxemia and pulmonary hypertension. *Arch. Path.* **71**: 447, 1961b.

Naeye, R. L.: Alveolar hypoventilation and cor pulmonale secondary to damage to the respiratory center. *Amer. J. Cardiol.* **8**: 416, 1961c.

Naeye, R. L.: Pulmonary vascular changes with chronic unilateral pulmonary hypoxia. *Circ. Res.* **17**: 160, 1965.

Naeye, R. L.: Alveolar hypoxia, differential effects on pulmonary arteries of varied size. *Exper. Biol. Med.* **132**: 558, 1969.

Nayak, N. C., Roy, S., and Narayanan, T. K.: Pathologic features of altitude sickness. *Amer. J. Path.* **45**: 381, 1964.

Peñaloza, D., Gamboa, R., Dyer, J., Echavarria, M., and Marticorena, E.: The influence of high altitudes on the electrical activity of the heart. I. Electrocardiographic and vectorcardiographic observations in the newborn, infants and children. *Amer. Heart J.* **59**: 111, 1960.

Peñaloza, D., Sime, F., Banchero, N., and Gamboa, R.: Pulmonary hypertension in healthy man born and living at high altitudes. *Med. Thorac.* **19**: 257, 1962.

Peñaloza, D., Sime, F., Banchero, N., Gamboa, R., Cruz, J., and Marticorena, E.: Pulmonary hypertension in healthy man born and living at high altitudes. *Amer. J. Cardiol.* **11**: 150, 1963.

Recavarren, S.: Editorial. The preterminal arterioles in the pulmonary circulation of high-altitude natives. *Circulation* **33**: 177, 1966.

Recavarren, S., and Arias-Stella, J.: Right ventricular hypertrophy in people born and living at high altitudes. *Brit. Heart J.* **26**: 806, 1964.

Reeves, J. T., Grover, E. B., and Grover, R. F.: Pulmonary circulation and oxygen transport in lambs at high altitude. *J. Appl. Physiol.* **18**: 560, 1963a.

Reeves, J. T., Grover, E. B., and Grover, R. F.: Circulatory responses to high altitude in the cat and rabbit. *J. Appl. Physiol.* **18**: 575, 1963b.

Reeves, J. T., and Leathers, J. E.: Hypoxic pulmonary hypertension of the calf with denervation of the lungs. *J. Appl. Physiol.* **19**: 976, 1964.

Reeves, J. T., Tucker, A., McMurtry, I., Alexander, A. F., Will, D. F., and Grover, R. F.: Lung mast cell hyperplasia at high altitude. *Circulation* **50** (suppl. 3): 50, 1974.

Riley, R. L., Himmelstein, A., Motley, H. L., Weiner, H. M., and Cournand, A.: Studies of the pulmonary circulation at rest and during exercise in normal individuals and in patients with chronic pulmonary disease. *Amer. J. Physiol.* **152**: 372, 1948.

Rotta, A., Canepa, A., Hurtado, A., Velasquez, T., and Chavez, R.: Pulmonary circulation at sea level and at high altitude. *J. Appl. Physiol.* **9**: 328, 1956.

Roy, S. B., Guleria, J. S., Khanna, P. K., Talwar, J. H., Manchanda, S. C., Pande, J. N., Kaushik, V. S., Subba, P. S., and Wood, J. E.: Immediate circulatory response to high altitude hypoxia in man. *Nature* **217**: 1177, 1968.

Roy, S. B., Guleria, J. S., Khanna, P. K., Manchanda, S. C., Pande, J. N., and Subba, P. S.: Haemodynamic studies in high altitude pulmonary oedema. *Brit. Heart J.* **31**: 52, 1969.

Saldana, M.: Normal cardiopulmonary structure and function and related clinical conditions in people native to high altitudes, In Liebow, A. A., and Smith, D. E., *The Lung.* Williams & Wilkins, Baltimore, 1968.

Saldana, M., and Arias-Stella, J.: Studies on the structure of the pulmonary trunk. II. The evolution of the elastic configuration of the pulmonary trunk in people native to high altitude. *Circulation* **27:** 1094, 1963a.

Saldana, M., and Arias-Stella, J.: Studies on the structure of the pulmonary trunk. III. The thickness of the media of the pulmonary trunk and ascending aorta in high altitude natives. *Circulation* **27:** 1101, 1963b.

Saldana, M. J., Salem, L. E., and Travezan, R.: High altitude hypoxia and chemodectomas. *Human Path.* **4:** 251, 1973.

Seide, M. J.: Heart failure due to extreme obesity. *New Engl. J. Med.* **257:** 1227, 1957.

Sieker, H. O., Estes, E. H., Kelser, G. A., and McIntosh, H. D.: A cardiopulmonary syndrome associated with extreme obesity. *J. Clin. Invest.* **34,** 916, 1955.

Silove, E. D., and Grover, R. F.: Effects of alpha adrenergic blockade and tissue catecholamine depletion on pulmonary vascular response to hypoxia. *J. Clin. Invest.* **47:** 274, 1968.

Sime, F., Peñaloza, D., and Ruis, L.: Bradycardia, increased cardiac output, and reversal of pulmonary hypertension in altitude natives living at sea level. *Brit. Heart J.* **33:** 647, 1971.

Singh, I.: High-altitude pulmonary edema. *Amer. Heart J.* **70:** 435, 1965.

Singh, I., Khanna, P. K., Lal, M., Hoon, R. S., and Rao, B. D. P.: High-altitude pulmonary hypertension. *Lancet* **2:** 146, 1965.

Singh, I., and Chohan, I. S.: Blood coagulation changes at high altitude predisposing to pulmonary hypertension. *Brit. Heart J.* **34:** 611, 1972.

Smith, D. J., and Coxe, J. W.: Reaction of isolated pulmonary blood vessels to anoxia, epinephrine, acetylcholine and histamine. *Amer. J. Physiol.* **167:** 732, 1951.

Smith, P., Moosavi, H., Winson, M., and Heath, D.: The influence of age and sex on the response of the right ventricle, pulmonary vasculature and carotid bodies to hypoxia in rats. *J. Path.* **112:** 11, 1974.

Staub, N.: Gas exchange vessels in the cat lung. *Fed. Proc.* **20:** 107, 1961.

Stroud, R. C., and Conn, H. L.: Pulmonary vascular effects of moderate and severe hypoxia in the dog. *Amer. J. Physiol.* **179:** 119, 1954.

Susmano, A., and Carleton, R. A.: Effect of antihistaminic drugs on hypoxic pulmonary hypertension. *Amer. J. Cardiol.* **31:** 718, 1973.

Talbot, S.: Cor pulmonale in ankylosing spondylitis. *Brit. J. Clin. Pract.* **25:** 491, 1971.

Tyler, T., Wallis, R., Leffler, C., and Cassin, S.: The effects of indomethacin on the pulmonary vascular response to hypoxia in the premature and mature newborn goat. *Proc. Soc. Exp. Biol. Med.* **150:** 695, 1975.

Urbanova, D., Ressl, J., Widimsky, J., Ostadal, B., Pelouch, V., and Prochazka, J.: Pulmonary vascular changes induced by intermittent altitude hypoxia and their reversibility in rat. *Beitr. Path.* **150:** 389, 1973.

Valdivia, E.: Right ventricular hypertrophy in guinea pigs exposed to simulated high altitude. *Circ. Res.* **5:** 612, 1957.

Valenca, L. M., Lincoln, J. C. R., Strieder, D. J., and Kazemi, H.: Pulmonary vascular response of the reimplanted dog lung to hypoxia. *J. Thorac. Cardiovasc. Surg.* **61:** 857, 1971.

Vogel, J. H. K., Weaver, W. F., Rose, R. L., Blount, S. G., and Grover, R. F.: Pulmonary hypertension on exertion in normal man living at 10,150 feet (Leadville, Colorado). *Med. Thorac.* **19:** 269, 1962.

Vogel, J. H. K., Pryor, R., and Blount, S. G.: The cardiovascular system in children from high altitude. *J. Pediatr.* **64:** 315, 1964.

Vogel, J. H. K., McNamara, D. G., and Blount, S. G.: Role of hypoxia in determining pulmonary vascular resistance in infants with ventricular septal defects. *Amer. J. Cardiol.* **20:** 346, 1967.

Von Euler, U. S., and Liljestrand, G.: Observations on the pulmonary arterial blood pressure in the cat. *Acta Physiol. Scand.* **12:** 301, 1946.

Wagenvoort, C. A., and Wagenvoort, N.: The pulmonary vasculature in normal cattle at sea level at different ages. *Path. Europ.* **4:** 265, 1969.

Wagenvoort, C. A., Wagenvoort, N., and Vogel, J. H. K.: The pulmonary vasculature in cattle in an altitude of 1600 metres with and without one-sided pulmonary arterial ligation. *J. Comparat. Path.* **79:** 517, 1969.

Wagenvoort, C. A., and Wagenvoort, N.: Hypoxic pulmonary vascular lesions in man at high altitude and in patients with chronic respiratory disease. *Path. Microbiol.* **39:** 276, 1973.

Wagenvoort, C. A., and Wagenvoort, N.: Pulmonary venous changes in chronic hypoxia. *Virch. Arch. A Path. Anat. Histol.* **1976** (in press).

Weir, E. K., Tucker, A., Reeves, J. T., Will, D. H., and Grover, R. F.: The genetic factor influencing pulmonary hypertension in cattle at high altitude. *Cardiovasc. Res.* **8:** 745, 1974.

Westcott, R. N., Fowler, N. O., Scott, R. C., Havenstein, V. D., and McGrure, J.: Anoxia and human pulmonary vascular resistance. *J. Clin. Invest.* **30:** 957, 1951.

Wilcox, B. R., Austen, G., and Bender, H. W.: Effect of hypoxia on pulmonary artery pressure of dogs. *Amer. J. Physiol.* **207:** 1314, 1964.

Will, J. A., and Kay, J. M.: Hypertensive pulmonary vascular disease associated with papain emphysema in rats. *Respiration* **31:** 208, 1974.

Will, D. H., Alexander, A. F., Reeves, J. T., and Grover, R. F.: High altitude-induced pulmonary hypertension in normal cattle. *Circ. Res.* **10:** 172, 1962.

Will, D. H., Horrell, J. F., Reeves, J. T., and Alexander, A. F.: Influence of altitude and age on pulmonary arterial pressure in cattle. *Proc. Soc. Exp. Biol. Med.* **150:** 564, 1975.

Wyss, S.: Lungenödem in Hochgebirge. *Cardiologia* **42:** 132, 1963.

Zakheim, R. M., Mattioli, L., Molteni, A., Mullis, K. B., and Bartley, J.: Prevention of pulmonary vascular changes of chronic alveolar hypoxia by inhibition of angiotensin I-converting enzyme in the rat. *Lab. Invest.* **33:** 57, 1975.

CHAPTER TWELVE

Pulmonary Hypertension in Lung Diseases

A great variety of lung conditions affect the pulmonary circulation and may cause pulmonary hypertension. This group of diseases is heterogeneous, not only in their etiology and in the mechanisms that cause the elevation of pulmonary arterial pressure but also with regard to the incidence of the resulting "cor pulmonale" and right cardiac insufficiency.

The term cor pulmonale often has had a confusing meaning. It has been defined by an expert committee of the World Health Organization (1961), which described it as "hypertrophy of the right ventricle resulting from diseases affecting the function and/or the structure of the lung, except when these pulmonary alterations are the result of diseases that primarily affect the left side of the heart or of congenital heart disease."

Although still widely used by the clinicians, for several reasons, the term cor pulmonale is not very satisfactory. It indicates a response of the right side of the heart to a large variety of diseases affecting the lungs, including such widely differing conditions as chronic bronchitis, tuberculosis, embolism, schistosomiasis, primary pulmonary hypertension, and pulmonary veno-occlusive disease. Although it is essentially a clinical term, the clinician usually can at best suspect right ventricular hypertrophy, which means that he is unable to make a firm diagnosis of cor pulmonale. At autopsy, the pathologist can adequately establish right ventricular hypertrophy, or—maybe better—an increased right ventricular mass, at least when he relies on the weights of free right and left ventricular walls and interventricular septum rather than on measurement of wall thickness, but he will not use the term cor pulmonale.

For the pathologist, another difficulty is that a clearly recognizable vascular pattern as plexogenic pulmonary arteriopathy should cause cor pulmonale when it is due to primary pulmonary hypertension or to hepatic injury but not when it is due to a cardiac left to right shunt. Also it is hard to visualize that perfectly healthy accli-matized individuals in high altitude regions should all suffer from cor pulmonale, since they tend to have right ventricular hypertrophy and changes in their lung vessels.

For these reasons it would be advisable that "cor pulmonale" be dismissed from our clinical terminology. Instead the clinician should speak of sustained pulmonary hypertension and the pathologist of right ventricular hypertrophy and pulmonary vascular alterations, while both should indicate the underlying cause, if known.

A number of diseases, falling under the above definition of chronic cor pulmonale, have been dealt with in previous chapters. In the remaining forms of lung disease, to be discussed in this chapter, pulmonary hypertension if it develops, is usually related to disturbances in respiratory function. These may result from obstruction to air flow within bronchi or bronchioli, to impairment of gas exchange by alterations in the alveolar walls, to a reduced ventilation-perfusion ratio in the presence of atelectasis or arteriovenous shunts, or to combinations of these disturbances. Moreover, in some cases the rise in pressure is due in part or entirely to involvement of the pulmonary arteries and arterioles or pulmonary veins. This is seen in some forms of vasculitis, usually as part of systemic diseases that also may affect the lungs. Malignant infiltration of the lungs in some instances also causes pulmonary vascular obstruction.

We therefore will consider in this chapter the following conditions.

   I. Chronic bronchitis and emphysema and bronchial asthma
  II. Bronchiectasis
III. Pulmonary granulomas and fibrosis
     A. Tuberculosis
     B. Interstitial fibrosis
        1. Pulmonary infections other than tuberculosis
        2. The various collagen diseases
        3. Lung diseases of unknown etiology
        4. Radiation fibrosis
        5. Chemical and toxic injury
     C. Pneumoconioses
 IV. Malignant infiltration

CHRONIC BRONCHITIS AND EMPHYSEMA

Among the most common forms of lung disease causing pulmonary hypertension are chronic bronchitis and emphysema, alone or in combination.

Chronic bronchitis is characterized clinically by chronic excessive bronchial mucus secretion and productive coughing and morphologically by an increase in goblet cells and mucous glands with infiltration of the bronchial walls by inflamma-tory cells. Swelling of the mucosa by inflammation, plugging by mucus and scarring of the bronchi and bronchioli, may cause narrowing of their lumina and thus obstruction of the airway, which is influenced little or not at all by bronchodilator drugs.

Emphysema, according to the definition of the World Health Organization (1961), is characterized anatomically by an abnormal increase in size of air spaces distal to the terminal bronchioles with destructive changes in their walls. Chronic airway obstruction is present in the more severe cases. These patients have progressively increasing dyspnea with or without chronic cough.

The reason that both conditions are dealt with together, is that many patients suffer from both chronic bronchitis and pulmonary emphysema at the same time, although there are patients with emphysema alone and even more with chronic bronchitis alone.

Right ventricular hypertrophy and cardiac failure commonly complicate chronic obstructive lung disease, although pulmonary hypertension is reversible (Harvey et al., 1951) and usually labile and mild except during attacks of acute respiratory infection with respiratory failure (Harris et al., 1968). It may be absent even in severe cases of panacinar emphysema (Spencer, 1968a). There is much controversy as to what causes elevation of pulmonary arterial pressure in patients with chronic bronchitis and emphysema. The problem is enhanced by the fact that there are two different clinical types of these patients—the "emphysematous" and the "bronchial" (Filley et al., 1968; Schüren and Hütteman, 1972).

In the first group morphologic emphysema is often severe with prominent overdistension of lung tissue and low diffusing capacity, while cough is usually slight. These patients tend to hyperventilate and often keep their oxygen saturation relatively normal. The patients in the second group usually have a history of recurrent respiratory infections with cough and production of abundant, often purulent, sputum. These have hypercapnia, severe hypoxemia, and cyanosis. The terms "pink puffers" and "blue bloaters" (Scadding, 1963; Mitchell et al., 1966) have been used to designate the two types. Right cardiac hypertrophy and failure are rare in the first and frequent in the second type (Burrows et al., 1964).

It has long been believed that in patients with pulmonary emphysema, the rise in pulmonary arterial pressure is caused by the destruction of alveolar capillaries. This concept, however, does not take into account the enormous number of capillaries within the lungs and the great reserve capacity of the pulmonary capillary bed. Even when there is marked loss of capillary networks, the majority of the pulmonary arterioles and venules remain patent and, although they may have lost many of their side-branches, these vessels apparently still supply and drain blood to and from the capillary bed (Reid and Heard, 1962, 1963). Also, whereas capillary networks disappear, some large flow capillaries may take over or may be formed, directing the flow to the pulmonary veins (Junghanss, 1959; Wyatt et al., 1961). Shunting at capillary level also was established by Oderr (1960).

There is no relationship between the degree of right ventricular hypertrophy and the severity of pulmonary emphysema (Cromie, 1961; Hicken et al., 1966a,b). Data collected by Heard (1969) gave the impression that the total heart weight tended to be less with increasing severity of emphysema. Thus it is clear that destruction of alveolar capillaries, although it probably contributes to the increased pulmonary vascular resistance in some severe cases of emphysema, is not a main factor in the production of pulmonary hypertension.

An increased cardiac output has been held responsible for the developing right ventricular hypertrophy in patients with pulmonary emphysema (Howarth et al.,

1947), but it has been shown that in many patients it is normal or even reduced and generally it does not seem to contribute to the elevated pressure (Wade and Bishop, 1962; Evans et al., 1963).

Thrombotic occlusion, primary or secondary to embolism, is found commonly in emphysematous lungs (McLean, 1958; Ryan, 1963; Bignon et al., 1970), but it is unlikely to be an important mechanism in raising the pulmonary arterial pressure. Kernen et al. (1958) found that the incidence of thromboembolism was the same in emphysematous patients with and without right ventricular hypertrophy. Dunnill (1961) believed that deformity and elongation of pulmonary arterial branches by pressure of adjacent emphysematous spaces is an important factor in elevating the pressure.

It seems likely that hypoxia plays a predominant part in the production of pulmonary hypertension (Harvey et al., 1951; Abraham et al., 1969). This would explain why right ventricular hypertrophy is observed more often in patients with the "bronchial" type of emphysema and also why it is far more common in centrilobular than in panacinar emphysema (Leopold and Gough, 1957). In centrilobular emphysema there is usually bronchiolitis, which in fact is regarded as the cause of this type of emphysema (Gough, 1965).

While there is a distinct correlation between chronic airway obstruction and pulmonary arterial pressure in patients with chronic bronchitis, there is no unanimity as to the significance of hypoxia for the increase in pulmonary vascular resistance. Administering pure oxygen produces little or no decrease in pulmonary arterial pressure (Denolin, 1961). Harris et al. (1968) believe that compression of blood vessels with displacement of the blood due to high alveolar and intrathoracic pressure rather than hypoxic vasoconstriction is basic to the rise in pressure. On the other hand, it has been shown that continuous administration of pure oxygen for periods from 4 to 8 weeks caused complete reversal of pulmonary hypertension in patients with chronic bronchitis (Abraham et al., 1968).

While these physiologic considerations are awaiting further clarification, it must be stated that from the morphologic point of view the pulmonary vascular alterations in chronic bronchitis and emphysema often resemble closely those found in various forms of chronic hypoxia.

Smoking

Cigarette smoking is an important factor in the etiology of chronic bronchitis (Thurlbeck and Angus, 1964). Even in the absence of clinical symptoms, heavy smoking is reported to cause pulmonary vascular changes that are not unlike those observed in chronic bronchitis (Auerbach et al., 1963; Naeye and Dellinger, 1971; Naeye et al., 1974).

Bronchial Asthma

Bronchial asthma is a recognized, although rare cause of cor pulmonale. If heart failure develops, it is usually in cases complicated by chronic bronchitis or recurrent respiratory infections. In these instances the morphology of the pulmonary vasculature is the same as in other patients with chronic obstructive airways disease.

Morphology

The pulmonary trunk in patients with pulmonary hypertension due to chronic bronchitis and/or emphysema is usually wider than the aorta and has a media that is thicker than normal and may match that of the aorta (Figure 12-1). The elastic configuration is of the "acquired" type (Heard, 1969). Also elastic pulmonary arteries within the lungs may show medial hypertrophy in addition to atheromatous patches. Dilatation of these arteries has been demonstrated in the postmortem arteriogram (Reid, 1967).

The muscular pulmonary arteries generally have a media that is within the normal range (Figure 12-2) or that is only slightly hypertrophied, even in patients with sustained pulmonary hypertension. This is surprising in view of the often pronounced right ventricular hypertrophy in the same patient.

It appears, however, that small muscular pulmonary arteries exhibit a considerable thickening of their walls, mainly due to medial hypertrophy, whereas numerous arterioles are muscularized (Figure 12-2) (James and Thomas, 1963). These small vessels are easily overlooked so that the pulmonary vasculature may erroneously be judged normal. The degree of muscularization of pulmonary arterioles is closely related to that of right ventricular hypertrophy (Hicken et al., 1965). Thus this feature is most commonly found in chronic bronchitis and in centrilobular emphysema.

Development of longitudinal smooth muscle fibers in the intima, particularly within a reduplication of the internal elastic lamina, frequently is found in patients with chronic bronchitis and emphysema. They are observed predominantly in small muscular pulmonary arteries (Figure 12-3) and arterioles (Figure 12-4) (Hicken et al., 1965; Wagenvoort and Wagenvoort, 1973).

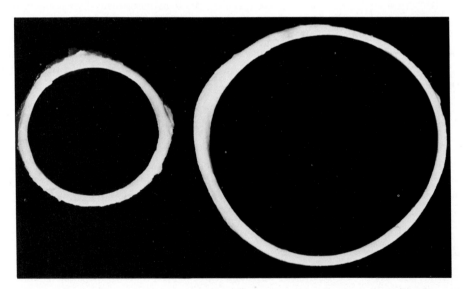

Figure 12-1. Transverse slices of aorta (*left*) and pulmonary trunk with hypertrophied media (*right*) after fixation in normally expanded state. In spite of pronounced dilatation, the wall of the pulmonary trunk has approximately the same thickness as that of the aorta. Man aged 69 years with chronic bronchitis and emphysema (×2).

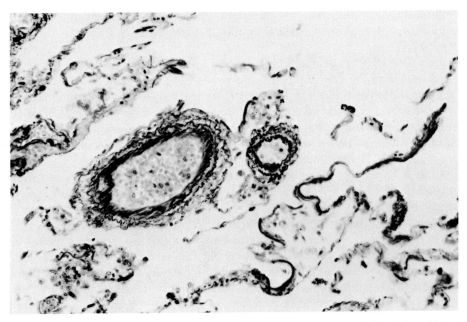

Figure 12-2. Muscular pulmonary artery and arteriole in a 66-year-old man with chronic bronchitis and emphysema. The muscular pulmonary artery has a normal medial thickness while the arteriole is muscularized (El.v.G., ×230).

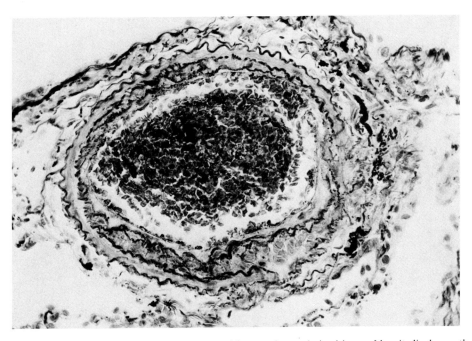

Figure 12-3. Small muscular pulmonary artery with a continuous intimal layer of longitudinal smooth muscle cells, shown in cross-section. Man aged 74 years with chronic bronchitis. (El.v.G., ×350).

The lesions just described, are identical to those found in individuals living at high altitude or with kyphoscoliosis and in other patients suffering from chronic hypoxia (Chapter 11).

Intimal fibrosis of the muscular pulmonary arteries is not an outstanding feature in patients with chronic bronchitis and emphysema. Particularly in chronic bronchitis, it is however more common and more marked (Figure 12-5) than in normal individuals of a comparable age group, although rarely widespread and occlusive. It is likely to result from organization of thrombi in areas of previous pneumonia or of pulmonary fibrosis (Wagenvoort and Wagenvoort, 1973). In some instances intimal fibrosis is caused by thromboembolism.

As we have seen (p. 262), the pulmonary alveolar capillaries are seriously affected in emphysema. Next to areas of total loss of capillaries, there are other regions in which the capillaries are scanty (Figure 12-6) and tend to differentiate into "flow capillaries" (Junghanss, 1959; Giese, 1960; Reid and Heard, 1962, 1963).

The pulmonary veins and venules in chronic bronchitis and emphysema have received less attention than the arteries and the capillaries. Although in centrilobular emphysema, the arteries that accompany the bronchioles initially will have a greater chance of being distorted by the emphysematous spaces than the veins that lie between the lobules, as could be expected, in many cases of emphysema the venules and veins do not escape altogether distortion and damage. Moreover, we found thickening of the venous media, intimal fibrosis (Figure 12-7), and even development

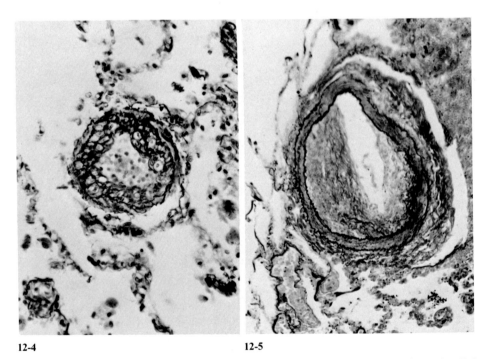

12-4   12-5

Figure 12-4.   Pulmonary arteriole with muscularization and thick intimal layer of smooth muscle cells in a 60-year-old man with chronic bronchitis and emphysema (El.v.G., ×230).

Figure 12-5.   Muscular pulmonary artery with marked eccentric intimal fibrosis in a 52-year-old woman with chronic bronchitis (El.v.G., ×140).

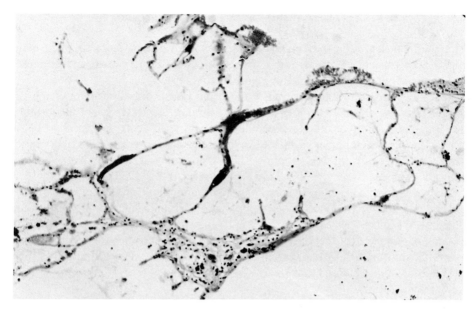

Figure 12-6. Lung tissue in a 62-year-old woman with pulmonary emphysema. The alveolar spaces are dilated and the alveolar walls are thin. Recognizable alveolar capillaries are scanty; however, there are some relatively wide "flow capillaries" (H. and E., ×90).

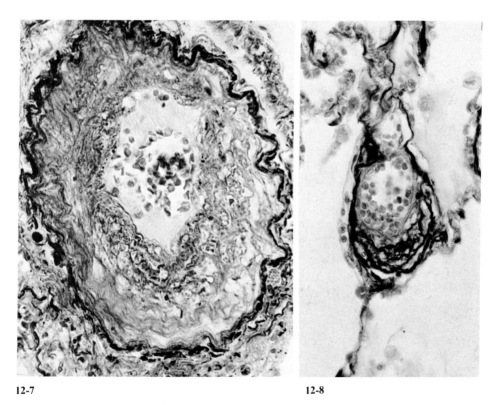

12-7   12-8

Figure 12-7. Pulmonary vein with severe intimal fibrosis in a 66-year-old man with chronic bronchitis and emphysema (El.v.G., ×350).
Figure 12-8. Pulmonary venule with a crescent-shaped layer of longitudinal smooth muscle cells in the intima, in a 59-year-old man with chronic bronchitis and emphysema (El.v.G., ×350).

of longitudinal smooth muscle fibers in the venous intima (Figure 12-8) in many patients with chronic obstructive lung disease (p. 240). These changes never caused marked obstruction and are probably related to hypoxia.

The bronchial arteries in patients with chronic bronchitis and emphysema are enlarged (Liebow et al., 1948) and tortuous (Florange, 1960). In cross section their walls have been reported to be thickened by medial hypertrophy and intimal fibrosis and also by the development of bundles of longitudinal smooth muscle fibers in the intima (Florange, 1960; Lee et al., 1971). The lumen is hereby narrowed and obliteration occurs commonly (Cudkowicz and Armstrong, 1953). Apparently there is much variation and medial hypertrophy and longitudinal smooth muscle bundles were not significantly increased as compared with control cases in the subjects studied by Wagenaar (1975).

Wide and enlarged bronchopulmonary arterial anastomoses were found by most authors (Liebow et al., 1948; Marchand et al., 1950; Cudkowicz and Armstrong, 1953), although Junghanss (1959) failed to detect an increased number in the postmortem angiogram.

The bronchial veins are dilated and so are their anastomoses with pulmonary veins. While normally the flow will be directed to the left atrium, reversal of the shunt is possible when the bronchial venous valves become insufficient following the pronounced dilatation (Liebow, 1953).

BRONCHIECTASIS

Right ventricular hypertrophy and cardiac failure are common complications in patients with bronchiectasis. Elevation of pulmonary arterial pressure and heart failure depend on the severity of the process rather than on the etiologic basis for the bronchiectasis, which may be postpneumonic, atelectatic, or congenital.

Both the pulmonary and the bronchial arteries are affected, although the changes in the latter vessels are more striking and have attracted particular attention. In a postmortem angiogram the pulmonary arteries in patients with bronchiectasis generally show a normal pattern (Gobbel et al., 1951), but in histologic sections they appear to have a hypertrophied media. Patchy intimal fibrosis (Figure 12-9) is common and not restricted to areas with ectatic bronchi. This intimal fibrosis is likely to result from organization of thrombi, since recognizable thrombosis is very common (Cockett and Vass, 1951). Also inflammatory reactions in the vascular wall often are found.

It has been shown that bronchial circulation is markedly increased in bronchiectasis. While normally the left ventricular output is only approximately one percent greater than the right ventricular output, in patients with bronchiectasis this difference may increase to close to 10 percent (Fritts et al., 1961).

Liebow et al. (1949) used the corrosion technique after vinylite injection of pulmonary and bronchial circulations to demonstrate enlargement and dilatation of bronchial arteries and a striking development of bronchopulmonary arterial anastomoses. These anastomoses may have a diameter of one mm or more.

The bronchial arteries often have a spiral course. Their caliber may become so large that they are sometimes the same size as the pulmonary artery that they join (Figure 12-10).

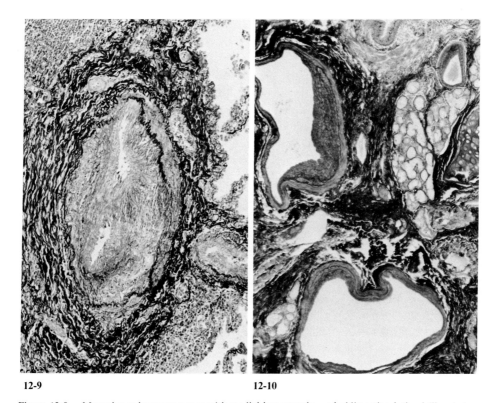

12-9   12-10

Figure 12-9. Muscular pulmonary artery with medial hypertrophy and obliterating intimal fibrosis in a 48-year-old woman with bronchiectasis and right ventricular hypertrophy (El.v.G., ×90).
Figure 12-10. Bronchial arteries of large caliber with some intimal fibrosis in a 38-year-old woman with bronchiectasis (El.v.G., ×50).

Aneurysmal dilatation of bronchial arteries occasionally causes hemoptysis (Cockett and Vass, 1951). The structural alterations of the wall of these arteries and of their anastomoses with pulmonary arteries are the same and include patches of intimal fibrosis and numerous bundles of longitudinal smooth muscle cells.

Although it has been assumed that the large arterial anastomoses (Figure 12-11) develop from preexisting vessels of this type (Marchand et al., 1950), it is more likely that these communications are formed by widening of newly formed channels within granulation tissue in areas of inflamed ectatic bronchi (Liebow et al., 1948).

The functional significance of the bronchopulmonary anastomoses is probably considerable. Liebow et al. (1949) expressed the opinion that they provide a shunting away from diseased areas of the lung toward healthy lung tissue, and that this accounts for the normal or almost normal oxygen saturation of the systemic arterial blood. Moreover, they believed that the large shunt along these anastomoses is responsible for the elevated pressure in the pulmonary arteries. While this shunt very likely contributes to a large extent to the pulmonary hypertension, there may be other factors as well, such as fibrosis of lung tissue and obliteration of many small arteries.

In patients with bronchiectasis on the basis of mucoviscidosis, the incidence of cardiac failure has risen with the increased life-span of these patients and appears to

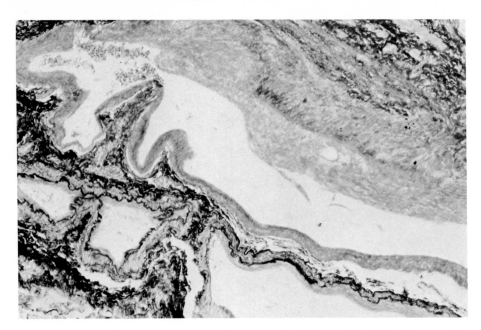

Figure 12-11.   Large bronchopulmonary arterial anastomosis with intimal fibrosis (top) about to join a pulmonary artery (bottom) in a 48-year-old woman with bronchiectasis and right ventricular hypertrophy (El.v.G., ×50).

be fairly large (Nadas et al., 1952; Goldring et al., 1964; Bowden et al., 1965; Wentworth et al., 1968; Ryland and Reid, 1975). In such cases hypoxia is probably the main cause of the pulmonary hypertension and the pulmonary vascular changes are identical to those observed in other forms of chronic hypoxia (Symchych, 1971). Even so, the bronchial arteries are dilated and tortuous around the affected bronchi.

PULMONARY GRANULOMAS AND FIBROSIS

There are many processes of widely varying etiology that cause changes in the lung tissue, which eventually may proceed to focal or interstitial fibrosis of the lungs. Sometimes the process begins with pulmonary edema or interstitial pneumonia or, in other instances, with the formation of granulomas. If large areas of lung tissue are involved in this fibrosis, there is loss of numerous alveolar capillaries, as well as of arterioles and venules. Even so, pulmonary hypertension is not common, and if it develops, it is usually mild at rest although it may become more severe at exercise. There is little doubt that the scarcity and relatively mild nature of the pulmonary hypertension in these cases, even in the presence of severe parenchymal alterations, reflect the marked adaptation and the large reserve of the pulmonary vascular bed.

The processes to be dealt with here, have in part an infectious origin such as tuberculosis; others belong to the groups of pneumoconioses, of auto-immune diseeases or of physico-chemical injuries. The cause of several conditions is unknown.

Tuberculosis

If pulmonary hypertension develops at all in patients with tuberculosis of the lungs, it is usually not severe, although there are exceptions. All types of lung vessels may become involved particularly when they are situated within or adjacent to areas of caseous necrosis or of fibrosis. Elastic and muscular pulmonary arteries as well as veins may become incorporated in areas of caseation, so that their walls become necrotic and their lumina obliterated (Brenner, 1935). In fibrotic areas the pulmonary arteries usually exhibit severe intimal fibrosis with narrowing or obliteration of the lumen (Figure 12-12). Thrombotic lesions often can be recognized (Cudkowicz, 1952).

In patients with cavernous tuberculosis, an elastic pulmonary artery lying in or in close proximity to a cavity may undergo weakening of its wall with the formation of an aneurysmal dilatation (Figure 12-13). These aneurysms of Rasmussen (1868) are often the source of fatal hemoptysis (Plessinger and Jolly, 1949).

Medial hypertrophy of muscular pulmonary arteries is often slight even in the presence of pulmonary hypertension (Heath and Best, 1958). Intimal fibrosis on the other hand is common, particularly in diseased areas of the lungs. The elastic laminae sometimes are incrusted with calcium and iron salts, which has been suggested to be due to chemotherapy (Gupta, 1962).

While all these changes may be considered as nonspecific reactions, a tuberculous vasculitis sometimes is observed with specific granulomas in the intima (Figure 12-14) and sometimes in media and adventitia (Figure 12-15) of both pulmonary

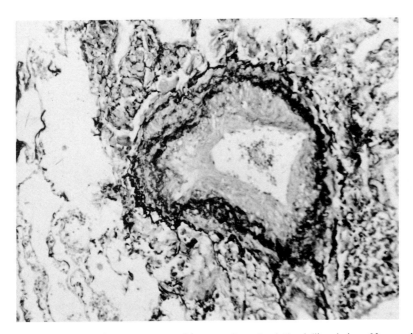

Figure 12-12. Muscular pulmonary artery with severe irregular intimal fibrosis in a 33-year-old man with pulmonary tuberculosis. This artery was immediately adjacent to an area of fibrosis and caseation (El.v.G., ×140).

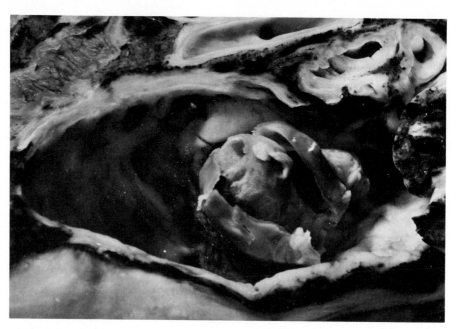

Figure 12-13. Aneurysm of Rasmussen in a 32-year-old man with pulmonary tuberculosis and fatal pulmonary hemorrhage. A ruptured aneurysm of a pulmonary artery, containing a thrombus, protrudes into a tuberculous cavity (×2).

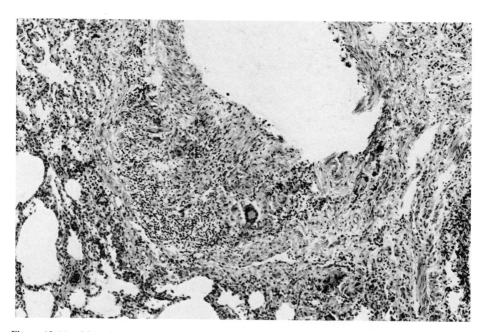

Figure 12-14. Muscular pulmonary artery with a tuberculous granuloma in its wall, in a 38-year-old man with pulmonary tuberculosis and right ventricular hypertrophy (H. and E., ×90).

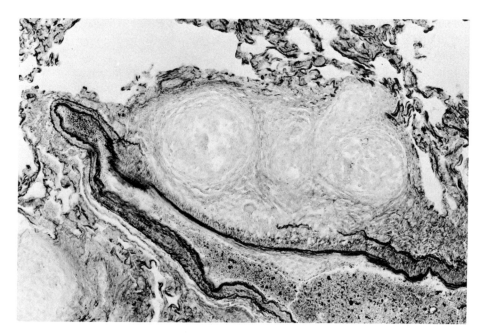

Figure 12-15. Muscular pulmonary artery with tuberculous granulomata in adventitia involving the media, from the same case as Figure 12-14 (El.v.G., ×90).

arteries and veins (Wagenvoort et al., 1964). Rarely is the pulmonary trunk thus affected (Gross, 1933).

The bronchial arteries in many cases of pulmonary tuberculosis are enlarged, dilated, and tortuous, while the bronchopulmonary arterial anastomoses are increased in number and size (Wood and Miller, 1938; Delarue et al., 1955). Cudkowicz (1952) believed that excessive dilatation of some bronchial arterioles was responsible for the formation of the aneurysms of Rasmussen, but this must be a misinterpretation in view of the size of the arteries in which these aneurysms occur.

Interstitial Fibrosis

The lungs respond in different ways to injury, one of which is interstitial fibrosis. Interstitial fibrosis is produced when the alveolar walls become thickened with deposition of reticulin and collagen fibers. This may happen in several ways (Spencer, 1967, 1968a).

In certain forms of pneumonia or pulmonary edema a fibrinous exudate may leak from the alveolar capillaries. If this exudate fails to be resorbed, alveolar epithelial cells grow over the new surface provided by this exudate, which is subsequently organized by fibroblasts derived from the interstitial cells of the alveolar wall. By this process plugs of connective tissue extending in the alveolar spaces are regularly formed.

Inhalation of fine particulate dust may damage the alveolar epithelium including its basement membrane. Alveolar macrophages accumulate at the sites of injury and are subsequently overgrown by proliferating epithelial cells. In these areas new reticulin and collagen fibers are formed in the alveolar walls, giving rise to interstitial fibrosis.

Interstitial edema, as occurs in chronically elevated pulmonary venous pressure and in increased alveolar capillary permeability, also may provoke collagen deposition and fibrosis.

From this description of the various ways in which interstitial fibrosis can develop, it becomes clear that it is a nonspecific alteration of the lung tissue with no more than limited significance for the diagnosis of its underlying cause.

Widely differing conditions like mitral stenosis (Chapter Nine), pulmonary venoocclusive disease (Chapter Ten), pneumoconioses, collagen diseases, viral pneumonias, and radiation all may give rise to interstitial fibrosis.

If interstitial fibrosis is severe and widespread throughout the lungs, it may affect the pulmonary circulation in various ways. The alveolar-capillary block with its impairment of alveolar oxygen exchange produces hypoxemia. The exchange of the far more diffusible carbon dioxide will remain normal or, if there is hyperventilation, may be increased. An elevated pulmonary vascular resistance may in part be hypoxic in nature.

However, there is also considerable destruction and loss of the alveolar capillary bed within the fibrotic alveolar walls, whereas many muscular pulmonary arteries in areas of fibrosis are narrowed or obstructed by reactive intimal fibrosis, while their media is often markedly thickened. In unaffected lung tissue the lung vessels are normal, although the alveolar capillaries usually are distended and engorged with blood (Spencer, 1968b). The bronchial arteries are enlarged as are their anastomoses with pulmonary arteries.

In some conditions, in addition to these nonspecific changes, there are also characteristic alterations, for instance granulomas that may affect the pulmonary vasculature.

If fibrosis of the lung proceeds and particularly when the terminal bronchioles and the respiratory bronchioles of the first order become involved, these tend to dilate to such an extent that they become cystic so that a honeycomb appearance is assumed. Honeycomb lung superficially may resemble centrilobular emphysema but can be distinguished by the greater size and thicker walls of the cysts. Since it is an end-result, in principle, it may be found in all conditions causing pulmonary fibrosis.

While all these mechanisms and alterations probably are involved, although to varying extents, the effect of interstitial fibrosis on pulmonary arterial resistance and pressure is usually mild. The pressure may be normal or may reach moderate levels. In most conditions leading to interstitial fibrosis, right cardiac failure is uncommon or has not been reported at all.

We will briefly discuss the various pulmonary diseases producing interstitial fibrosis, although only in so far as they are recognized as producing, if only occasionally, marked pulmonary hypertension.

Pulmonary Infections

Pulmonary infections, other than tuberculosis or those associated with chronic bronchitis and bronchiectasis, do not commonly cause marked elevation of the pulmonary arterial pressure. Heath et al. (1968) described a patient who developed honeycomb lung and congestive cardiac failure following pneumonia, the cause of which was not specified. Slight medial hypertrophy of muscular pulmonary and of bronchial arteries was observed.

Pulmonary hypertension following unilateral lung reimplantation and contralateral pneumonectomy in dogs also has been attributed in some instances to chronic inflammatory reactions (Wagenvoort et al., 1973).

Viral infections of the lung often are characterized by interstitial pneumonia which may result in interstitial fibrosis. If the lungs are severely affected, the pulmonary arterial pressure may be raised but rarely to a great extent.

Collagen Diseases

Scleroderma or progressive systemic sclerosis may affect many organs. If the lungs are involved, usually in a later stage of the disease (Weaver et al., 1968), the alveolar walls become thickened first by interstitial edema and subsequently by fibrosis. The alveolar capillaries initially are dilated but gradually become more and more lost in the process of progressive fibrosis and disruption of alveolar walls (Getzowa, 1945). When these walls rupture cystic spaces are formed, eventually leading to the picture of a honeycomb lung. In these cystic and fibrotic areas the bronchioles are regularly narrowed or obstructed (Spencer, 1968a).

The blood vessels in these severely damaged lungs are usually distinctly affected. Medial hypertrophy and particularly patchy intimal fibrosis (Figure 12-16) based on organized thrombi are most marked in the fibrotic areas. Sometimes a new circular layer of smooth muscle cells is formed in the thickened intima directly under the endothelium, so that the appearance of a double muscular coat is produced (Wagenvoort, et al., 1964). Also the pulmonary veins in these areas are often thick-walled with marked intimal fibrosis. None of these lesions are specific for scleroderma. Bronchiolar obstruction is probably responsible for some of the vascular changes known to occur in hypoxic pulmonary hypertension. Vasculitis sometimes is observed, even in the absence of pulmonary hypertension.

When the lungs are involved in scleroderma, pulmonary hypertension occasionally is observed. Sometimes it is severe (Conner and Bashour, 1961; Oram and Stokes, 1961; Degeorges and Slama, 1962; Naeye, 1963; Pace et al., 1963). Various factors play a part in the elevation of pulmonary vascular resistance, such as the loss of capillaries and arterioles, the narrowing and obliteration of many muscular pulmonary arteries and of pulmonary veins and their inability to dilate in fibrotic areas. Moreover, hypoxic vasoconstriction due to bronchiolar obstruction and impaired gas exchange, and the development of intrapulmonary shunts causing hypoxemia may all be involved (Naeye, 1963).

Sometimes pulmonary hypertension in progressive systemic sclerosis is associated with Raynaud's phenomenon (p. 134) (Linenthal and Talkov, 1941; Trell and Lindström, 1971). In these instances the full picture of plexogenic pulmonary arteriopathy may develop.

Dermatomyositis sometimes causes pulmonary changes closely resembling those of scleroderma and occasionally progressing to honeycomb lung. The vascular changes are essentially similar to those in scleroderma, although usually less frequent and less pronounced. Severe pulmonary hypertension and right cardiac failure do occur (Caldwell and Aitchison, 1956; Hyun et al., 1962), though rarely.

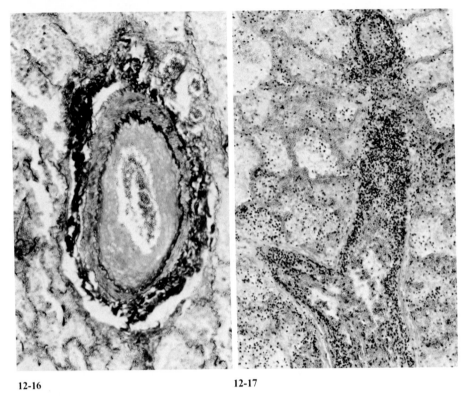

12-16   12-17

Figure 12-16. Muscular pulmonary artery with medial hypertrophy and pronounced intimal fibrosis in a 50-year-old woman with diffuse fibrosis of lungs due to scleroderma and pulmonary hypertension (El.v.G., ×90).

Figure 12-17. Necrotizing pulmonary arteritis due to disseminated lupus erythematodes in a 29-year-old woman. There was right ventricular hypertrophy (H. and E., ×140).

Disseminated lupus erythematodes is sometimes associated with pleuritis and interstitial pneumonia resulting in interstitial fibrosis. The thickened alveolar septa are lined by prominent cuboidal epithelium. Pulmonary vascular changes include fibrosis and necrotizing vasculitis of smaller and larger muscular pulmonary arteries (Figure 12-17) and thrombotic obliteration of these vessels (Klemperer et al., 1941; Aitchison and Williams, 1956; Liebow and Carrington, 1966). "Wire-loop" capillaries with thickened basal membranes, staining positively with the periodic acid-Schiff reagent like those in glomerular capillaries, have been described (Kapancy and Chamay, 1967).

Even though pulmonary or pleural involvement has been described in up to 50 percent of the patients with this disease (Fricsay-von Telbisz, 1956; Hejtmancik et al., 1964), the alterations in the lung vessels are mild as compared to those in scleroderma (Gross et al., 1972; Olsen and Lever, 1972). Pulmonary hypertension and cardiac failure are rare sequences of the condition (Degeorges and Slama, 1962; Slama et al., 1967).

Rheumatoid disease, if affecting the lungs, is another rare cause of pulmonary hypertension. Since it was realized that rheumatoid disease is a condition not limited to the joints but a systemic disease, reports on its pulmonary manifestations multiplied. Spencer (1968a) divided the pulmonary changes in pleural lesions, interstitial pneumonitis and fibrosis, and modified pneumoconiotic changes, the so-called Caplan's lesions. Granulomatous lesions and nodular amyloidosis may be added to the picture while the changes may proceed to honeycombing (Liebow and Carrington, 1966; Liebow, 1975).

The pulmonary vascular changes, affecting both pulmonary and bronchial arteries, are nonspecific (Christie, 1954). Pulmonary arteritis is common and patients who developed pulmonary hypertension and right cardiac failure have been described (Gardner et al., 1957; Heath et al., 1968; Walker and Wright, 1968), although Patterson et al. (1965) could find only three cases with pulmonary hypertension among over 700 patients with rheumatoid arthritis.

Polyarteritis nodosa is one of the collagen diseases that rarely affects the pulmonary parenchyma. Fibrotic and granulomatous reactions have been reported however (Sweeney and Baggenstoss, 1949; Spencer, 1957). Pulmonary arterial lesions in these instances are particularly observed as part of a generalized vascular involvement. Foci of acute necrotizing arteritis with an inflammatory exudate consisting first of polymorphonuclear and eosinophilic granulocytes, and later of lymphocytes and plasma cells, may extend well beyond the walls of the arteries into the pulmonary parenchyma (Figure 12-18). The bronchial arteries also are often involved.

It is questionable whether polyarteritis nodosa ever leads to pulmonary hypertension and right cardiac failure. Such cases have been described (Old and Russell, 1947; Braunstein, 1955; Gloor and Huber, 1962) but were complicated by other causes of pulmonary hypertension or were examples of pulmonary arteritis due to pulmonary hypertension, erroneously diagnosed as polyarteritis nodosa.

Also other forms of vasculitis, like *allergic arteritis* or arteritis in *Wegener's syn-*

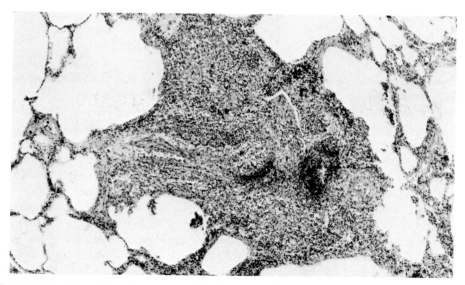

Figure 12-18. Necrotizing pulmonary arteritis due to generalized polyarteritis nodosa in a 75-year-old woman (H. and E., ×140).

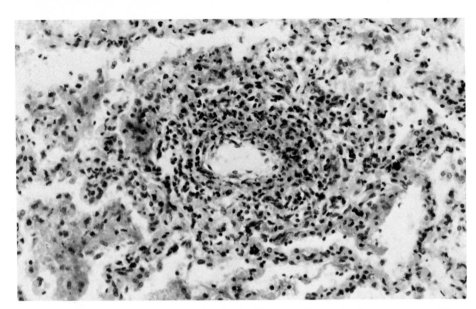

Figure 12-19.   Necrotizing pulmonary arteritis due to Wegener's disease affecting the lungs in a 26-year-old woman (H. and E., ×230).

drome (Figure 12-19), even though sometimes involving many pulmonary arteries, as far as we are aware, do not give rise to significant elevation of pulmonary arterial pressure. In *Takayasu's disease,* a form of arteritis of unknown etiology affecting predominantly the thoracic aorta and its branches, occasionally the pulmonary arteries are involved (Mitov et al., 1971). In some instances this gave rise to pulmonary hypertension (Clin. Path. Conf. 1969; Ishihama et al., 1973). The histologic picture of the lung vessels included an inflammatory infiltrate of lymphocytes and histiocytes with an occasional plasma cell.

Lung Diseases of Unknown Etiology

Hamman-Rich lung, so called after the authors who first described this condition (1944), is a form of progressive chronic interstitial fibrosis of the lungs and is encountered with increasing frequency. Its cause is unknown. Although confined to the lungs and not affecting other organs, it has much in common with some of the collagen diseases (Spencer, 1968a).

This disease is characterized clinically by progressive dyspnea, chest pain, cyanosis, an unproductive cough, and sometimes by hemoptysis. In later stages occasionally pulmonary hypertension develops (Muschenheim, 1961).

The early microscopic lesions are pulmonary edema and interstitial edema accompanied by diapedesis of erythrocytes, desquamation of histiocytes, and sometimes by hyalin membranes. Gradually a diffuse fibrosis of the alveolar walls, which become lined by cuboidal epithelial cells, develops. In the later stages destruction of alveoli and of respiratory bronchioles may lead to the picture of honeycomb lung (Rubin and Lubliner, 1957). In severe cases much of the alveolar capillary bed and many pulmonary arterioles are lost, while larger arteries often are narrowed or obliterated by patchy intimal fibrosis. These changes, together with a marked hypoxic factor due to the alveolar-capillary block, are responsible for the pulmonary hypertension often encountered in these patients.

Desquamative interstitial pneumonia is an uncommon condition first described by Liebow et al. (1965) and regarded as a new entity, although others believe it to be a stage in the evolution of interstitial pneumonia (Spencer, 1975). In this condition thickening of the alveolar septa is observed combined with a scanty, diffuse infiltrate of eosinophils and plasma cells. Moveover there are some focal accumulations of lymphocytes. The most characteristic alteration is the desquamation of numerous granular pneumocytes into the alveolar spaces. In late stages honeycomb lung develops (McCann and Brewer, 1974). Although pulmonary vascular changes and particularly intimal fibrosis of muscular pulmonary arteries (Figure 12-20) and veins (Figure 12-21) are common, pulmonary hypertension and cardiac failure are rare (Liebow et al., 1965).

Idiopathic pulmonary hemosiderosis, first described by Ceelen (1931), is an uncommon condition affecting mainly children. The extensive deposition of hemosiderin in the lung tissue is due to numerous and diffuse intra-alveolar hemorrhages which in turn are probably based on vascular damage. Destruction of elastic

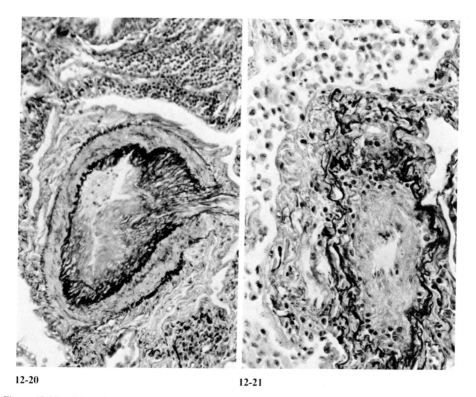

12-20   12-21

Figure 12-20. Muscular pulmonary artery with medial hypertrophy and obliteration by intimal fibrosis in a 61-year-old man with fibrosis of the lung due to desquamative interstitial pneumonia. There was mild elevation of pulmonary arterial pressure (El.v.G., × 140).

Figure 12-21. Pulmonary vein with subtotal obliteration by intimal fibrosis from the same case as Figure 12-20. Alveolar spaces are filled with desquamated granular pneumocytes (El.v.G., ×230).

fibers with subsequent impregnation by calcium and iron precedes the formation of siderotic nodules. These are associated with many foreign body giant cells and hemosiderin-laden phagocytes.

The vessels of the lung may undergo progressive narrowing and obliteration by intimal fibrosis, and pulmonary hypertension is a rare and late complication (Soergel and Sommers, 1962).

Histiocytic reticulosis including Letterer-Siwe's disease, eosinophilic granuloma, and Hand-Schüller-Christian disease, may affect the lungs and may sometimes produce pulmonary hypertension and right heart failure. In all these conditions the rise in pressure is caused by various mechanisms. Fibrosis and granulomatous reactions produce loss of alveolar capillaries and arterioles. Honeycomb lung is commonly the end-result. Moreover, perivascular proliferation of histiocytic cells with infiltration in the arterial adventitia causes narrowing and endarteritis (Spencer, 1968a).

Sarcoidosis is a disease of unknown etiology in which the lungs often are involved. If this happens, the lung function commonly is disturbed, and the pulmonary circulation also may be impaired with right cardiac failure as a serious and sometimes fatal complication.

The characteristic lesion is a granuloma with little or no central necrosis (Figure 12-22). By coalescence of these granulomas, palpable and visible nodules are produced in the lung tissue and particularly around bronchi and lung vessels. There is a strong tendency for lesions to heal resulting in fibrosis and eventually in the appearances of honeycomb lung. Interstitial fibrosis (Michaels et al., 1960) and bronchostenosis (Honey and Jepson, 1957) are further impediments to the gas exchange.

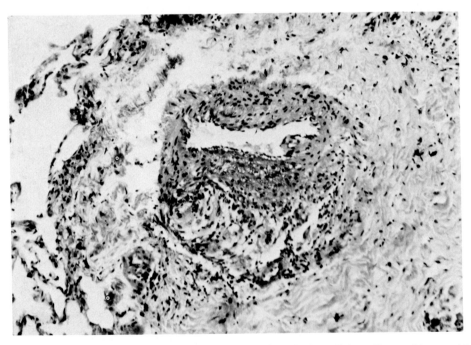

Figure 12-22. Muscular pulmonary artery with a granuloma in its wall in a 64-year-old man with pulmonary sarcoidosis (H. and E., ×140).

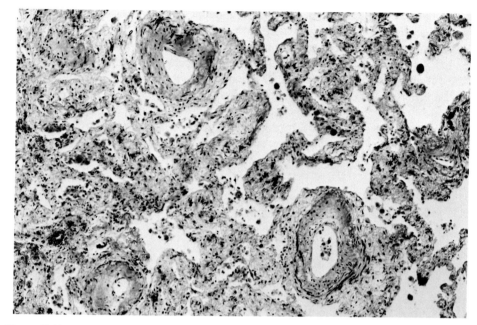

Figure 12-23. Interstitial fibrosis of lung tissue and intimal fibrosis of multiple muscular pulmonary arteries due to radiation for bronchial carcinoma in a 56-year-old man (H. and E., ×90).

The granulomas and subsequent fibrosis around the pulmonary vasculature cause narrowing and nonspecific intimal fibrosis. Moreover the vessels may become obstructed by granuloma's in the intima. Extensive granulomatous arteritis does occur (Michaels et al., 1960) though uncommonly.

Radiation Fibrosis

When lungs are exposed to excessive radiation, as may happen particularly during radiotherapy for tumors of lungs, mammary glands, thyroid, or esophagus, the first signs of damage consist of pulmonary edema and petechial hemorrhages. This is followed by a gradual and progressive interstitial fibrosis and fibroelastosis of the lungs (Jennings and Arden, 1962), associated with damage to bronchi and bronchioles.

The blood vessels of the lungs usually are involved (Figure 12-23) since particularly the small pulmonary arteries and veins develop medial hypertrophy and intimal fibrosis. Thrombotic changes are also common. The lymph vessels may become injured as well, causing disturbance of the lymphatic drainage. Right cardiac failure is uncommonly observed, possibly because the underlying condition necessitating radiation often will cause death before pulmonary hypertension becomes a problem.

Chemical and Toxic Injury

Various chemical agents may produce pulmonary edema with subsequent pulmonary fibrosis. In the case of paraquat, this is usually an intra-alveolar fibrosis and the concomitant pulmonary vascular lesions such as medial hypertrophy and development of longitudinal smooth muscle bundles in the small pulmonary arteries suggest that these are due to hypoxia (Smith and Heath, 1974).

Several drugs, used in the treatment of hypertension like apresoline and hexamethonium (Doniach et al., 1954), or of chronic myeloid leukemia like busulphan (Oliner et al., 1961; Littler et al., 1969), are known to produce interstitial pulmonary fibrosis, if only occasionally and probably only in patients who have a hypersensitivity for these substances. Although pulmonary vascular lesions, including proliferative endarteritis have been described in these instances (Oliner et al., 1961), we are not aware that unequivocal pulmonary hypertension has been reported in these patients.

Pneumoconioses

There are various forms of pneumoconiosis that directly or indirectly affect the pulmonary circulation and in this way cause elevation of pulmonary arterial pressure and right cardiac failure. Such a course of events is particularly seen in silicosis.

Silicosis is characterized by more of less massive fibrosis of lung tissue rather than by interstitial fibrosis. The minute silica particles initially are taken up by the alveolar epithelial cells and by alveolar macrophages and subsequently deposited in the peribronchial and perivascular connective tissue. Silicotic nodules coalescing to form fibrotic areas, therefore, are observed particularly around bronchi and vessels. Pulmonary arteries and veins undergo marked changes in these areas with fragmentation and loss of elastic membranes, fibrosis of adventitia and media, and gradual obliteration by intimal fibrosis (Geever, 1947; Nicod, 1949; Rüttner and Gassman, 1957). Even large elastic pulmonary arteries sometimes are affected in this way, while aneurysmal dilatation and rupture in other areas are occasional findings (Schepers, 1955).

Also many alveolar capillaries and pulmonary lymphatics are obstructed and lost, while there is an increase in bronchopulmonary arterial anastomoses. Alveolar hypoventilation is another factor which may contribute to an increased pulmonary vascular resistance and pressure.

Berylliosis may cause a form of chronic lung disease in workers who handle beryllium or its compounds. It produces essentially a granulomatous and fibrotic reaction in the lungs with secondary changes in the pulmonary vasculature. In advanced cases pulmonary hypertension may develop, though this is uncommon.

MALIGNANT INFILTRATION

A primary neoplasm in the lungs will not affect the pulmonary vascular resistance and pressure significantly, since it is a localized process. Even so, the pulmonary arteries in the lobe in which the tumor is situated usually exhibit marked medial hypertrophy and intimal fibrosis (Wagenvoort and Wagenvoort, 1965). This is probably related to the development of a pronounced collateral circulation between these vessels and the bronchial arteries known to supply the tumor area (Wood and Miller, 1938; Cudkowicz and Armstrong, 1953).

Diffuse lymphatic spread of carcinoma gives sometimes rise to pulmonary hypertension and acute or subacute right heart failure. The chance of the patient surviving long enough to develop chronic cardiac insufficiency is minimal. Pulmonary hypertension has been reported particularly in patients with primary carcinoma of the stomach and the mammary gland, although occasionally the primary growth was located in lung, pancreas, or other organs (Greenspan, 1934; Brill and Robertson, 1937; Morgan, 1949; Storstein, 1951; Altemus and Lee, 1967; Kane et al., 1975).

The mechanism of pulmonary vascular obstruction in these instances is probably only partly related to the distension of the perivascular lymphatics by tumor cells. Multiple neoplastic nodules arond the lung vessels (Figure 12-24) may well impair their distension and lead to reactive intimal fibrosis. It is likely, however, that tumor emboli (p. 163) and particularly the thrombotic and fibrotic reaction elicited by these intravascular tumor cells are essentially responsible for rapid and pronounced vascular obstruction (Morgan, 1949). Rarely tumor growth and associated intravascular thrombosis is observed along the pulmonary veins (Schiller and Madge, 1970) but pulmonary hypertension has not been described in such cases.

Obstruction of the pulmonary trunk and main arteries by primary or secondary sarcomas of these vessels is rare although the number of case reports is rapidly increasing. The histologic types of these primary tumors include fibrosarcoma (Wolf et al., 1960), fibromyxosarcoma (Busch and Ziebarth-Schroth, 1972), and leiomyosarcoma (Figure 12-25) (Wackers et al., 1969; Thys et al., 1974). The tumor mass may extend far into the intrapulmonary arteries (Jaques and Barclay, 1960;

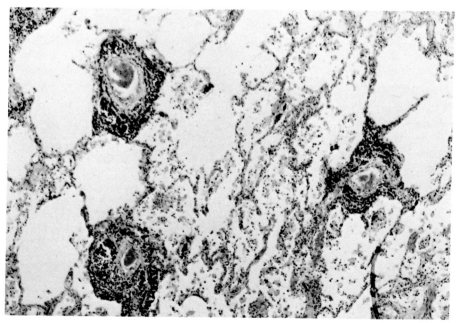

Figure 12-24. Lung tissue in a 68-year-old man with an anaplastic carcinoma of the bronchus and right ventricular hypertrophy. There is extensive spread of tumor along periarterial lymphatics (H. and E., ×90).

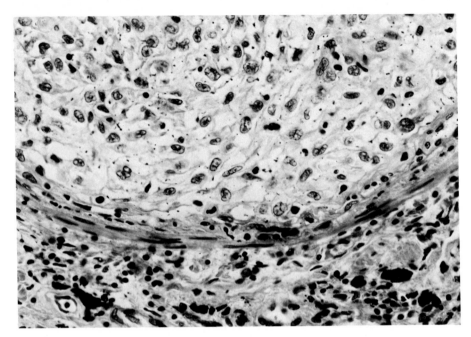

Figure 12-25. Large muscular pulmonary artery obstructed by tumor in a 69-year-old man with a primary leiomyosarcoma of the pulmonary trunk (H. and E., ×350).

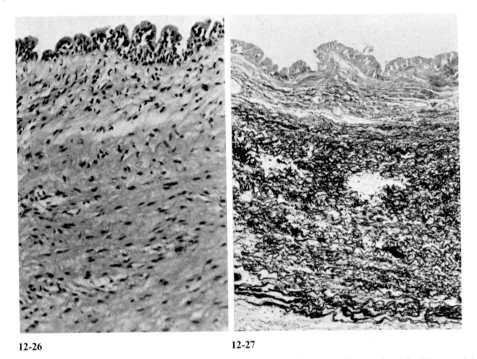

12-26   12-27

Figure 12-26. Pulmonary trunk in a 58-year-old man with carcinoma of the renal pelvis. The arterial intima is replaced by a layer of tumor cells (H. and E., ×140).

Figure 12-27. Left main pulmonary artery from the same case as Figure 12-26. The intima is lined by tumor cells but the media is unaffected (El.v.G., ×90).

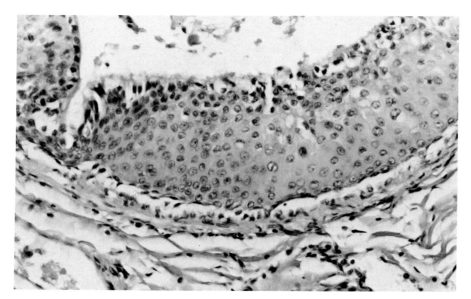

Figure 12-28. Muscular pulmonary artery in a 39-year-old man with carcinoma of the renal pelvis. The arterial wall is lined by a layer of tumor cells (H. and E., ×230).

Chatelanat, 1962). Right ventricular hypertrophy and heart failure is the usual cause of death in these patients.

Even more uncommon is the lining of pulmonary trunk, main arteries and intrapulmonary arteries by metastatic carcinoma (Figures 12-26, 12-27, and 12-28). In two cases of renal pelvic carcinoma it was found that tumor cells after hematogenous spread, progressively replaced the endothelial lining far into small pulmonary arterial branches with gradually increasing obstruction of their lumina (Wagenvoort et al., 1961, 1964).

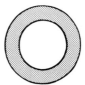 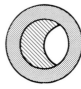

Hypertensive vascular lesions in lung diseases: Usually medial hypertrophy and eccentric intimal fibrosis in arteries and veins. Hypoxic vascular lesions also may be present.

REFERENCES

Abraham, A. S., Cole, R. B., and Bishop, J. M.: Reversal of pulmonary hypertension by prolonged oxygen administration to patients with chronic bronchitis. *Circ. Res.* **23:** 147, 1968.

Abraham, A. S., Cole, R. B., Green, I. D., Hedworth-Whitty, R. B., Clarke, S. W., and Bishop, J. M.: Factors contributing to the reversible pulmonary hypertension of patients with acute respiratory failure studied by serial observation during recovery. *Circ. Res.* **24:** 51, 1969.

Aitchison, J. D., and Williams, A. W.: Pulmonary changes in disseminated lupus erythematosus. *Ann. Rheum. Dis.* **15:** 26, 1956.

Altemus, L. R., and Lee, R. E.: Carcinomatosis of the lung with pulmonary hypertension. *Arch. Int. Med.* **119**: 32, 1967.

Auerbach, O., Stout, A. P., Hammond, E. C., and Garfinkel, L.: Smoking habits and age in relation to pulmonary changes. Rupture of alveolar septums, fibrosis and thickening of walls of small arteries and arterioles. *New Engl. J. Med.* **269**: 1045, 1963.

Bignon, J., Pariente, R., and Brouet, G.: Fréquence autopsique des thrombo-embolies pulmonaires au stade terminal des bronchopneumopathies chroniques obstructives. *Bull. Physio-Path. Resp.* **6**: 405, 1970.

Bowden, D. H., Fisher, V. W., and Wyatt, J. P.: Cor pulmonale in cystic fibrosis: A morphometric analysis. *Amer. J. Med.* **38**: 226, 1965.

Braunstein, H.: Periarteritis nodosa limited to the pulmonary circulation. *Amer. J. Path.* **31**: 837, 1955.

Brenner, O.: Pathology of the vessels of the pulmonary circulation. Tuberculosis of the pulmonary vessels. *Arch. Int. Med.* **56**: 1189, 1935.

Brill, J. C., and Robertson, T. D.: Subacute cor pulmonale. *Arch. Int. Med.* **60**: 1043, 1937.

Burrows, B., Niden, A. H., Fletcher, C. M., and Jones, N. L.: Clinical types of chronic obstructive lung disease in London and in Chicago. *Amer. Rev. Resp. Dis.* **90**: 14, 1964.

Busch, W., and Ziebart-Schroth, A.: Ein weiterer Fall von primärem Sarkom der A. pulmonalis. *Zbl. Allg. Path.* **116**: 300, 1972.

Caldwell, I. W., and Aitchison, J. D.: Pulmonary hypertension in dermatomyositis. *Brit. Heart J.* **18**: 273, 1956.

Ceelen, W.: Die Kreislaufstörungen der Lunge. In Henke, F., and Lubarsch, O., *Handbuch der Speziellen Path. Anatomie,* III, Springer, Berlin, 1931.

Chatelanat, F.: Fibromyxosarcoma des valvules pulmonaires et son extension dans les poumons. *Path. Microbiol.* **25**: 366, 1962.

Christie, G. S.: Pulmonary lesions in rheumatoid arthritis. *Australasian Ann. Med.* **3**: 49, 1954.

Clin. Path. Conference: A case of aortitis with nephrotic syndrome. *Brit. Med. J.* **II**: 359, 1969.

Cockett, F. B., and Vass, C. C. N.: A comparison of the role of the bronchial arteries in bronchiectasis and in experimental ligation of the pulmonary artery. *Thorax* **6**: 268, 1951.

Conner, P. K., and Bashour, F. A.: Cardiopulmonary changes in sclerodermia. A physiologic study. *Amer. Heart J.* **61**: 494, 1961.

Cromie, J. B.: Correlation of anatomic pulmonary emphysema and right ventricular hypertrophy. *Amer. Rev. Resp. Dis.* **84**: 657, 1961.

Cudkowicz, L.: The blood supply of the lung in pulmonary tuberculosis. *Thorax* **7**: 270, 1952.

Cudkowicz, L., and Armstrong, J. B.: The bronchial arteries in pulmonary emphysema. *Thorax* **8**: 46, 1953.

Degeorges, M., and Slama, R.: Les localisations cardiaques et vasculaires de la lupo-érythémato-viscérite. *Sem. Hôp.* **38**: 10, 1962.

Delarue, J., Sors, C., Mignot, J., and Paillas, J.: Lésions bronchopulmonaires et modifications circulatoires. *Presse Méd.* **63**: 173, 1955.

Denolin, H.: Contribution à l'étude de la circulation pulmonaire en clinique. *Acta Cardiol.* **16** (suppl. 10), 1961.

Doniach, I., Morrison, B., and Steiner, R. E.: Lung changes during hexamethonium therapy for hypertension. *Brit. Heart J.* **16**: 101, 1954.

Dunnill, M. S.: An assessment of the anatomical factor in cor pulmonale in emphysema. *J. Clin. Path.* **14**: 246, 1961.

Evans, T. O., Van der Reis, L., and Selzer, A.: Circulatory effects of chronic pulmonary emphysema. *Amer. Heart J.* **66**: 741, 1963.

Filley, G. F., Dart, G. A., and Mitchell, R. S.: Emphysema and chronic bronchitis: Clinical manifestations and their physiological significance. In *Current Research in Chronic Airways Obstruction.* Public Health Service Public. no. 1717, 1968, p. 339.

Florange, W.: Anatomie und Pathologie der Arteria bronchialis. *Ergebn. Allg. Path.* **39**: 152, 1960.

Fricsay-v.Telbisz, M.: Die pulmonale Form des Lupus erythematosus disseminatus acutus. *Schweiz. Med. Wschr.* **86**: 269, 1956.

Fritts, H. W., Harris, P., Chidsey, C. A., Clauss, R. H., and Cournand, A.: Estimation of flow through bronchial-pulmonary vascular anastomoses with use of T-1284 dye. *Circulation* **23:** 390, 1961.

Gardner, D. L., Duthie, J. R., McLeod, J., and Allen, W. S. A.: Pulmonary hypertension in rheumatoid arthritis: report of a case with intimal sclerosis of the pulmonary and digital arteries. *Scott. Med. J.* **2:** 183, 1957.

Geever, E. F.: Pulmonary vascular lesions in silicosis and related pathologic changes. *Amer. J. Med. Sci.* **214:** 292, 1947.

Getzowa, S.: Cystic and compact pulmonary sclerosis in progressive scleroderma. *Arch. Path.* **40:** 99, 1945.

Giese, W.: Die Atemorgane. In Kaufmann, *Lehrbuch der speziellen pathologischen Anatomie,* ed. 2, vol. II. De Gruyter & Co., Berlin, 1960.

Gloor, B., and Huber, J.: Isolierte Periarteriitis nodosa der Lungen, kombiniert mit alter Lungenembolie. *Schweiz. Med. Wschr.* **92:** 273, 1962.

Gobbel, W. G., Gordon, J., and Digman, G. J.: The pulmonary artery in bronchiectasis. *J. Thorac. Surg.* **21:** 385, 1951.

Goldring, R. M., Fishman, A. P., Turino, G. M., Cohen, H. I., Denning, C. R., and Andersen, D. H.: Pulmonary hypertension and cor pulmonale in cystic fibrosis of the pancreas. *J. Pediat.* **65:** 501, 1964.

Gough, J.: Pathological changes in the lungs associated with cor pulmonale. *Bull. N. Y. Acad. Sci.* **41:** 927, 1965.

Greenspan, E. B.: Carcinomatous endarteritis of the pulmonary vessels resulting in failure of the right ventricle. *Arch. Int. Med.* **54:** 625, 1934.

Gross, M., Esterly, J. R., and Earle, R. H.: Pulmonary alterations in systemic lupus erythematosus. *Amer. Rev. Resp. Dis.* **105:** 572, 1972.

Gross, P.: Tuberculous vegetations of the trunk of the pulmonary artery. *Amer. J. Path.* **9:** 17, 1933.

Gupta, I. M.: Mineralising elastosis in blood vessels in resected lungs from patients undergoing prolonged chemotherapy. *J. Path. Bact.* **83:** 13, 1962.

Hamman, L., and Rich, A. R.: Acute diffuse interstitital fibrosis of the lungs. *Bull. J. Hopk. Hosp.* **74:** 177, 1944.

Harris, P., Segel, N., Green, I., and Housley, E.: The influence of the airways resistance and alveolar pressure on the pulmonary vascular resistance in chronic bronchitis. *Cardiovasc. Res.* **2:** 84, 1968.

Harvey, R. M., Ferrer, M. I., Richards, D. W., and Cournand, A.: Influence of chronic pulmonary disease of the heart and circulation. *Amer. J. Med.* **10:** 719, 1951.

Heath, D., and Best, P. V.: The tunica media of the arteries of the lung in pulmonary hypertension. *J. Path. Bact.* **76:** 165, 1958.

Heath, D., Gillund, T. D., Kay, J. M., and Hawkins, C. F.: Pulmonary vascular disease in honeycomb lung. *J. Path. Bact.* **95:** 423, 1968.

Heard, B. E.: *Pathology of Chronic Bronchitis and Emphysema.* Churchill, Ltd., London, 1969.

Hejtmancik, M. R., Wright, J. C., Quint, R., and Jennings, F. L.: The cardiovascular manifestations of systemic lupus erythematosus. *Amer. Heart J.* **68:** 119, 1964.

Hicken, P., Heath, D., Brewer, D. B., and Whitaker, W.: The small pulmonary arteries in emphysema. *J. Path. Bact.* **90:** 107, 1965.

Hicken, P., Heath, D., and Brewer, D.: The relation between the weight of the right ventricle and the percentage of abnormal air space in the lung in emphysema. *J. Path. Bact.* **92:** 519, 1966a.

Hicken, P., Brewer, D., and Heath, D.: The relation between the weight of the right ventricle of the heart and the internal surface area and number of alveoli in the human lung in emphysema. *J. Path. Bact.* **92:** 529, 1966b.

Honey, M., and Jepson, E.: Multiple bronchostenoses due to sarcoidosis. *Brit. Med. J.* **ii:** 1330, 1957.

Howarth, S., McMichael, J., and Sharpey-Schafer, E. P.: Effects of oxygen, venesection and digitalis in chronic heart failure from disease of the lungs. *Clin. Sc.* **6:** 187, 1947.

Hyun, B. H., Diggs, C. L., and Toone, E. C.: Dermatomyositis with cystic fibrosis (honeycombing) of the lung. *Dis. Chest* **42:** 449, 1962.

Ishihama, Y., Iwasaki, T., Onga, H., Yoshida, H., Yorifuji, S., Tomomatsu, T., and Funabiki, N.: An autopsy case of Takayasu's arteritis with pulmonary hypertension. *Japan. Circ. J.* **37**: 647, 1973.

Jacques, J. E., and Barclay, R.: The solid sarcomatous pulmonary artery. *Brit. J. Dis. Chest* **54**: 217, 1960.

James, W. R. L., and Thomas, A. J.: Right ventricular hypertrophy and the small pulmonary arteries in chronic lung disease. *Brit. Heart J.* **25**: 583, 1963.

Jennings, F. L., and Arden, A.: Development of radiation pneumonitis. Time and dose factors. *Arch. Path.* **74**: 351, 1962.

Junghanss, W.: Das Lungenemphysem im postmortalen Angiogramm. *Virch. Arch. Path. Anat.* **332**: 538, 1959.

Kane, R. D., Hawkins, H. K., Miller, J. A., and Noce, P. S.: Microscopic pulmonary tumor emboli associated with dyspnea. *Cancer* **36**: 1473, 1975.

Kapancy, Y., and Chamay, A.: Lésions en anse de fil de fer des capillaires pulmonaires dans le lupus érythemateux disseminé (L.E.D.). *Virch. Arch. Path. Anat.* **342**: 236, 1967.

Kernen, J. A., O'Neal, R. M., and Edwards, D. L.: Pulmonary arteriosclerosis and thromboembolism in chronic pulmonary emphysema. *Arch. Path.* **65**: 471, 1958.

Klemperer, P., Pollack, A. D., and Baehr, G.: Pathology of disseminated lupus erythematosus. *Arch. Path.* **32**: 569, 1941.

Lee, B. Y., Trainor, F. S., Schulz, R. Z., Forestiere, J. A., and Madden, J. L.: Pulmonary vascular alterations in diseases of the lungs. *Surg. Gynec. Obstet.* **132**: 3, 1971.

Leopold, J. G., and Gough, J.: Centrilobular form of hypertrophic emphysema and its relation to chronic bronchitis. *Thorax* **12**: 219, 1957.

Liebow, A. A.: The bronchopulmonary venous collateral circulation with special reference to emphysema. *Amer. J. Path.* **29**: 251, 1953.

Liebow, A. A.: Definition and classification of interstitial pneumonias in human pathology. *Progr. Resp. Res.* **8**: 1, 1975.

Liebow, A. A., Hales, M. R., and Lindskog, G. E.: Enlargement of the bronchial arteries and their anastomoses with the pulmonary arteries in chronic pulmonary disease. *Amer. J. Path.* **24**: 691, 1948.

Liebow, A. A., Hales, M. R., and Lindskog, G. E.: Enlargement of the bronchial arteries and their anastomoses with the pulmonary arteries in bronchiectasis. *Amer. J. Path.* **25**: 211, 1949.

Liebow, A. A., Steer, A., and Billingsley, J. G.: Desquamative interstitial pneumonia. *Amer. J. Med.* **39**: 369, 1965.

Liebow, A. A., and Carrington, C. B.: Hypersensitivity reactions involving the lung. *Trans. Stud. Coll. Phys. Philad.* **34**: 47, 1966.

Linenthal, H., and Talkov, R.: Pulmonary fibrosis in Raynaud's disease. *New Engl. J. Med.* **224**: 682, 1941.

Littler, W. A., Kay, J. M., Hasleton, P. S., and Heath, D.: Busulphan lung. *Thorax* **24**: 639, 1969.

Marchand, P., Gilroy, J. C., and Wilson, V. H.: An anatomical study of the bronchial vascular system and its variations in disease. *Thorax* **5**: 207, 1950.

McCann, B. G., and Brewer, D. B.: A case of desquamative interstitial pneumonia progressing to "honeycomb lung." *J. Path.* **112**: 199, 1974.

McLean, K. H.: The significance of pulmonary vascular changes in emphysema. *Australasian Ann. Med.* **7**: 69, 1958.

Michaels, L., Brown, N. J., and Cory-Wright, M.: Arterial changes in pulmonary sarcoidosis. *Arch. Path.* **69**: 741, 1960.

Mitchell, R. S., Ryan, S. F., Petty, T. L., and Filley, G. F.: The significance of morphologic chronic hyperplastic bronchitis. *Amer. Rev. Resp. Dis.* **93**: 720, 1966.

Mitov, A., Solakov, P., and Peeva, I.: A rare case of Takayasu disease affecting abdominal aorta and pulmonary artery. *Cor et Vasa* **13**: 147, 1971.

Morgan, A. D.: The pathology of subacute cor pulmonale in diffuse carcinomatosis of the lungs. *J. Path. Bact.* **61**: 75, 1949.

Muschenheim, C.: Some observations on the Hamman-Rich disease. *Amer. J. Med. Sci.* **241**: 279, 1961.

Nadas, A. S., Cogan, G., Landing, B. H., and Schwachman, H.: Studies in pancreatic fibrosis: Cor pulmonale: clinical and pathological observations. *Pediatrics* **10**:319, 1952.

Naeye, R. L.: Pulmonary vascular lesions in systemic scleroderma. *Dis. Chest* **44**: 368, 1963.

Naeye, R. L., and Dellinger, W. S.: Pulmonary arterial changes with age and smoking. *Arch. Path.* **92**: 284, 1971.

Naeye, R. L., Greenberg, S. D., and Valdivia, E.: Small pulmonary vessels in advanced pulmonary emphysema. *Arch. Path.* **97**: 216, 1974.

Nicod, J. L.: Les lésions vasculaires dans de poumon silicotique et leurs relations avec la tuberculose. *Schweiz. Z. Path. Bact.* **12**: 157, 1949.

Oderr, C. P.: Emphysema, soot, and pulmonary circulation; macroscopic studies of aging lungs. *J.A.M.A.* **172**: 1991, 1960.

Old, J. W., and Russell, W. O.: Congenital heart disease with necrotizing arteritis (periarteritis nodosa) limited to the pulmonary arteries: report of case with necropsy. *Amer. J. Path.* **23**: 903, 1947.

Oliner, H., Schwartz, R., Rubio, F., and Dameshek, W.: Interstitial pulmonary fibrosis following busulphan therapy. *Amer. J. Med.* **31**: 134, 1961.

Olsen, E. G. J., and Lever, J. V.: Pulmonary changes in systemic lupus erythematosus. *Brit. J. Dis. Chest* **66**: 71, 1967.

Oram, S., and Stokes, W.: The heart in scleroderma. *Brit. Heart J.* **23**: 243, 1961.

Pace, W. R., Decker, J. L., and Martin, C. J.: Polymyositis: report of two cases with pulmonary function studies suggestive of progressive systemic sclerosis. *Amer. J. Med. Sci.* **245**: 322, 1963.

Patterson, C. D., Harville, W. E., and Pierce, J. A.: Rheumatoid lung disease. *Ann. Int. Med.* **62**: 685, 1965.

Plessinger, V. A., and Jolly, P. N.: Rasmussen's aneurysms and fatal hemorrhage in pulmonary tuberculosis. *Amer. Rev. Tuberc.* **60**: 589, 1949.

Rasmussen, V.: On haemoptyse, navnlig den lethale, i anatomisk og klinisk henseende. *Hospitals-Tidende* **11**: 33, 1868.

Reid, J. A., and Heard, B. E.: Preliminary studies of the pulmonary capillaries by India ink injection. *Med. Thorac.* **19**: 220, 1962.

Reid, J. A., and Heard, B. E.: The capillary network of normal and emphysematous human lungs studied by injection of Indian ink. *Thorax* **18**: 201, 1963.

Reid, L.: *The Pathology of Emphysema.* Lloyd-Luke Ltd., London, 1967.

Rubin, E. H., and Lubliner, R.: The Hamman-Rich syndrome: review of the literature and analysis of 15 cases. *Medicine* **36**: 397, 1957.

Rüttner, J. R., and Gassman, R.: Lungengefässveränderungen bei Silikose. *Schweiz. Zschr. Allg. Path.* **20**: 737, 1957.

Ryan, S. F.: Pulmonary embolism and thrombosis in chronic obstructive emphysema. *Amer. J. Path.* **43**: 767, 1963.

Ryland, D., and Reid, L.: The pulmonary circulation in cystic fibrosis. *Thorax* **30**: 285, 1975.

Scadding, J. G.: Meaning of diagnostic terms in broncho-pulmonary disease. *Brit. Med. J.* **ii**: 1425, 1963.

Schepers, G. W. H.: Comparative vascular pathology of occupational chest diseases. *Arch. Industr. Health* **12**: 7, 1955.

Schiller, H. M., and Madge, G. E.: Neoplasms within the pulmonary veins. *Chest* **58**: 535, 1970.

Schüren, K. P., and Hütteman, U.: Chronisches Cor pulmonale bei obstruktiven Lungenerkrankungen: Korrelation der gestörten Atmungsfunktion zur Hämodynamik des Lungenkreislaufs und kontraktilen Funktion des rechten Ventrikels. *Verh. Dtsch. Ges. Kreislaufforsch.* **38**: 205, 1972.

Slama, R., Crevelier, A., Coumel, P., and Snanoudj, S.: Hypertension artérielle pulmonaire primitive et lupus érythemateux disséminé. *Presse Méd.* **75**: 961, 1967.

Smith, P., and Heath, D.: Paraquat lung: a reappraisal. *Thorax* **29**: 643, 1974.

Soergel, K. H., and Sommers, S. C.: Idiopathic pulmonary hemosiderosis and related syndromes. *Amer. J. Med.* **32**: 499, 1962.

Spencer, H.: Pulmonary lesions in polyarteritis nodosa. *Brit. J. Tuberc.* **51**: 123, 1957.

Spencer, H.: Interstitial pneumonia. *Ann. Rev. Med.* **18:** 423, 1967.

Spencer, H.: *Pathology of the Lung.* Pergamon Press, Ltd., Oxford, London, 1968a.

Spencer, H.: In Liebow, A. A., and Smith, D. E., *The Lung.* Williams & Wilkins, Baltimore, 1968b.

Spencer, H.: Pathogenesis of interstitial fibrosis of the lung. *Progr. Resp. Res.* **8:** 34, 1975.

Storstein, O.: Circulatory failure in metastatic carcinoma of the lung. A physiologic and pathologic study of its pathogenesis. *Circulation* **4:** 913, 1951.

Sweeney, A. R., and Baggenstoss, A. H.: Pulmonary lesions of periarteritis nodosa. *Proc. Staff Meet. Mayo Clin.* **24:** 35, 1949.

Symchych, P. S.: Pulmonary hypertension in cystic fibrosis. *Arch. Path.* **92:** 409, 1971.

Thurlbeck, W. M., and Angus, G. E.: A distribution curve for chronic bronchitis. *Thorax* **19:** 436, 1964.

Thijs, L. G., Kroon, T. A. J., and Van Leeuwen, T. M.,: Leiomyosarcoma of the pulmonary trunk associated with prericardial effusion. *Thorax* **29:** 490, 1974.

Trell, E., and Lindström, C.: Pulmonary hypertension in systemic sclerosis. *Ann. Rheum. Dis.* **30:** 390, 1971.

Wackers, F. J. T., van der Schoot, J. B., and Hampe, J. F.: Sarcoma of the pulmonary trunk associated with hemorrhagic tendency. A case report and review of the literature. *Cancer* **23:** 339, 1969.

Wade, O. L., and Bishop, J. M.: *Cardiac Output and Regional Blood Flow.* Blackwell, Oxford, 1962, p. 150.

Wagenaar, S. S.: Histologie en histopathologie van bronchiale arterien. Thesis, Amsterdam, 1975.

Wagenvoort, C. A., Morrow, G. W., and Ten Cate, H. W.: Squamous cell carcinoma of the renal pelvis with muco-epidermoid metastasis. *J. Urol.* **85:** 727, 1961.

Wagenvoort, C. A., Heath, D., and Edwards, J. E.: *The Pathology of the Pulmonary Vasculature.* Charles C Thomas, Springfield, Ill., 1964.

Wagenvoort, C. A., and Wagenvoort, N.: Pulmonary arteries in bronchial carcinoma. *Arch. Path.* **79:** 529, 1965.

Wagenvoort, C. A., and Wagenvoort, N.: Hypoxic pulmonary vascular lesions in man at high altitude and in patients with chronic respiratory disease. *Path. Microbiol.* **39:** 276, 1973.

Wagenvoort, C. A., Wagenvoort, N., and Wildevuur, C. R. H.: Morphological changes in long-term denervated and reimplanted lungs. In Wildevuur, C. R. H., *Morphology in Lung Transplantation.* Karger, Basel, 1973.

Walker, W. C., and Wright, V.: Pulmonary lesions and rheumatoid arthritis. *Medicine* **47:** 501, 1968.

Weaver, A. L., Brundage, B. H., Nelson, R. A., and Bischoff, M. B.: Pulmonary involvement in polymyositis: report of a case with response to corticosteroid therapy. *Arthr. Rheum.* **11:** 765, 1968.

Wentworth, P., Gough, J., and Wentworth, J. E.: Pulmonary changes and cor pulmonale in mucoviscidosis. *Thorax* **23:** 582, 1968.

W.H.O. Report. Chronic cor pulmonale. Report of an expert committee, Geneva, 1961.

Wolf, P. L., Dickenman, R. C., and Langston, J. D.: Fibrosarcoma of the pulmonary artery, masquerading as a pheochromocytoma. *Amer. J. Clin. Path.* **34:** 146, 1960.

Wood, D. A., and Miller, M.: The rôle of the dual pulmonary circulation in various pathologic conditions of the lungs. *J. Thorac. Surg.* **7:** 649, 1938.

Wyatt, J. P., Fischer, V. W., and Sweet, H.: Centrilobular emphysema. *Lab. Invest.* **10:** 159, 1961.

CHAPTER THIRTEEN

Pulmonary Hypertension in Congenital Malformation of Pulmonary Vessels

Congenital cardiovascular anomalies involving the pulmonary vasculature are uncommon but often produce pulmonary hypertension. A brief discussion of these conditions is therefore necessary.

The mechanism by which the rise in pulmonary arterial pressure is produced varies widely in these anomalies. Hyperkinetic pulmonary hypertension with a large flow through the pulmonary circulation and direct transmission of systemic pressure is present in those malformations that include a wide communication between aorta and pulmonary vasculature, as in many cases of persistent truncus arteriosus or aorticopulmonary septal defect.

An increased pulmonary arterial resistance sometimes is provided by multiple congenital stenoses of the branches of the pulmonary artery, while pulmonary venous hypertension is produced by similar obstruction of pulmonary veins or sometimes by anomalous pulmonary venous drainage.

PULMONARY ARTERIES

Persistent Truncus Arteriosus

In the anomaly called persistent truncus arteriosus, only a single arterial vessel leaves the ventricular part of the heart. Failure of the truncoconal septum to develop is basic to this malformation. Since there is almost always an associated ventricular septal defect (Van Praagh and Van Praagh, 1965), the truncus arteriosus usually overrides this defect and thus takes its origin from both ventricles or, if the ventricular septum is completely absent, from a single ventricle. The truncus arteriosus sometimes may arise from the right ventricle and rarely from the left.

Collett and Edwards (1949) classified four types. In type I (48 percent) both the ascending aorta and a single pulmonary trunk arise from the truncus arteriosus. The pulmonary trunk divides into left and right main pulmonary arteries. In type II (29 percent) there is no pulmonary trunk but left and right main pulmonary arteries have origins from the dorsal part of the truncus arteriosus, immediately adjacent to each other. Type III (10 percent) represents the situation in which there is an independent origin of the main pulmonary arteries from either side of the truncus arteriosus, while in type IV (13 percent) the main pulmonary arteries as well as the ductus arteriosus are absent. In these latter instances the lungs are supplied only by bronchial arteries, which originate from the descending aorta.

The origin of the pulmonary arteries may be stenotic, and in this way the pulmonary circulation may be protected from the high pressure prevailing in the truncus arteriosus. If, however, in types I, II, or III these arteries are wide, hyperkinetic pulmonary hypertension usually is present and the well-known picture of plexogenic pulmonary arteriopathy (Chapter Four) develops. In cases with unilateral stenosis the muscular pulmonary arteries (Figure 13-1) and arterioles (Figure 13-2) may be normal on the side of the stenosis, while on the contralateral side marked medial hypertrophy (Figure 13-3) and intimal fibrosis (Figure 13-4) may occur.

Aorticopulmonary Septal Defect

This rare malformation, also called aortopulmonary window, is a form of partial persistence of the truncus arteriosus (Edwards, 1968). It provides a situation not

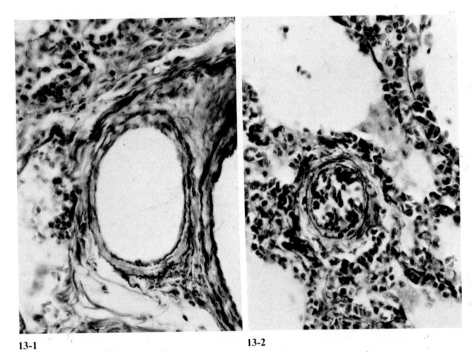

13-1   13-2

Figure 13-1. Normal muscular pulmonary artery from the right lung of a 2½-year-old girl with persistent truncus arteriosus. This lung was protected by a stenosis in the initial portion of the right pulmonary artery (El.v.G., ×230).

Figure 13-2. Normal pulmonary arteriole from the right lung of the same case as Figure 13-1. Smooth muscle cells are present in part of the vascular circumference (El.v.G., ×230).

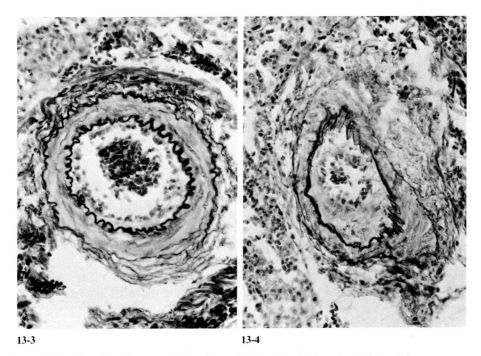

13-3   13-4

Figure 13-3. Muscular pulmonary artery with medial hypertrophy from the left lung of the same case as Figure·13-1. There was unilateral left-sided pulmonary hypertension (El.v.G., ×230).
Figure 13-4. Muscular pulmonary artery with medial hypertrophy and cellular intimal proliferation from the left lung of the same case as Figure 13-1 (El.v.G., ×230).

unlike that in a wide patent ductus arteriosus, which it may resemble clinically, but a continuous murmur is usually absent (Morrow et al., 1962).

In this anomaly the pulmonary trunk and ascending aorta arise from their ostia separately but shortly above the ostia there is a defect of variable size in the aorticopulmonary septum. Sometimes this defect is immediately adjacent to the ostia but even then there are normal pulmonary and aortic valves by which the condition can be separated from a persistent truncus arteriosus (Neufeld et al., 1962). Moreover, a ventricular septal defect usually is absent (Binet et al., 1973).

Pulmonary hypertension almost always complicates this anomaly with the pattern of plexogenic pulmonary arteriopathy (Chapter Four). This makes an early diagnosis and early corrective surgery of the defect imperative (Thibert and Simon, 1974).

Unilateral Absence of Pulmonary Artery

In this rare anomaly the pulmonary trunk, instead of bifurcating, runs as a single pulmonary artery to one of the lungs. The other lung, in the absence of a pulmonary artery, is supplied by a branch from the aorta. This branch arises from the ascending aorta, from one of the large branches of the aortic arch, from the aortic arch itself, or from the descending aorta.

Cucci et al. (1964) suggested that such a malformation is caused by the dorsal shifting of one of the two ridges responsible for the septation of the truncus arteriosus. This would result in incorporation of the sixth arch on the side of the dorsorotated truncal ridge into the ascending aorta. Such a view, however, would not be consistent with the modern concepts on the development of pulmonary trunk and ascending aorta (p. 17).

Pool and associates (1962) collected 98 cases including 4 of their own, from the world literature and gave an extensive review of the subject. In 78 of these cases full data were available. In 40 of these the left and in 38 the right pulmonary artery was absent. The ages ranged from infancy up to 63 years.

Absence of one pulmonary artery often is associated with other cardiovascular shunts such as a patent ductus arteriosus or a ventricular septal defect. In these instances pulmonary hypertension occurs in 88 percent of the patients, while this incidence is 19 percent in isolated cases (Pool et al., 1962).

In the absence of cardiac shunts it is remarkable that pulmonary hypertension should be present in the lung receiving its blood supply from the pulmonary artery, since in adults ligation of one pulmonary artery or pneumonectomy does not result in a significant elevation of pulmonary arterial pressure (p. 9). It must be assumed that the thick-walled fetal pulmonary arteries, when exposed to the stimulus of the full cardiac output, react more vigorously than those in an adult and in this way keep up a high vascular resistance.

If pulmonary hypertension develops in unilateral absence of a pulmonary artery, it is usually at an early age. Most of these patients die young from right heart failure, although some reach adulthood. On the other hand, there are also patients with isolated unilateral pulmonary arterial absence who develop pulmonary hypertension only during exercise (Elder et al., 1958) or who even may remain entirely asymptomatic (Pool et al., 1962). It is likely that in patients with this malformation an individual hypo- or hyper-reactivity of the lung vessels is decisive for the development of pulmonary hypertension.

Since the hemodynamic situation is essentially different in both lungs, the lung vessels also may show a different pattern in left and right lung. This difference is of course accentuated when there is unilateral pulmonary hypertension and even more so when there is stenosis of the systemic artery to the contralateral lung. In such a case there may be a marked contrast between the severely hypertrophic media of the muscular pulmonary arteries in the one lung and the atrophic media of those in the other lung (Wagenvoort et al., 1961).

Pulmonary hypertension also may occur in the lung supplied by the systemic artery so that in some instances hypertensive pulmonary vascular lesions may be found in both lungs (Schubert and Ruickoldt, 1955; DuShane et al., 1960).

In unilateral agenesis of a lung there is of course also absence of one pulmonary artery (Ferguson and Neuhauser, 1944; Ferencz, 1961), which in principle may have the same hemodynamic consequences.

Absent Left Pulmonary Artery

In the absence of the left pulmonary artery the systemic arterial blood supply is never derived from the ascending aorta. A patent ductus arteriosus is present only in exceptional cases (Wu et al., 1964). On the other hand, for unknown reasons there is a close association with the tetralogy of Fallot. In 17 patients with the association of tetralogy of Fallot with unilateral absence of a pulmonary artery, this vessel was absent on the left side in 16, while the only patient with an absent right pulmonary artery had a dextrocardia (Pool et al., 1962). Other cardiac malformations such as septal defects are uncommon and have no preference for agenesis of left or right pulmonary artery. Stenosis of the single right pulmonary artery also has been reported (Baxter et al., 1961; Chesler and Duckworth, 1964).

Absent Right Pulmonary Artery

In 7 out of 40 cases of absent right pulmonary artery the systemic artery to the right lung arose from the ascending aorta (Pool et al., 1962). In these instances it may be assumed that the proximal part of the sixth aortic arch was interrupted, while the distal end, which normally disappears, remained intact, so that the right pulmonary artery was completely derived from the ascending aorta. The finding of ductal tissue in the proximal course of a narrowed right pulmonary artery originating from the ascending aorta, suggests that a right ductus arteriosus participated in the formation of this vessel. It is likely, therefore, that such an artery represents a right pulmonary artery originating from the aorta (Wagenvoort et al., 1961).

An absence of a right pulmonary artery is commonly associated with a patent ductus arteriosus but not with a tetralogy of Fallot.

Localized Pulmonary Arterial Stenosis

Congenital stenosis of the pulmonary artery distal to the pulmonary valve, or of its branches, may be a cause of pulmonary hypertension. Originally, it was believed to be a very rare occurrence, but since the descriptions of Shumacker and Lurie (1953) of one case and of Søndergaard (1954) of three cases, it has become clear that this condition is not extremely uncommon, although often unrecognized clinically and at autopsy. In 1965, McCue et al. reviewed 319 cases from the literature, adding 20 of their own. D'Cruz et al. (1964) reported on 84 patients, 32 with unilateral and 52 with bilateral stenoses, and Eldredge et al. (1972) on 70 patients, of whom 17 underwent serial catheterization.

A characteristic clinical feature in many cases is a continuous murmur, and such a murmur also has been produced in dogs by experimental graded constriction of a large pulmonary arterial branch (Eldredge et al., 1972). Others insist that the murmur is systolic rather than continuous (LeBauer and Perloff, 1967) or believe that if there is a continuous murmur, this results from abnormally increased bronchial arterial flow accompanying obstruction of a pulmonary artery (Lees and Dother, 1965).

Pulmonary hypertension varies according to the number of branches that are stenotic and to the degree of obstruction. The systolic pressure is elevated with rapid fall to diastolic levels (LeBauer and Perloff, 1967).

It is now well documented that congenital stenosis of pulmonary arteries is often part of a postrubella syndrome. It is then often associated with patent ductus arteriosus, valvular pulmonic stenosis, coarctation of the aorta, or combination of such anomalies (Rowe, 1963; Emmanouilides et al., 1964; Hartmann et al., 1967;

Wasserman et al., 1968; Tang et al., 1971). The association of multiple pulmonary arterial stenoses with other congenital anomalies either of the cardiovascular system or of other organs, is also common. Familial occurrence has been described (McDonald et al., 1969; Watson and Miller, 1973).

A congenital stenosis may be found in the pulmonary trunk as a membranous stenosis immediately above the pulmonary valve or as a calcified ring around the artery.

The bifurcation may be the site of stenosis with narrowing of the proximal parts of both left and right pulmonary arteries. For these cases the term "coarctation of the pulmonary artery" has been used (Søndergaard, 1954). In one of his cases fibrous bands extended from the ligamentum arteriosum to both branches.

The stenoses may be located more distally in the course of one or both main pulmonary arteries and in the intrapulmonary primary, or even in peripheral branches. Tubular hypoplasia rather than focal stenosis also has been reported (Belcher and Pattinson, 1957).

Classifications of this condition have been based on anatomic (Smith, 1958), clinical (Delaney and Nadas, 1964) or roentgenologic (Gay et al., 1963) features.

In a case of multiple stenoses of intrapulmonary arteries MacMahon et al. (1967) described marked thickening of the intima and media as well as of the adventitia in the affected segment. In one of our own cases in which there was a localized stenosis of the pulmonary trunk (Figures 13-5 and 13-6), this vessel was narrowed by a thick

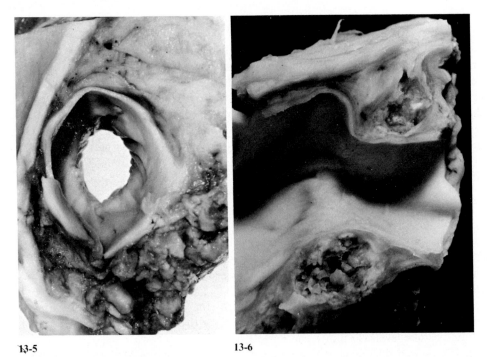

13-5   13-6

Figure 13-5.   Localized stenosis of the pulmonary trunk in a 74-year-old man with right ventricular hypertrophy. The patient died of myocardial infarction.
Figure 13-6.   Longitudinal section of pulmonary trunk from the same case as Figure 13-5. There is a calcified ring around the stenotic area.

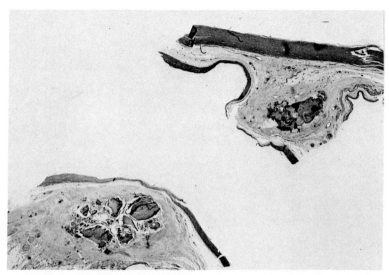

Figure 13-7. Histologic section of the pulmonary trunk from the same case as Figure 13-5. Calcified ring in cross section in the adventitia. The media is intact but thinned in the area of stenosis. Wall of aorta at top (H. and E., ×3.5).

calcified ring in the adventitia, while there was thinning of the media in this area (Figure 13-7).

Pulmonary Sequestration

The term pulmonary sequestration describes a congenital anomaly of the lung characterized by a mass of nonfunctioning, often cystic lung tissue, resembling a hamartoma, that is supplied by one or more abnormal systemic arteries, while the remaining lung tissue is normally supplied by the pulmonary artery.

Extralobar and intralobar sequestrations are recognized. In the extralobar sequestration, the abnormal mass of lung tissue is isolated, usually on the left, and presents as an accessory lung and often as a cyst containing lung tissue and cystic bronchi (Heath and Watts, 1957).

The intralobar sequestration, which is the more common variety, has a characteristic position in the posterior basic segment of one of the lower lobes (Figure 13-8). The anomalous systemic artery or arteries usually are derived from the lower thoracic aorta, less often from the upper abdominal aorta, and rarely from other systemic arteries. Sometimes this area receives branches from the pulmonary artery as well (Wagenvoort et al., 1964).

Pulmonary sequestration does not cause elevation of pressure in the pulmonary circulation and the vessels within the lung tend to be normal with the exception of the sequestrated area. In this area the tissue is exposed to systemic pressures, and in some cases hypertensive vascular changes can be observed. These range from atherosclerosis of the aberrant artery and its branches (Johnston, 1956) to medial hypertrophy and necrotizing arteritis (Heath and Watts, 1957), while in some instances even plexiform lesions have been described (Ostrow et al., 1973). In most

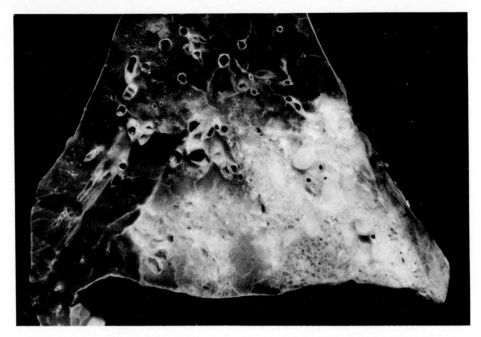

Figure 13-8. Lower lobe of left lung with intralobar sequestration in a 7-year-old boy. The area of sequestration is pale as a result of inflammation and contains cystic bronchi filled with mucus.

cases, however, the pulmonary arteries are either normal or exhibit intimal fibrosis (Figure 13-9) secondary to the inflammatory alterations, usually accompanying these malformations. A proportion of the arteries supplying the sequestrated area have a structure intermediate between pulmonary and bronchial arteries (Figure 13-10). These are called "hybrid" arteries.

Pulmonary Arteriovenous Fistulae

Pulmonary arteriovenous fistula or aneurysm is a relatively common malformation of the lung vessels. These fistulae vary in size from minute teleangiectatic areas to large vascular malformations measuring up to 8 × 6 × 4 cm (Hepburn and Dauphinee, 1942). They usually are situated in the lower lobe and often immediately adjacent to the pleura (Figures 13-11, 13-12, 13-13 and 13-14). One or more tortuous pulmonary arterial branches feed these fistulae, usually without bronchial arterial contribution. They are drained by large, wide pulmonary veins.

These fistulae are often multiple and may be an expression of Rendu-Osler's disease. They may cause cerebral abscess and thrombosis, systemic hypoxia, and sometimes fatal pulmonary hemorrhage, but pulmonary hypertension as a rule does not occur, nor would it be expected.

Even so there are some reports of pulmonary hypertension as in the cases of Sapru et al. (1969) and Javier et al. (1970). The cause of the pulmonary hypertension in these cases has remained obscure, although Javier et al. (1970) attributed the mild elevation of pressure in their case to a left to right bronchial artery shunt. One

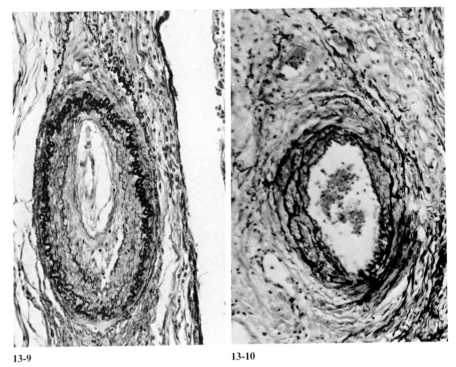

13-9   13-10

Figure 13-9. Muscular pulmonary artery with marked intimal fibrosis in an area of lung sequestration in a 45-year-old woman (El.v.G., ×230).

Figure 13-10. "Hybrid" artery of a type intermediate between a pulmonary and a bronchial artery in an area of lung sequestration, in a 23-year-old man (El.v.G., ×140).

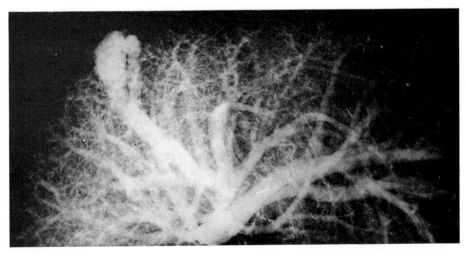

Figure 13-11. Postmortem arteriogram of the lung of a 20-year-old woman with Rendu-Osler's disease and multiple arteriovenous fistulae. One of these is visible directly under the pleura (top, left).

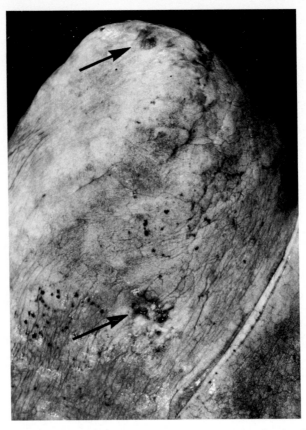

Figure 13-12. Apex of left lung with multiple arteriovenous fistulae under the pleura (arrows). Same case as Figure 13-11.

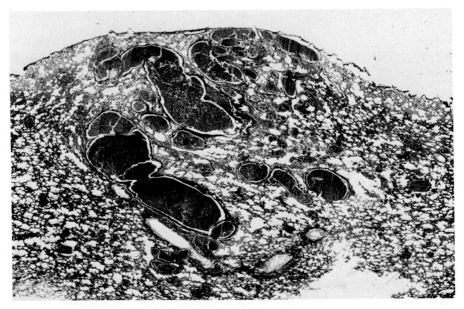

Figure 13-13. Arteriovenous fistula from the same case as Figure 13-11. It consists of wide, tortuous channels representing in part arteries and in part veins (El.v.G., ×12).

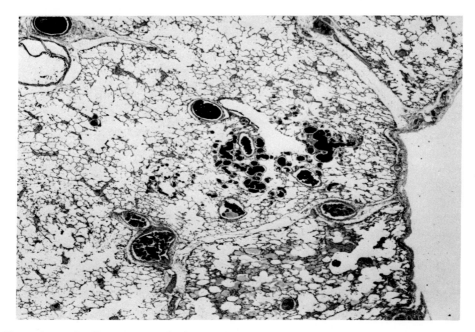

Figure 13-14. Small arteriovenous fistula from the same case as Figure 13-11. Such small fistulae were fairly numerous in both lungs (H. and E., ×20).

would expect that in severe elevation of pulmonary arterial pressure the arteriovenous fistula would act as a safety valve. This apparently happened in the patient described by Le Roux et al. (1970). The patient, a girl with pulmonary hypertension due to schistosomiasis, died of heart failure following resection of an arteriovenous fistula.

Trell et al. (1972) reported of two sisters with Rendu-Osler's disease and intrahepatic arteriovenous fistulae with systemic-pulmonary arterial anastomoses who developed severe pulmonary hypertension. The pulmonary vasculature showed pronounced changes that reportedly included alterations suggestive of plexiform lesions, although this is not borne out by their illustrations.

PULMONARY VEINS

Anomalous Pulmonary Venous Connection

Partial anomalous pulmonary venous connection implies that some pulmonary veins do not communicate with the left atrium, while the others have a normal connection. The right lung is much more often involved than the left. The anomalous veins, that may drain a whole lung or part of it, connect directly with the right atrium or indirectly after merging with a systemic vein. An atrial septal defect usually but not always is present (Edwards, 1968).

The right atrium and the pulmonary trunk usually are dilated and the right ventricle may be hypertrophied. If most of the pulmonary veins are connected in this way, which is rare, the condition resembles total anomalous pulmonary venous connection.

In total anomalous pulmonary venous connection, none of the pulmonary veins communicate with the left atrium and the blood carried by these veins is directed toward the right atrium. Sometimes, when the pulmonary veins are normally connected with the left atrium, they drain their blood to the right atrium if there is an atrial septal defect. The physiologic effect is then the same as when there is an abnormal anatomic connection with the right atrium. In these instances the term "anomalous pulmonary venous drainage," which includes this situation, is advisable (Edwards, 1968).

The communication of the pulmonary veins with the right atrium may happen in various ways. A supracardiac connection may occur into the remnant of the left superior vena cava or directly into the right superior vena cava. A direct communication with the right atrium, eventually by way of the coronary sinus, is another common variation. Infracardiac connections are less frequent. In these instances a common anomalous pulmonary vein perforates the diaphragm and joins the ductus venosus, the left gastric vein, the inferior vena cava, a hepatic vein, or the portal system. All sorts of combinations of these varieties occur (Edwards and Helmholtz, 1956; Darling et al., 1957; Burroughs and Edwards, 1960; Blake et al., 1965).

In all forms of total anomalous pulmonary venous connection, all the pulmonary venous blood eventually arrives in the right atrium. There is always a communication between both atria, either as a patent foramen ovale or as an atrial septal defect, so that, in principle, the atria and the ventricles all contain blood with equal oxygen saturation. Some difference between pulmonary and systemic arterial oxygenation may result from the preferential flow from the inferior vena cava through the patent foramen ovale so that in the infracardiac connections of the pulmonary veins, the systemic oxygen saturation is usually somewhat greater than in the other forms.

The hemodynamic and clinical implications of the anomaly have been described by Snellen and Albers (1952), Burchell (1956) and Swan et al. (1956). One of the consequences may be pulmonary hypertension. Sometimes it is not clear why the pulmonary vascular resistance is increased but in many instances localized stenoses of the anomalous pulmonary veins, particularly when they have a connection with veins below the diaphragm, are likely to be the cause (Edwards, 1960; Hauck et al., 1960). Moreover, the whole anomalous vein may be the site of increased resistance by its length and small caliber (Carey and Edwards, 1963).

In our own experience, if the pattern of pulmonary vascular lesions in patients with anomalous pulmonary venous connection is abnormal, it usually is the same as in cases of chronic pulmonary venous hypertension. In infants with this condition the small pulmonary veins often show pronounced arterialization (Figure 13-15), while the pulmonary arteries exhibit medial hypertrophy (Figure 13-16). Moreover, there may be pronounced diffuse lymphangiectasy (Figure 13-17). Indeed, these findings suggest that an obstruction at the venous level is basic to the elevated pressure.

Scimitar Syndrome

The underlying malformation in the scimitar syndrome is a complex one, usually involving the heart, the lungs and the pulmonary arteries and veins. The heart

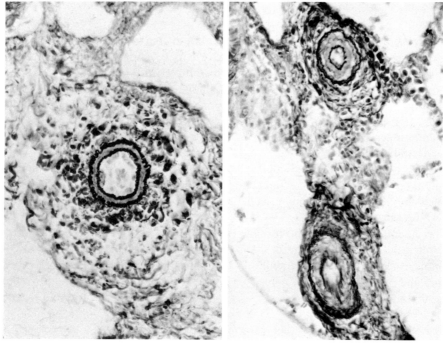

13-15   13-16

Figure 13-15. Pulmonary vein with pronounced medial hypertrophy and arterialization in a 2-month-old male infant with total anomalous pulmonary venous connection (El.v.G., ×230).

Figure 13-16. Muscular pulmonary arteries with pronounced medial hypertrophy from the same case as Figure 13-15 (El.v.G., ×230).

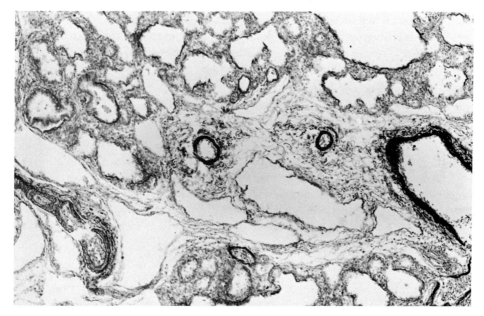

Figure 13-17. Lung tissue with medial hypertrophy of pulmonary arteries (left) and pulmonary veins (middle and right) and lymphangiectasis, in a 6-month-old female infant with total anomalous pulmonary venous connection (El.v.G., ×90).

generally shows dextrorotation and dextroposition, but as a rule, it is otherwise normal. Usually the right lung is hypoplastic and consists of only two lobes. Bronchiectasis sometimes is described in this lung (Kittle and Crockett, 1962). In one case the condition was associated with a "horseshoe lung" (Dische et al., 1974).

Commonly the right lung is supplied by one or more large systemic pulmonary arteries originating directly from the descending aorta. The right pulmonary artery is usually much smaller in caliber than the left (Sanger et al., 1963), or it may be absent (Hollis, 1964).

The most characteristic and constant feature, however, is anomalous drainage of the pulmonary veins from the right lung or more frequently from the right lower lobe to the abdominal inferior vena cava, by way of a single venous trunk which penetrates the diaphragm.

This anomalous vein can be recognized on a chest roentgenogram as a more or less vertical but crescent-shaped shadow resembling a curved Turkish sword, or scimitar. Because the venous anomaly is the most constant characteristic of the syndrome and even has led to its name, we prefer to discuss this syndrome in connection with anomalous pulmonary venous connections, of which it represents a partial form.

The scimitar syndrome is not extremely rare since more and more cases are recognized, usually in infants or children but also often in adults. Both sexes are affected equally. The great variety of its symptoms is reflected in many reports (Park, 1912; Dotter et al., 1949; Jue et al., 1966; Massumi et al., 1967; Trell et al., 1971; Kuiper-Oosterwal and Moulaert, 1973; Farnsworth and Ankeney, 1974).

Pulmonary hypertension is uncommon in the scimitar syndrome, although hypertensive pulmonary vascular changes may be observed in the right lung or right lower lobe supplied by anomalous systemic arteries. In the case of Glancy et al. (1968) pulmonary hypertension was due to an associated patent ductus but Neill et al. (1960) described pulmonary hypertension with extensive vascular changes, including plexiform lesions, and in the absence of associated anomalies, in one patient, whose father exhibited the same syndrome.

Atresia of Common Pulmonary Vein

A very rare malformation related to total anomalous pulmonary venous connection is atresia of the common pulmonary vein (Lucas et al., 1962a). In this condition the pulmonary veins form a blind pouch without any connection with the atria. Small branches of mediastinal veins may permit some flow to the systemic veins but severe pulmonary venous obstruction is characteristic.

Levoatrial Cardinal Vein

Levoatrial cardinal vein represents a rare anomaly that essentially is an example of an abnormal connection of the pulmonary veins. It is observed in infants with mitral atresia or aortic atresia, particularly in the absence of a wide interatrial communication (Lucas et al., 1962b; Shone and Edwards, 1964).

In these instances there is a severe outflow obstruction to the left atrium and thus to the pulmonary veins, even though these normally are connected with the left atrium. A collateral vein, serving as an escape route, runs from a pulmonary to a systemic vein. Since during development, the distal portion of the pulmonary veins is incorporated into the left atrium, this collateral channel also may connect the left atrium with a systemic vein. It is regarded as a retained primitive connection with the cardinal venous system (Edwards and DuShane, 1950).

Obviously, pulmonary hypertension in patients with levoatrial cardinal vein is due to the associated malformations of the mitral or aortic valves and is congestive in nature.

Congenital Stenosis of Pulmonary Veins

Narrowing of a pulmonary vein either by a localized stenosis or by tubular hypoplasia generally is considered a rare condition but it is likely that this malformation is often overlooked by the pathologist.

As we have seen (p. 302), anomalous pulmonary veins may be affected by both focal stenosis and tubular hypoplasia, but pulmonary veins with a normal connection also may be stenotic. In some patients all or almost all veins are stenotic (Reye, 1951; Bernstein et al., 1959; Edwards, 1960; Shone et al., 1962). In others a single vein or some veins are involved (Ferencz and Dammann, 1957). Sometimes these malformations are unilateral (Emslie-Smith et al., 1955; Binet et al., 1972; Nasrallah et al., 1975). The obstruction may be located in the course of the veins but also at their junction with the left atrium (Figure 13-18) (Sherman et al., 1958; Becker et al., 1970).

Stenosis of pulmonary veins may be associated with other congenital cardiac anomalies (Becu et al., 1955) and even with congenital stenosis of pulmonary arteries (Diamond, 1958). This is one reason to assume that the venous obstruction is congenital (Edwards, 1960) although in occasional cases an acquired origin has been suggested (Contis et al., 1967). The differential diagnosis with pulmonary veno-occlusive disease has been discussed in Chapter Ten.

Pulmonary hypertension is a common complication of this condition, particularly when the stenoses are multiple. The picture of the lung vessels conforms to that observed in pulmonary venous hypertension, including marked medial hypertrophy and arterialization of pulmonary veins (Figure 13-19). There is the additional feature of a pronounced development of collateral channels within the lungs (Becu et al., 1955).

Cor Triatriatum

Cor triatriatum is a malformation consisting of a bi-partitioning of the left atrium so that there is an accessory chamber superimposed upon this atrium and connected with it by an opening of varying size. The pulmonary veins all join this accessory chamber (Borst, 1905; Grondin et al., 1964). It is likely that the cause of this malformation is the inability of the common pulmonary vein to become incorporated into the left atrium. The accessory chamber may be viewed as part of the pulmonary

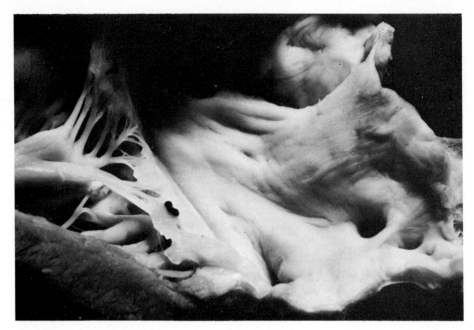

Figure 13-18. Left atrium with stenotic orifice of left pulmonary veins (right) in a female stillborn infant. There was complete obstruction of the right-sided pulmonary venous orifice.

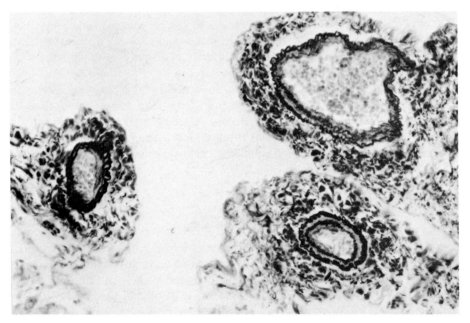

Figure 13-19. Pulmonary veins with marked medial hypertrophy and arterialization from the same case as Figure 13-18. There is also pronounced lymphangiectasis (El.v.G., ×230).

venous system with an opening, usually stenotic, into the atrium. Therefore, it is justified to discuss this condition in connection with pulmonary venous stenoses.

Since the pulmonary venous outflow often is obstructed, pulmonary hypertension commonly occurs and may be severe (Magidson, 1962; Jegier et al., 1963).

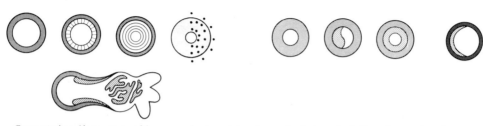

Congenital malformations of lung vessels: A variety of vascular lesions, including plexogenic pulmonary arteriopathy and congestive hypertensive vascular lesions, dependent upon the nature of the malformation.

REFERENCES

Baxter, C. F., Booth, R. W., and Sirak, H. D.: Surgical correction of congenital stenosis of the right pulmonary artery accompanied by agenesis of the left pulmonary artery. *J. Thorac. Cardiovasc. Surg.* **41:** 796, 1961.

Becker, A. E., Becker, M. J., and Edwards, J. E.: Occlusion of pulmonary veins, "mitral" insufficiency, and ventricular septal defect. *Amer. J. Dis. Child.* **120:** 557, 1970.

Becu, L. M., Tauxe, W. N., DuShane, J. W., and Edwards, J. E.: Anomalous connection of pulmonary veins with normal pulmonary venous drainage. Report of case associated with pulmonary venous stenosis and cor triatriatum. *Arch. Path.* **59:** 463, 1955.

Belcher, J. R., and Pattinson, J. N.: Hypoplasia of the lobar pulmonary arteries. *J. Thorac. Surg.* **34:** 357, 1957.

Bernstein, J., Nolke, A. C., and Reed, J. O.: Extrapulmonary stenosis of the pulmonary veins. *Circulation* **19:** 891, 1959.

Binet, J. P., Bouchard, F., Langlois, J., Chetochine, F., Conso, J. F., and Pottemain, M.: Unilateral congenital stenosis of the pulmonary veins. A very rare cause of pulmonary hypertension. *J. Thorac. Cardiovasc. Surg.* **63:** 397, 1972.

Binet, J. P., Langlois, J., Planche, C., Conso, J. F., and Gayral, F.: Fistules aorto-pulmonaires (étude de 10 cas opérés). *Arch. Malad. Coeur* **66:** 963, 1973.

Blake, H. A., Hall, R. J., and Manion, W. C.: Anomalous pulmonary venous return. *Circulation* **32:** 406, 1965.

Borst: Ein Cor triatriatum. *Verh. Dtsch. Ges. Path.* **9:** 178, 1905.

Burchell, H. B.: Total anomalous pulmonary venous drainage; clinical and physiologic patterns. *Proc. Staff Meet. Mayo Clin.* **31:** 161, 1956.

Burroughs, J. T., and Edwards, J. E.: Total anomalous pulmonary venous connection. *Amer. Heart J.* **59:** 913, 1960.

Carey, L. S., and Edwards, J. E.: Severe pulmonary venous obstruction in total anomalous pulmonary venous connection to the left innominate vein. *Amer. J. Roentgenol.* **90:** 593, 1963.

Chesler, E., and Duckworth, W. C.: Congenital absence of left pulmonary artery with coarctation of right pulmonary artery. *Brit. Heart J.* **26:** 705, 1964.

Collett, R. W., and Edwards, J. E.: Persistent truncus arteriosus: A classification according to anatomic types. *Surg. Clin. N. Amer.* **29:** 1245, 1949.

Contis, G., Fung, R. H., Vawter, G. F., and Nadas, A. S.: Stenosis and obstruction of the pulmonary veins associated with pulmonary artery hypertension. *Amer. J. Cardiol.* **20:** 718, 1967.

Cucci, C. E., Doyle, E. F., and Lewis, E. W.: Absence of a primary division of the pulmonary trunk. An ontogenetic theory. *Circulation* **29:** 124, 1964.

Darling, R. C., Rothney, W. B., and Craig, J. M.: Total pulmonary venous drainage into right side of heart. *Lab. Invest.* **6:** 44, 1957.

D'Cruz, I. A., Agustsson, M. H., Bicoff, J. P., Weinberg, M., and Arcilla, R. A.: Stenotic lesions of the pulmonary arteries: Clinical and hemodynamic findings in 84 cases. *Amer. J. Cardiol.* **13:** 441, 1964.

Delaney, T. B., and Nadas, A. S.: Peripheral pulmonic stenosis. *Amer. J. Cardiol.* **13:** 451, 1964.

Diamond, I.: The Hamman-Rich syndrome in childhood: Report of a case with unilateral pulmonary arterial and venous stenosis and arteriovenous occlusion. *Pediatrics* **22:** 279, 1958.

Dische, M. B., Teixeira, M. L., Winchester, P. H., and Engle, M. A.: Horseshoe lung associated with a variant of the "scimitar" syndrome. *Brit. Heart J.* **36:** 617, 1974.

Dotter, C. T., Hardisty, N. M., and Steinberg, I.: Anomalous right pulmonary vein entering the inferior vena cava: two cases diagnosed during life by angiocardiography and cardiac catheterization. *Amer. J. Med. Sci.* **218:** 31, 1949.

DuShane, J. W., Weidman, W. H., Ongley, P. A., Swan, H. J. C., Kirklin, J. W., Edwards, J. E., and Schmutzler, H.: Origin of right pulmonary artery from aorta. *Amer. Heart J.* **59:** 782, 1960.

Edwards, J. E.: Congenital stenosis of pulmonary veins. Pathologic and developmental considerations. *Lab. Invest.* **9:** 46, 1960.

Edwards, J. E.: Congenital malformations of the heart and great vessels. In Gould, S. E., *Pathology of the Heart and Blood Vessels*, ed. 3. Charles C Thomas, Springfield, Ill., 1968.

Edwards, J. E., and DuShane, J. W.: Thoracic venous anomalies. I. Vascular connection between the left atrium and the left innominate vein (levoatriocardinal vein) associated with mitral atresia and premature closure of the foramen ovale (Case 1). II. Pulmonary veins draining wholly into the ductus venosus (Case 2). *Arch. Path.* **49:** 517, 1950.

Edwards, J. E., and Helmholtz, H. F.: A classification of total anomalous pulmonary venous connection based on developmental considerations. *Proc. Staff Meet. Mayo Clin.* **31:** 151, 1956.

Elder, J. C., Brofman, B. L., Kohn, P. M., and Charms, B. L.: Unilateral pulmonary artery absence or hypoplasia. Radiographic and cardiopulmonary studies in five patients. *Circulation* **17:** 557, 1958.

Eldredge, W. J., Tingelstad, J. B., Robertson, L. W., Mauck, H. P. and McCue, C. M.: Observation on the natural history of pulmonary artery coarctations. *Circulation* **45:** 404, 1972.

Emmanouilides, G. C., Linde, L. M., and Crittenden, I. H.: Pulmonary artery stenosis associated with ductus arteriosus following maternal rubella. *Circulation* **29:** 514, 1964.

Emslie-Smith, D., Hill, I. G. W., and Lowe, K. G.: Unilateral membranous pulmonary venous occlusion, pulmonary hypertension and patent ductus arteriosus. *Brit. Heart J.* **17:** 79, 1955.

Farnsworth, A. E., and Ankeney, J. L.: The spectrum of the scimitar syndrome. *J. Thorac. Cardiovasc. Surg.* **68:** 37, 1974.

Ferencz, C.: Congenital abnormalities of pulmonary vessels and their relation to malformations of the lung. *Pediatrics* **28:** 993, 1961.

Ferencz, C., and Dammann, J. F.: Significance of the pulmonary vascular bed in congenital heart disease: V. Lesions of the left side of the heart causing obstruction of the pulmonary venous return. *Circulation* **16:** 1046, 1957.

Ferguson, C. F., and Neuhauser, E. B. D.: Congenital absence of the lung (agenesis) and other anomalies of the tracheobronchial tree. *Amer. J. Roentgenol.* **52:** 459, 1944.

Gay, B. B., Franch, R. H., Shuford, W. H., and Rogers, J. V.: The roentgenologic features of single and multiple coarctations of the pulmonary artery and branches. *Amer. J. Roentgenol.* **90:** 599, 1963.

Glancy, D. I., Braunwald, N. S., O'Brien, K. P., and Roberts, W. C.: Scimitar syndrome associated with patent ductus arteriosus, aortic coarctation and irreversible pulmonary hypertension. *J. Hopk. Med. J.* **123:** 297, 1968.

Grondin, C., Leonard, A. S., Anderson, R. C., Amplatz, K., and Edwards, J. E.: Cor triatriatum: A diagnostic surgical enigma. *J. Thorac. Cardiovasc. Surg.* **48:** 527, 1964.

Hartmann, A. F., Goldring, D., and Elliott, L. P.: Course of peripheral pulmonary stenosis in children. *Circulation* **34:** (suppl. 2) 135, 1967.

Hauck, A. J., Rudolph, A. M., and Nadas, A. S.: Pulmonary venous obstruction in infants with anomalous pulmonary venous drainage. *Circulation* **22:** 761, 1960.

Heath, D., and Watts, G. T.: The significance of vascular changes in an accessory lung presenting as a diaphragmatic cyst. *Thorax* **12**: 142, 1957.

Hepburn, J., and Dauphinee, J. A.: Successful removal of hemangioma of the lung followed by the disappearance of polycythemia. *Amer. J. Med. Sci.* **204**: 681, 1942.

Hollis, W. J.: The scimitar anomaly with absent right pulmonary artery. *Amer. J. Cardiol.* **14**: 262, 1964.

Javier, R. P., Hildner, F. J., and Samet, P.: Pulmonary arteriovenous fistulae with bidirectional shunting. *Chest* **58**: 623, 1970.

Jegier, W., Gibbons, J. E., and Wiglesworth, F. W.: Cor triatriatum: Clinical, hemodynamic and pathological studies: Surgical correction in early life. *Pediatrics* **31**: 255, 1963.

Johnston, D. G.: Inflammatory and vascular lesions of bronchopulmonary sequestration. *Amer. J. Clin. Path.* **26**: 636, 1956.

Jue, K. L., Amplatz, K., Adams, P., and Anderson, R. C.: Anomalies of great vessels associated with lung hypoplasia. The scimitar syndrome. *Amer. J. Dis. Child.* **111**: 35, 1966.

Kittle, C. F., and Crockett, J. E.: Vena cava bronchovascular syndrome. A triad of anomalies involving the right lung: anomalous pulmonary vein, abnormal bronchi and systemic pulmonary arteries. *Ann. Surg.* **156**: 222, 1962.

Kuiper-Oosterwal, C. H., and Moulaert, A.: The scimitar syndrome in infancy and childhood. *Europ. J. Cardiol.* **1**: 55, 1973.

LeBauer, E. J., and Perloff, J. K.: Auscultatory manifestations of isolated bilateral pulmonary artery stenosis: a phonocardiographic, hemodynamic, and angiographic correlative study. *Circulation* **34**: (Suppl. 2) 170, 1967.

Lees, M. H., and Dotter, C. T.: Bronchial circulation in severe multiple peripheral pulmonary artery stenosis. Case report illustrating the origin of continuous murmur. *Circulation* **31**: 759, 1965.

Le Roux, B. T., Gibb, B. H., and Wainwright, J.: Pulmonary arteriovenous fistula with bilharzial pulmonary hypertension. *Brit. Heart J.* **32**: 571, 1970.

Lucas, R. V., Woolfrey, B. F., Anderson, R. C., Lester, R. G., and Edwards, J. E.: Atresia of the common pulmonary vein. *Pediatrics* **29**: 729, 1962a.

Lucas, R. V., Lester, R. G., Lillehei, C. W., and Edwards, J. E.: Mitral atresia with levoatriocardinal vein. A form of congenital pulmonary venous obstruction. *Amer. J. Cardiol.* **9**: 607, 1962b.

MacMahon, H. E., Lee, H. Y., and Stone, P. A.: Congenital segmental coarctation of pulmonary arteries. An anatomic study. *Amer. J. Path.* **50**: 15, 1967.

Magidson, A.: Cor triatriatum. Severe pulmonary arterial hypertension and pulmonary venous hypertension in a child. *Amer. J. Cardiol.* **9**: 603, 1962.

Massumi, R. A., Alwan, A. O., Hernandez, T. J., Just, H. G., and Tawakkol, A. A.: The scimitar syndrome. A physiologic explanation for the associated dextroposition of the heart, maldevelopment of the right lung and its artery, and for the systemic collateral supply to the lung. *J. Thorac. Cardiovasc. Surg.* **53**: 623, 1967.

McCue, C. M., Robertson, L. W., Lester, R. G., and Mauck, H. P.: Pulmonary artery coarctations. *J. Pediat.* **67**: 222, 1965.

McDonald, A. H., Gerlis, L. M., and Sommerville, J.: Familial arteriopathy with associated pulmonary and systemic stenoses. *Brit. Heart J.* **31**: 375, 1969.

Morrow, A. G., Greenfield, L. J., and Braunwald, E.: Congenital aortopulmonary septal defect. Clinical and hemodynamic findings, surgical technic, and results of operative correction. *Circulation* **25**: 463, 1962.

Nasrallah, A. T., Mullins, C. E., Singer, D., Harrison, G., and McNamara, D. G.: Unilateral pulmonary vein atresia: Diagnosis and treatment. *Amer. J. Cardiol.* **36**: 969, 1975.

Neill, C. A., Ferencz, C., Sabiston, D. C., and Sheldon, H.: The familial occurrence of hypoplastic right lung with systemic arterial supply and venous drainage "scimitar syndrome." *Bull. J. Hopk. Hosp.* **107**: 1, 1960.

Neufeld, H. N., Lester, R. G., Adams, P., Anderson, R. C., and Lillehei, C. W.: Aorticopulmonary septal defect. *Amer. J. Cardiol.* **9**: 12, 1962.

Ostrow, P. T., Salyer, W. R., White, J. J., Haller, J. A., and Hutchins, G. M.: Hypertensive pulmonary vascular disease in intralobar sequestration. *Amer. J. Path.* **70**: 33a, 1973.

Park, E. A.: Defective development of the right lung, due to anomalous development of the right pulmonary artery and vein, accompanied by dislocation of the heart simulating dextrocardia. *Proc. N.Y. Path. Soc.* **12:** 88, 1912.

Pool, P. E., Vogel, J. H. K. and Blount, S. G.: Congenital unilateral absence of a pulmonary artery. *Amer. J. Cardiol.* **10:** 706, 1962.

Reye, R. D. K.: Congenital stenosis of pulmonary veins in their extrapulmonary course. *Med. J. Aust.* **1:** 801, 1951.

Rowe, R. D.: Maternal rubella and pulmonary artery stenoses. *Pediatrics* **32:** 180, 1963.

Sanger, P. W., Taylor, F. H., and Robicsek, F.: The "scimitar syndrome." *Arch. Surg.* **86:** 580, 1963.

Sapru, R. P., Hutchison, D. C. S., and Hall, J. L.: Pulmonary hypertension in patients with pulmonary arteriovenous fistulae. *Brit. Heart J.* **31:** 559, 1969.

Schubert, W., and Ruickoldt, E.: Ein Beitrag zu den Missbildungen der Arteria pulmonalis. *Arch. Kinderheilk.* **151:** 52, 1955.

Sherman, F. E., Stengel, W. F., and Bauersfeld, S. R.: Congenital stenosis of pulmonary veins at their atrial junctions. *Amer. Heart J.* **56:** 908, 1958.

Shone, J. D., Amplatz, K., Anderson, R. C., Adams, P., and Edwards, J. E.: Congenital stenosis of individual pulmonary veins. *Circulation* **26:** 574, 1962.

Shone, J. D., and Edwards, J. E.: Mitral atresia associated with pulmonary venous anomalies. *Brit. Heart J.* **26:** 241, 1964.

Shumacker, H. B., and Lurie, P. R.: Pulmonary valvotomy. Description of a new operative approach with comments about diagnostic characteristics of pulmonary valvular stenosis. *J. Thorac. Surg.* **25:** 173, 1953.

Smith, W. G.: Pulmonary hypertension and continuous murmur due to multiple peripheral stenoses of the pulmonary arteries. *Thorax* **13:** 194, 1958.

Snellen, H. A., and Albers, F. H.: Clinical diagnosis of anomalous pulmonary venous drainage. *Circulation* **6:** 801, 1952.

Søndergaard, T.: Coarctation of the pulmonary artery. *Danish Med. Bull.* **1:** 46, 1954.

Swan, H. J. C., Toscano-Barboza, E., and Wood, E. H.: Hemodynamic findings in total anomalous pulmonary venous drainage. *Proc. Staff Meet. Mayo Clin.* **31:** 177, 1956.

Tang, J. S., Kauffman, S. L. and Lynfield, J.: Hypoplasia of the pulmonary arteries in infants with congenital rubella. *Amer. J. Cardiol.* **27:** 491, 1971.

Thibert, M., and Simon, G.: Fistules aorto-pulmonaires (à propos de 13 observations). *Arch. Malad. Coeur* **67:** 251, 1974.

Trell, E., Johansson, B. W., Andren, L., and Ohlsson, N. M.: The scimitar syndrome with particular reference to its pathogenesis. *Z. Kreislaufforsch.* **60:** 880, 1971.

Trell, E., Johansson, B. W., Linell, F., and Ripa, J.: Familial pulmonary hypertension and multiple abnormalities of large systemic arteries in Osler's disease. *Amer. J. Med.* **53:** 50, 1972.

Van Praagh, R., and Van Praagh, S.: The anatomy of common aorticopulmonary trunk (truncus arteriosus communis) and its embryologic implications. A study of 57 necropsy cases. *Amer. J. Cardiol.* **16:** 406, 1965.

Wagenvoort, C. A., Neufeld, H. N., Birge, R. F., Caffrey, J. A., and Edwards, J. E.: Origin of right pulmonary artery from ascending aorta. *Circulation* **23:** 84, 1961.

Wagenvoort, C. A., Heath, D., and Edwards, J. E.: *The Pathology of the Pulmonary Vasculature.* Charles C Thomas, Springfield, Ill., 1964.

Wasserman, M. P., Varghese, P. J., and Rowe, R. D.: The evolution of pulmonary arterial stenosis associated with congenital rubella. *Amer. Heart J.* **76:** 638, 1968.

Watson, G. H., and Miller, V.: Arterio-hepatic dysplasia. Familial pulmonary arterial stenosis with neonatal liver disease. *Arch. Dis. Childh.* **48:** 459, 1973.

Wu, C., Balcon, R., Kurtzman, R. S., and Wendt, V. E.: Absent left pulmonary artery, right-sided aortic arch and patent ductus arteriosus with right to left shunt. *Amer. J. Cardiol.* **14:** 702, 1964.

CHAPTER FOURTEEN

Postoperative Pulmonary Hypertension in Tetralogy of Fallot

In tetralogy of Fallot, as it is now usually defined, there is an obstruction to the right ventricular outflow tract and a ventricular septal defect with a right to left shunt if not at rest then at least at exercise. This results in a diminished pulmonary flow. The pressure in the pulmonary artery is normal or subnormal, and pulmonary hypertension is not a feature of this malformation.

This may be different after surgery. Sometimes, although uncommonly, pulmonary hypertension appears to be present, or to develop over the years, after the surgical creation of a shunt between systemic and pulmonary circulations or after a reparative operation. The mechanisms involved in the elevation of the pulmonary arterial pressure may vary but the consequences often are serious and this warrants a discussion of these complications in a separate chapter.

Since in tetralogy of Fallot the pulmonary vessels exhibit some peculiar features, even in the absence of pulmonary hypertension, we will first outline the changes generally observed in this condition.

There are several varieties of Fallot's tetralogy and also some other congenital cardiac malformations resulting in cyanosis and diminished pulmonary flow for which the same consequences with regard to the pulmonary circulation after surgery apply.

PULMONARY VASCULATURE IN TETRALOGY OF FALLOT

The pulmonary trunk in cases of diminished pulmonary flow is usually of small caliber as compared to the aorta (Sunderland et al., 1973). Sometimes it is dilated (D'Cruz et al., 1964) and often it has a thin wall, containing very little elastic tissue. This has been regarded as a form of disuse atrophy (Heath et al., 1959).

One of the most constant features of the muscular pulmonary arteries in tetralogy of Fallot, and to a lesser extent in isolated pulmonary stenosis, is thinning of the vascular wall or medial atrophy (Figure 14-1). Since in the normal lung the media is thin, this may escape attention, and this may explain why the media of these arteries sometimes is considered to be within normal limits (Civin and Edwards, 1950; Dammann and Ferencz, 1956). Others found the media to be thinner than normal, sometimes even absent in arteries that normally would contain a distinct muscular coat (Valenzuela et al., 1954; Best and Heath, 1958; Fragoyannis and Kardalinos, 1962; Wagenvoort et al., 1964; Wagenvoort et al., 1967). Even in infants with pulmonic stenosis or atresia, the media may be thinner than in the normal newborn infant (Naeye, 1961; Wagenvoort and Edwards, 1961). In some instances it was likely that medial atrophy started even before birth.

Moreover, the pulmonary arteries usually are dilated and wide in tetralogy of Fallot (Giampalmo and Schoenmackers, 1952; Wagenvoort et al., 1967; Harms et al., 1973). This is also evident in the postmortem arteriogram, which shows a "moss-like" appearance by its very marked filling.

The reason for this widening is not clear. It is probably not or not only a poststenotic dilatation since all peripheral vessels are involved; even capillaries and veins are usually wider than normal. Possibly it is an expression of increased blood volume in these cases.

In such lungs it is not uncommon to find occasional muscular pulmonary arteries that are thick-walled and apparently constricted. The significance of this is unknown. They usually are so scarce that they have little influence on the mean medial thickness of the pulmonary arteries, established by morphometry.

Conspicuous intimal changes are due to intravascular thrombosis. There is a distinct tendency to pulmonary vascular thrombosis in tetralogy of Fallot based on the anoxemia with cyanosis, compensatory polycythemia, and increased viscosity of the blood, in combination with the diminished pulmonary flow (Rich, 1948; Best and Heath, 1958; Heath et al., 1958; Ferencz, 1960a; McGonigle and Rosenau, 1964; Thomas, 1964).

The thrombotic lesions find their expression in various ways. Recent thrombi without or with early organization are relatively common in both medium-sized and small pulmonary arteries. Their organization results in patches of intimal fibrosis (Figure 14-2) and sometimes in total or subtotal occlusion of the vessels.

Recanalization of the organized thrombi is not only common but also peculiar since it generally results in the formation of intravascular fibrous septa (Figure 14-3). These septa, which may become very delicate, are lined by endothelium and divide the lumen into multiple compartments. The intravascular septa are particularly observed in tetralogy of Fallot (Rich, 1948; Giampalmo and Schoenmackers, 1952) but also may occur in pulmonic stenosis with intact ventricular septum and in pulmonic atresia (Cain, 1958) as well as in tricuspid atresia.

Generally, in such patients with diminished pulmonary flow, the channels of recanalization in these vessels are much wider, and thereby the septa much thinner, than in other conditions in which recanalization of thrombi occurs. It is likely that the tendency to form these thin septa and wide recanalization channels rests on the same principles that cause the vessels in tetralogy of Fallot to be wide and thin-walled.

On the other hand, this form of septal recanalization cannot be considered pathognomonic for cases of cyanotic heart disease, since it occasionally is observed in

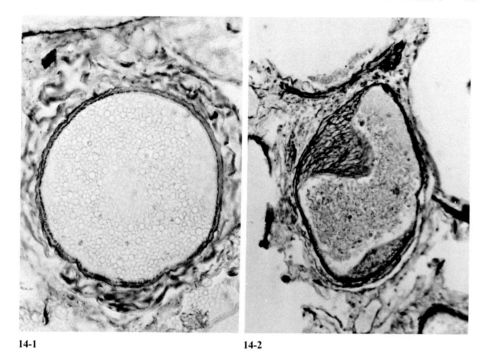

14-1   14-2

Figure 14-1. Muscular pulmonary artery with medial atrophy and wide lumen in a 5-year-old boy with tetralogy of Fallot (El.v.G., ×230).

Figure 14-2. Muscular pulmonary artery with medial atrophy and eccentric intimal fibrosis due to organization of thrombi in the same case as Figure 14-1 (El.v.G., ×140).

patients with other forms of cardiac malformation and also in chronic thromboembolism.

While in tetralogy of Fallot the septal recanalization is probably due to local thrombosis in the great majority of the cases, there are indications that sometimes the same structures result from thromboembolism. In patients with an associated endocarditis of pulmonic or tricuspid valves, intravascular septa often are particularly numerous and also especially localized in the lower lobes (Wagenvoort, 1959). Septal recanalization sometimes has been misinterpreted as plexiform lesions which they may resemble (p. 160).

Thrombotic lesions, whether recent or organized, may occur at any age and have been described in newborn infants with pulmonic atresia (Wagenvoort and Edwards, 1961; Naeye, 1963). The intravascular septa have been found in infants as young as 6 weeks (Wagenvoort and Edwards, 1961) and 4 months (Ferrier, 1955), but there is little doubt that they are much more numerous in older children and adults (Heath et al., 1958; Ferencz, 1960a). Marquis (1956) described them in a 64-year-old woman with Fallot's tetralogy.

Alveolar capillaries are usually wide in tetralogy of Fallot and often engorged with blood in spite of the diminished flow. The pulmonary veins and venules tend to be wide and dilated. Thrombotic lesions and intravascular fibrous septa may be present (Figure 14-4) (Best and Heath, 1958) but are much less numerous than in the arteries (Wagenvoort, 1959; Ferencz, 1960a).

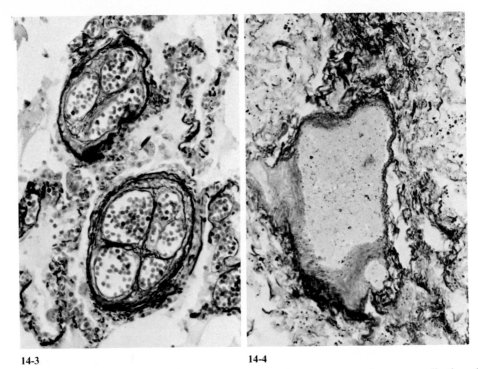

14-3   14-4

Figure 14-3. Muscular pulmonary arteries with intravascular fibrous septa due to recanalization of thrombi in a 9-year-old boy with tetralogy of Fallot (El.v.G., ×230).

Figure 14-4. Pulmonary vein with intravascular fibrous septa in the same case as Figure 14-3 (El.v.G., ×90).

Bronchial arteries are wide in tetralogy of Fallot and to a varying extent are a source for collateral arteries. These collateral arteries develop not only from bronchial but also from other systemic arteries such as intercostal arteries, the internal mammary artery, and the mediastinal plexus (Hales and Liebow, 1948). They communicate with pulmonary arteries with fairly large anastomoses (Collister et al., 1953). Such anastomoses also may occur near the hilum (Edwards, 1968).

This collateral circulation supplies blood to the lungs to a greatly varying extent but in many instances this supply is greater than that from the bronchial arteries. Collateral circulation may provide the only blood supply in cases of pulmonic atresia. The development of collaterals is usually greater in older children and adults than in young children (Bing et al., 1947; Thomas, 1964).

The structure of the collateral arteries corresponds to that of the bronchial arteries. Intimal fibrosis is common and recanalized thrombi occasionally are present.

POSTOPERATIVE PULMONARY HYPERTENSION

Surgical intervention in patients with tetralogy of Fallot or comparable cardiac malformations is aimed either at the creation of a shunt between systemic and pulmonary circulations or at complete correction of the anomaly by excision of the pulmonic stenosis and closure of the ventricular septal defect.

Anastomotic Operations

The effect of an anastomotic operation usually has a distinct beneficial effect for the patient since the pulmonary flow becomes increased and more blood becomes fully oxygenated.

In several instances, however, the shunt becomes inadequate as a result of subsequent thrombosis or during the child's growth. Therefore, these procedures are now more and more limited to complicated or severe cases such as pulmonic atresia or to young infants as a temporary and palliative measure.

One of the problems arising in the various forms of anastomotic operations is the size of the anastomosis. If the shunt is too small, its effect is insufficient. If, on the other hand, the shunt is too large, its hemodynamic effect becomes that of a widely patent ductus arteriosus with pulmonary hypertension as a consequence.

The situation even may be more unfortunate for these patients than for the ones with patency of the ductus, since in the latter cases the pulmonary circulation was adapted from birth with medial hypertrophy of the muscular pulmonary arteries, while in the former no adaptation is presented to the suddenly increased flow. As we have seen, the pulmonary arteries are thin-walled.

The lungs of patients dying in heart failure within the first week after an anastomotic operation for tetralogy of Fallot, almost always show severe congestion, distension of pulmonary vessels, engorgement of capillaries, and pulmonary edema. Frequently there is rupture of capillaries or of arterioles with hemorrhage (Ferencz, 1960b). These alterations may all be present even if the size of the anastomosis is adequate. It is likely that similar or even more severe changes are present in those patients in whom the anastomosis has been made too wide.

If the pulmonary circulation is able to cope with the immediate effects of too large a shunt, the patients may do well for a long time. We agree with Fragoyannis and Kardalinos (1962) that the muscular pulmonary arteries in the lung at the side of the Blalock-Taussig anastomosis often have a thicker media than those in the other lung.

In the long run, and sometimes only after many years, sustained pulmonary hypertension and hypertensive pulmonary vascular lesions may develop. Although such a course is unusual, several well-documented cases have proved that pulmonary hypertension is a distinct hazard after a shunt operation.

An anastomosis according to Potts, involving a shunt between descending aorta and pulmonary arteries, probably carries a high risk for pulmonary hypertension as a late complication (Leeds, 1958; Ross et al., 1958; Wagenvoort et al., 1960; Von Bernuth et al., 1971). The same applies to the Waterston operation in which an anastomosis is made between ascending aorta and pulmonary artery (Soyer et al., 1971; Bercot and Piwnica, 1973; Jaques and Singleton, 1973). Although an indirect communication between aorta and pulmonary artery, as in the Blalock-Taussig procedure in which a subclavian artery is anastomosed with the pulmonary artery, is likely to be less hazardous, several cases resulting in pulmonary hypertension are on record (Epstein and Naji, 1960; Ferencz, 1960b; Paul et al., 1961; McGaff et al., 1962). The time lag between the creation of too large a shunt and the clinical signs of pulmonary hypertension is in the range of 2 to 10 years.

The changes in the pulmonary arteries are the same as in other cases of a shunt between systemic and pulmonary circulations. Plexogenic pulmonary arteriopathy with medial hypertrophy, concentric-laminar intimal fibrosis (Figure 14-5), necrotizing arteritis (Figure 14-6), and plexiform lesions (Figure 14-7) develop (Ross, 1958). In the case of Wagenvoort et al. (1960) such lesions were present in association with late thrombotic alterations such as intravascular fibrous septa. Epstein and Naji (1960) described the development of a pulmonary arterial aneurysm in their case.

Surgical Correction

In patients in whom a complete repair for tetralogy of Fallot has been carried out, the hemodynamic situation in principle is the same as after an adequate shunt operation. The lung vessels must withstand a marked increase in pulmonary flow, and if

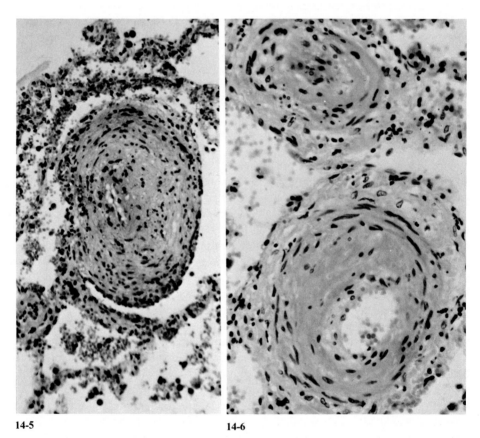

14-5   14-6

Figure 14-5. Muscular pulmonary artery with concentric-laminar intimal fibrosis in a 23-year-old woman with tetralogy of Fallot and pulmonary hypertension, who died 19 years after creation of a Potts' anastomosis (H. and E., ×140).

Figure 14-6. Muscular pulmonary arteritis with fibrinoid necrosis in the same case as Figure 14-5 (H. and E., ×230).

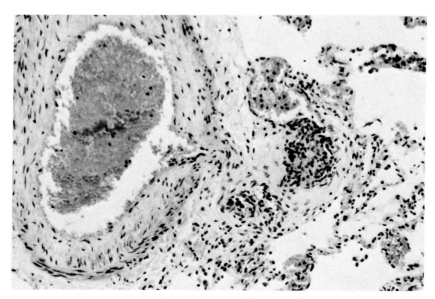

Figure 14-7. Muscular pulmonary artery with mild concentric-laminar intimal fibrosis and a plexiform lesion in a branch (right) in the same case as Figure 14-5 (H. and E., ×140).

they fail to do so, the patient may die with pulmonary congestion, edema, and hemorrhage, while the pulmonary vessels are generally distended. These hazards are mainly confined to the first postoperative week.

It appears however, that there are some patients who develop pulmonary hypertension for various reasons and who may eventually die from this complication. Kinsley et al. (1974) gave a survey of the mechanisms involved.

One of the causes of pulmonary hypertension in these patients is residual ventricular septal defect, including reopening of the defect after initial adequate closure. Since the pulmonary arteries are now no longer protected by the pulmonic stenosis which has been excised, these patients are at a considerable risk of developing pulmonary hypertension. In one case, studied by us, a boy with tetralogy of Fallot who died 2½ months after surgical repair, there was a reopening of the defect while the pulmonary arteries exhibited marked medial hypertrophy and early cellular proliferation of the intima (Wagenvoort et al., 1964).

Another cause is absence of a pulmonary artery, usually of the left pulmonary artery, which as we have discussed before (p. 294) sometimes may result in elevation of pulmonary arterial pressure (Kinsley et al., 1974). Localized stenosis of pulmonary arteries, either congenital or acquired at the site of stitches or grafts, are occasionally the cause of pulmonary hypertension.

Rarely does pulmonary hypertension result from the sequelae of pulmonary vascular thrombosis. Rich (1948), in his description of thrombotic lesions and particularly of septal recanalization in pulmonary arteries in patients with tetralogy of Fallot, commented on the extraordinary large numbers of these changes in some cases. He suggested that these might cause considerable obstruction to the pulmonary flow. It is also our experience that in some patients practically all pulmonary arterial branches contain these lesions (Figures 14-8, 14-9, 14-10, and 14-11).

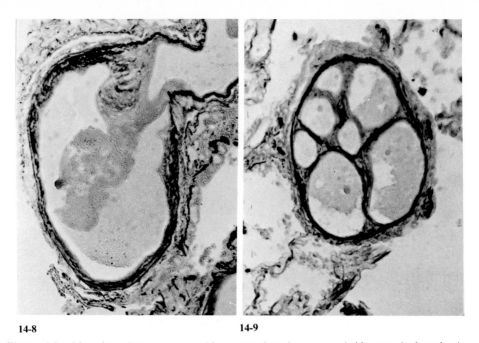

14-8   14-9

Figure 14-8. Muscular pulmonary artery with a recent thrombus on top of older organized patches in a 19-year-old woman with tetralogy of Fallot with pulmonary hypertension (El.v.G., ×90).
Figure 14-9. Muscular pulmonary artery with multiple delicate intravascular fibrous septa from the same case as Figure 14-8 (El.v.G., ×140).

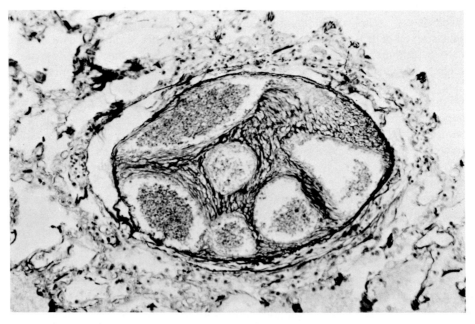

Figure 14-10. Muscular pulmonary artery with rather coarse intravascular fibrous septa containing much elastic tissue from the same case as Figure 14-8 (El.v.G., ×140).

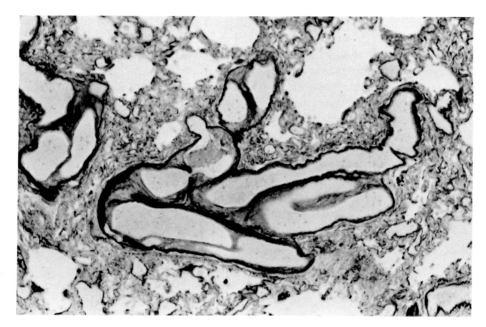

Figure 14-11. Large muscular pulmonary arteries with multiple intravascular fibrous septa causing obstruction of their branches in the same case as Figure 14-8 (El.v.G., ×55).

It is indeed surprising that this does not lead regularly to pulmonary hypertension. It is true that organization and recanalization may restore much of the original pathway. On the other hand, we could demonstrate by serial reconstruction of arteries thus affected, that large numbers of their branches were sealed off by these septa (Figure 14-12) (Wagenvoort, unpublished data). Ferencz (1964) suggested that the septa may disappear in the presence of a large flow, such as may result from

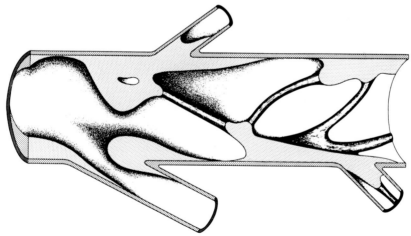

Figure 14-12. Schematic representation of segment of muscular pulmonary artery, with organized thrombi and intravascular fibrous septa, reconstructed from serial sections, from the same case as Figure 14-8. The orifices of its branches are narrowed or obstructed.

anastomotic or corrective surgical procedures. This may happen occasionally but it is certainly not the most common course of event in our experience.

In spite of the apparently severe blockage of the pulmonary circulation by thrombotic alterations, there usually is no indication of an elevated pressure. We have seen one patient, however, in whom pulmonary hypertension following adequate surgical repair was most likely caused by the numerous septa in the pulmonary arteries (Wagenvoort et al., 1964). Similar cases have been described by Kinsley et al. (1974), and this complication was one of the arguments of Bonchek et al. (1973) to advocate early total correction in patients with tetralogy of Fallot.

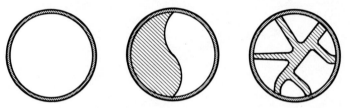

Hypertensive vascular lesions in tetralogy of Fallot: Arteries with thin media, eccentric intimal fibrosis, and extensive intravascular fibrous septa. Sometimes plexogenic pulmonary arteriopathy.

REFERENCES

Bercot, M., and Piwnica, A.: Hypertension artérielle pulmonaire après anastomose aorte-artère pulmonaire droite pour tétralogie de Fallot. Réparation complète. *Nouv. Presse Méd.* **2**: 967, 1973.

Best, P. V., and Heath, D.: Pulmonary thrombosis in cyanotic congenital heart disease without pulmonary hypertension. *J. Path. Bact.* **75**: 281, 1958.

Bonchek, L. I., Starr, A., Sunderland, C. O., and Menashe, V. D.: Natural history of tetralogy of Fallot in infancy. Clinical and therapeutic implications. *Circulation* **48**: 392, 1973.

Bing, R. J., Vandam, L. D., and Gray, F. D.: Physiological studies in congenital heart disease. II. Results of pre-operative studies in patients with tetralogy of Fallot. *Bull. J. Hopk. Hosp.* **80**: 121, 1947.

Cain, H.: Die Lungenstrombahn bei angeborener Pulmonalstenose und Pulmonalatresie. *Zbl. Allg. Path.* **97**: 329, 1958.

Civin, W. H., and Edwards, J. E.: Pathology of the pulmonary vascular tree. I. A comparison of the intra-pulmonary arteries in the Eisenmenger complex and in stenosis of ostium infundibuli associated with biventricular origin of the aorta. *Circulation* **2**: 545, 1950.

Collister, R. M., Dankmeijer, J., Snellen, H. A., and Van der Wel, H. A.: Postmortem X-ray studies of congenital malformations of the heart. *Arch. Path.* **55**: 31, 1953.

Dammann, J. F., and Ferencz, C.: The significance of the pulmonary vascular bed in congenital heart disease. I. Normal lungs, II. Malformations of the heart in which there is pulmonary stenosis. *Amer. Heart J.* **52**: 7, 1956.

D'Cruz, I. A., Arcilla, R. A., and Agustsson, M. H.: Dilatation of the pulmonary trunk in stenosis of the pulmonary valve and of the pulmonary arteries in children. *Amer. Heart J.* **68**: 612, 1964.

Edwards, J. E.: Congenital malformations of the heart and great vessels. B. Malformations of ventricular septal complex. In Gould, S. E., *Pathology of the Heart and Blood Vessels*. Charles C Thomas, Springfield, Ill., 1968.

Epstein, S., and Naji, A. F.: Pulmonary artery aneurysm with dissection after Blalock operation for tetralogy of Fallot. *J. Cardiol.* **5**: 560, 1960.

Ferencz, C.: The pulmonary vascular bed in tetralogy of Fallot. I. Changes associated with pulmonic stenosis. *Bull. J. Hopk. Hosp.* **106**: 81, 1960a.

Ferencz, C.: The pulmonary vascular bed in tetralogy of Fallot. II. Changes following a systemic-pulmonary arterial anastomosis. *Bull. J. Hopk. Hosp.* **106**: 100, 1960b.

Ferencz, C.: Pulmonary vascular changes in tetralogy of Fallot. *Dis. Chest* **46:** 664, 1964.

Ferrier, P.: Endofibrose des artérioles pulmonaires en cas de "maladie bleue." *Presse Méd.* **63:** 453, 1955.

Fragoyannis, S., and Kardalinos, A.: Congenital heart disease with pulmonary ischemia. A study of the pulmonary vascular lesions before and after systemic pulmonary anastomosis. *Amer. Heart J.* **63:** 335, 1962.

Giampalmo, A., and Schoenmackers, J.: Die Lunge bei Morbus caeruleus. *Beitr. Path. Anat.* **112:** 387, 1952.

Hales, M. B., and Liebow, A. A.: Collateral circulation to the lungs in congenital pulmonic stenosis. *Bull. Int. Ass. Med. Museums* **28:** 1, 1948.

Harms, D., Hansen, P., Fischer, K., and Bernhard, A.: Pathologische Anatomie der "Fallot-Lunge". Qualitative und quantitative Untersuchungen nach Korrektur Fallotischer Vitien. *Virch. Arch. Path. Anat.* **361:** 77, 1973.

Heath, D., DuShane, J. W., Wood, E. H., and Edwards, J. E.: The etiology of pulmonary thrombosis in cyanotic congenital heart disease with pulmonary stenosis. *Thorax* **13:** 213, 1958.

Heath, D., Wood, E. H., DuShane, J. W., and Edwards, J. E.: The structure of the pulmonary trunk at different ages and in cases of pulmonary hypertension and pulmonary stenosis. *J. Path. Bact.* **77:** 44, 1959.

Jaques, W., and Singleton, L.: Pulmonary vascular changes in the right lung of a child with a Waterston shunt for 6 years. *Amer. J. Path.* **70:** 28a, 1973.

Kinsley, R. H., McGoon, D. C., Danielson, G. K., Wallace, R. B., and Mair, D. D.: Pulmonary arterial hypertension after repair of tetralogy of Fallot. *J. Thorac. Cardiovasc. Surg.* **67:** 110, 1974.

Leeds, S. E.: The tetralogy of Fallot in older persons up to the fifth decade. Results of subclavian pulmonary anastomosis with a five-to-ten year follow-up. *Amer. J. Surg.* **96:** 234, 1958.

Marquis, R. M.: Longevity and the early history of the tetralogy of Fallot. *Brit. Med. J.* **i:** 819, 1956.

McGaff, C. J., Ross, R. S., and Braunwald, E.: The development of elevated pulmonary vascular resistance in man following increased pulmonary blood flow from systemic pulmonary anastomoses. *Amer. J. Med.* **33:** 201, 1962.

McGonigle, D., and Rosenau, W.: Lesions of pulmonary vessels in tetralogy of Fallot. *Arch. Path.* **78:** 165, 1964.

Naeye, R. L.: Perinatal changes in the pulmonary vascular bed with stenosis and atresia of the pulmonic valve. *Amer. Heart J.* **61:** 586, 1961.

Naeye, R. L.: Arteriosclerosis in congenital heart disease. *Arch. Path.* **75:** 162, 1963.

Paul, M. H., Miller, R. A., and Potts, W. J.: Long-term results of aortic-pulmonary anastomosis for tetralogy of Fallot: An analysis of the first 100 cases eleven to thirteen years after operation. *Circulation* **23:** 525, 1961.

Rich, A. R.: A hitherto unrecognized tendency to the development of widespread pulmonary vascular obstruction in patients with congenital pulmonary stenosis (Tetralogy of Fallot). *Bull. J. Hopk. Hosp.* **82:** 389, 1948.

Ross, R. S., Taussig, H. B., and Evans, M. H.: Late hemodynamic complications of anastomotic surgery for treatment of the tetralogy of Fallot. *Circulation* **18:** 553, 1958.

Soyer, R., Rioux, C., Passelecq, J., Guérin, L., Briotet, J. M., Bouvier, M., and Dubost, C.: Anastomose de Waterston compliquée d'hypertension artérielle pulmonaire grave. Réparation complète— Guérison. *Ann. Chir. Thor. Cardio-vasc.* **10:** 149, 1971.

Sunderland, C. O., Matarazzo, R. G., Lees, M. H., Menashe, V. D., Bonchek, L. I., Rosenberg, J. A., and Starr, A.: Total correction of tetralogy of Fallot in infancy. Postoperative hemodynamic evaluation. *Circulation* **48:** 398, 1973.

Thomas, M. A.: Pulmonary vascular changes in pulmonary stenosis with and without ventricular septal defect. *Brit. Heart J.* **26:** 655, 1964.

Valenzuela, C. T., Toriello, J., and Thomas, W. A.: Structural changes in intrapulmonary arteries exposed to systemic pressures from birth. *Arch. Path.* **47:** 51, 1954.

Von Bernuth, G., Ritter, D. G., Frye, R. L., Weidman, W. H., Davis, G. D., and McGoon, D. C.: Evaluation of patients with tetralogy of Fallot and Potts anastomosis. *Amer. J. Cardiol.* **27:** 259, 1971.

Wagenvoort, C. A.: Vaatafwijkingen in de long bij de tetralogie van Fallot. *Nederl. Tijdschr. Geneesk.* **103:** 2530, 1959.

Wagenvoort, C. A., DuShane, J. W., and Edwards, J. E.: Cardiac clinics 151. Hypertensive pulmonary arterial lesions as a late result of anastomosis of systemic and pulmonary circulations. *Proc. Staff Meet. Mayo Clin.* **35:** 186, 1960.

Wagenvoort, C. A., and Edwards, J. E.: The pulmonary arterial tree in pulmonic atresia. *Arch. Path.* **71:** 646, 1961.

Wagenvoort, C. A., Heath, D., and Edwards, J. E.: *The Pathology of the Pulmonary Vasculature.* Charles C Thomas, Springfield, Ill., 1964.

Wagenvoort, C. A., Nauta, J., Van der Schaar, P. J., Weeda, H. W. H., and Wagenvoort, N.: Vascular changes in pulmonic stenosis and tetralogy of Fallot in lung biopsies. *Circulation* **36:** 924, 1967.

CHAPTER FIFTEEN

Regression of Pulmonary Vascular Lesions

The changes in the pulmonary vasculature in pulmonary hypertension are in part an adaptation to the altered hemodynamic situation and in part the sequelae of injury to the vascular wall. Often these changes tend to be severely progressive as for instance in patients with a congenital cardiac shunt, while in some patients with pulmonary venous hypertension, they may remain stationary over long periods.

The questions to be considered in this chapter are whether and to what extent pulmonary vascular changes will regress after the cause of the pulmonary hypertension is removed. One has to realize that this cause is often not simple and uncomplicated. A ventricular septal defect may be the cause of a rise in pulmonary arterial pressure but in the course of time irreversible hypertensive pulmonary vascular changes with obstruction of the pulmonary vascular bed may develop. Removal of the original cause, that is closure of the ventricular septal defect, may not result in alleviation of pulmonary hypertension, which is now due to vascular obstruction.

Another consideration is that regression of pulmonary hypertension and of vascular lesions are not the same and do not necessarily run parallel. There is often an immediate effect of the closure of a defect or of valvotomy in mitral stenosis in the sense of an abrupt fall in pulmonary arterial pressure. It is obvious that the alterations in the lung vessels could not have changed in so short a period.

Reversibility of vascular lesions can be studied only in some forms of pulmonary hypertension. In unexplained plexogenic pulmonary arteriopathy and pulmonary veno-occlusive disease the cause is obscure and, as far as we know, there are no well-documented reports of spontaneous regression. Various lung diseases, if they have reached the stage in which they produce pulmonary hypertension, are usually incurable and the same applies to severe hepatic injury.

Therefore, it is understandable that, as to regression of pulmonary hypertension and pulmonary vascular lesions, we are best informed with regard to those conditions in which we are able to remove the cause or otherwise to decrease the pulmonary arterial pressure. To the first group belongs hypoxic pulmonary hypertension, particularly when it results from living at high altitudes or from obstruction of upper respiratory airways, and furthermore all forms of congenital or acquired cardiac disease amenable to surgical correction, such as ventricular septal defect and mitral stenosis. The second group comprises those patients in whom the surgical creation of a pulmonic stenosis produces alleviation of pulmonary hypertension.

Moreover, information has been gained from experimental production of elevated pulmonary arterial pressure in animals, followed by removal of the cause of the pulmonary hypertension.

CONGENITAL CARDIAC SHUNTS

The type of pulmonary vascular disease generally occurring in congenital cardiac defects with a shunt associated with pulmonary hypertension is plexogenic pulmonary arteriopathy. As we have seen in Chapter Four, this consists of a pattern of changes which in its complete form comprises medial hypertrophy, cellular intimal proliferation, concentric-laminar intimal fibrosis, necrotizing arteritis, and plexiform lesions. These alterations, however, are not necessarily all present at the same time. Necrotizing arteritis and plexiform lesions indicate the later and often terminal stages of the disease. In the early stages vascular changes may be limited to medial hypertrophy.

Regression of Pulmonary Hypertension

It is clear that there is a close relationship between the stage of the vascular disease and reversibility of pulmonary hypertension. In ventricular septal defect, for instance, there is usually a high pulmonary blood flow in the early stages. With increasing obstruction of the vascular bed by intimal fibrosis the flow becomes controlled and finally reduced (Dammann and Ferencz, 1956). The development of necrotizing arteritis and plexiform lesions has an ominous prognostic significance since these lesions contribute considerably to flow reduction and usually can be taken as an indication that pulmonary hypertension has become irreversible, although in their absence, widespread and severe intimal fibrosis alone also can produce severe obstruction.

In all these instances, the high resistance of the vascular bed is no longer labile since it has acquired a distinct organic basis. This phase of severely reduced flow with pulmonary arterial pressures sometimes approaching or exceeding systemic pressures also has been termed "high resistance, low reserve vascular bed" (Edwards, 1957) and "Eisenmenger syndrome" (Wood, 1958).

In the earlier stages of the vascular disease, the elevation of the pressure is usually less pronounced and is due in part to the high flow prevailing at that time and also to a functional factor in the sense of constriction of arterial smooth muscle. Since this constriction, although it results in an increased resistance, is potentially reversible, Edwards (1957) used the term "high resistance, high reserve vascular bed" to indicate this phase. If the disease has not progressed beyond this stage, pulmonary hypertension may be expected to regress upon closure of the defect and the patient's prognosis is good.

Distinction must be made between the immediate and the long-term regression of pulmonary hypertension after closure of a cardiac shunt. *Immediate regression* can be expected when pulmonary hypertension is due mainly or entirely to a large pulmonary flow in the presence of a left to right shunt, which is eliminated as soon as the defect is closed. In patients who have severe obliterative lesions in their lung vessels, no immediate response to correction of the cardiac condition is likely to occur. These patients, who will keep a high pulmonary arterial pressure, will benefit little from the operation. It is even likely that their condition will deteriorate immediately following this procedure.

There are also many transitional cases in which the pulmonary vascular resistance is partly reversible. According to Heath et al. (1958), if there is medial hypertrophy alone or associated with moderate intimal fibrosis, the systolic pulmonary arterial pressure falls immediately to normal or near normal values. In the transitional cases, morphologically characterized as a rule by marked forms of intimal fibrosis, this fall is distinctly less complete, while in the patients with plexiform lesions in their lung vessels, there is usually no decrease in pressure at all.

Others (Burchell, 1959; Lucas et al., 1961; Reeve et al., 1966) found that in cases of congenital cardiac defect, pulmonary hypertension is largely irreversible. It is clear, however, that much depends on the degree of the organic lesions in the pulmonary vascular bed.

Also *long-term regression* of pulmonary hypertension depends largely on the degree of severity of the hypertensive pulmonary vascular changes. Sometimes pulmonary arterial resistance may fall considerably, as Beck et al. (1959) demonstrated, over periods from 3 to 34 months after closure of an atrial septal defect. Similar findings have been reported in ventricular septal defect (Leachman and Pereyo, 1968). Over a 5- to 10-year period Nadas et al. (1960) found little tendency to progression of pulmonary hypertension when the operation was performed in early age.

In the long run, pulmonary hypertension most likely will regress to a limited degree in some but will remain stationary or even become progressive in many other patients. Long-term regression of pulmonary hypertension is probably closely related to the reversibility of the vascular changes (Wagenvoort et al., 1964).

Regression of Pulmonary Vascular Lesions

Few data about reversibility of hypertensive lesions in the pulmonary vasculature have been derived from patients in whom a congenital cardiac defect has been closed. This is understandable because it is very unusual that comparison of lung tissue in the same patient before and after closure is possible. If a lung biopsy is taken at the time of surgical closure—and unfortunately this is far from a standard procedure—the chances are slight that lung tissue will become available at a later time. Usually the patients do well but if a second procedure should be necessary or the patient should die as a result of the cardiac condition, it is unlikely that the changes would have regressed in these instances.

The banding operation of the pulmonary artery, or in other words, the surgical creation of a pulmonic stenosis, has provided an opportunity to compare lung tissue before and after the correction of the congenital cardiac shunt. The principle of this operation was suggested by Civin and Edwards (1950). The technic was developed and described by Dammann (1951) and Muller and Dammann (1952). The banding operation is essentially a temporary procedure aimed at protecting the pulmonary vasculature from the effects of high pulmonary flow and pressure. It has been used particularly in infants and young children with a ventricular septal defect, when closure of the defect was technically difficult and risky. At a later time, when the children were old enough to undergo a corrective operation, the banding is relieved.

The indications have been broadened subsequently to include older children who developed progressive pulmonary vascular disease and also those with congenital malformations like single ventricle, who were considered unsuitable for corrective operation. Although pulmonary arterial banding is still advocated (Grainger et al., 1967; Reid et al., 1968), there is a growing tendency to perform a one-stage corrective operation in infancy before hypertensive pulmonary vascular changes have developed (Kirklin, 1971; Breckenridge et al., 1973).

The banding operation provides the pathologist with an opportunity to study a lung biopsy at the time of the banding, while another biopsy may become available at the time of the closure of the defect, often several years later. Dammann and his coworkers (1961) were the first to use this opportunity. They studied biopsies at the time of the banding operation and later at corrective surgery in 10 patients. All patients had initially medial hypertrophy which regressed to normal or to near normal in 8. In 2, there was residual hypertrophy; in 3, there was initially some intimal thickening that was absent in the second biopsy. It is of course possible that cellular proliferation may be completely reversible, although it is more likely that remnants of intimal fibrosis would show up at a later period.

Our own experience concerns 20 patients in whom a lung biopsy was taken at the time of the banding operation and a second one, $2\frac{1}{2}$ to 11 years later, at the time of corrective surgery. Medial hypertrophy, assessed by morphometry, was present in all first biopsies (Figure 15-1) and often was very pronounced. Without exception the medial thickness was decreased in the second biopsy (Figure 15-2). In some cases this decrease was mild and even not significant, but in most it was considerable and in 11 children medial hypertrophy had regressed to normal or near normal values.

Cellular intimal proliferation or intimal fibrosis was observed in the initial lung biopsy in seven children. In four of these the degree of severity of the intimal changes has remained virtually unchanged in the second biopsy. In three it was distinctly reduced. In all seven children, however, there was a distinct change in the type of intimal fibrosis. In the initial biopsy cellular proliferation (Figure 15-3) was the most characteristic intimal alteration with only occasional deposition of collagen. In the later biopsy the intimal thickening consisted of dense collagen-rich fibrous tissue usually with pronounced retraction and with widening of the lumen as a consequence (Figure 15-4). In the four children in whom there was no notable regression of intimal lesions, the same type of compact fibrosis was seen but there were several vessels in the second biopsy with complete obliteration and shrinkage of the whole vessel. Apparently, if there is no residual lumen left, retraction of collagen does not lead to restoration of the lumen.

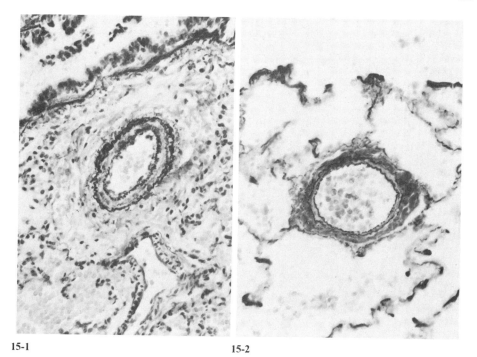

15-1   15-2

Figure 15-1.   Muscular pulmonary artery with medial hypertrophy in a 5-year-old boy with a ventricular septal defect. Biopsy taken at the time of a banding operation (El.v.G., ×230).
Figure 15-2.   Muscular pulmonary artery with normal media from the same patient as in Figure 15-1, 10 years after banding of the pulmonary artery (El.v.G., ×230).

These findings therefore indicate that medial hypertrophy tends to regress after the creation of a pulmonary stenosis, so that the normal medial thickness may be restored in some instances. Early intimal lesions also may regress in the sense that, while becoming more compact and retracted, they cause less obstruction of the lumen as long as this was not obliterated before the banding.

In experiments in which pulmonary hypertension was induced in dogs by creation of a systemic-pulmonary shunt, the regression of the vascular lesions has been studied after closure of this shunt. Ferguson et al. (1955) stated that regression of pulmonary vascular lesions under these circumstances is slow. Restoration of luminal diameter was brought about mainly by a process of recanalization. They even observed intravascular fibrous septa. It seems likely that somehow thrombosis developed in the arteries in their cases. This, however, is not what is observed in patients after banding of a pulmonary artery.

Blank et al. (1959, 1961) found an increased lumen-to-wall ratio of the pulmonary arteries in dogs following a reversal operation and some residual evidence of intimal fibrosis. Geer et al. (1965) reported regression of medial hypertrophy and of minimal to moderate degrees of intimal fibrosis but there was no change with regard to marked intimal fibrosis nor of plexiform lesions.

Very little is known about the reversibility of necrotizing arteritis and plexiform lesions. As we have seen the prognosis is poor when these changes are present in the lung vessels. The incidental findings of either type of lesion in lung biopsies of

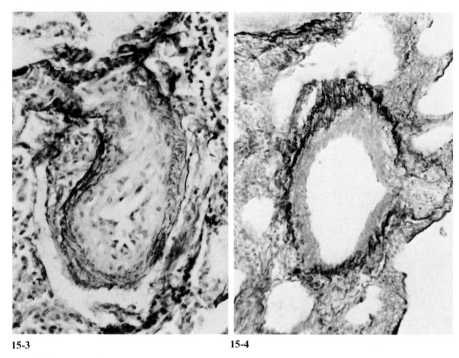

15-3   15-4

Figure 15-3. Muscular pulmonary artery with subtotal occlusion by cellular intimal proliferation in a 4-year-old boy with a ventricular septal defect. Biopsy taken at the time of a banding operation (El.v.G., ×230).

Figure 15-4. Muscular pulmonary artery with thin media and with a layer of intimal fibrosis from the same patient as in Figure 15-3, 7 years after banding of the pulmonary artery. The lumen is largely patent (El.v.G., ×140).

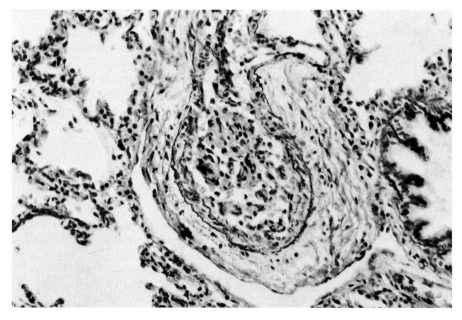

Figure 15-5. Muscular pulmonary artery with early plexiform lesion in a 4-year-old boy with a ventricular septal defect. Biopsy taken at the time of a banding operation. The patient was well at the time of surgical closure of the defect 10 years later, and a biopsy at this time revealed only some intimal fibrosis (H. and E., ×230).

patients who responded well to corrective surgery (p. 87) (Figure 15-5) demonstrates that the presence of these lesions, as long as they are scarce, does not preclude recovery, but the ultimate fate of the lesions themselves is unknown (Wagenvoort and Wagenvoort, 1974).

HYPOXIC PULMONARY HYPERTENSION

The reversibility of hypoxic pulmonary hypertension has been studied particularly in individuals living or staying at high altitudes, in whom pulmonary arterial pressure dropped after administration of oxygen or return to sea level. This has been discussed in Chapter Eleven (p. 237 and 248). Such a regression is also known from children with upper airway obstruction following tonsillectomy or adenoidectomy (p. 251).

The characteristic pulmonary vascular lesions to be found in these circumstances, notably medial hypertrophy of small pulmonary arteries and arterioles and longitudinal smooth intimal muscle bundles disappear in experimental animals when they are returned to normal atmospheric conditions (p. 237) (Figure 15-6). Also right ventricular hypertrophy, medial hypertrophy of pulmonary trunk, and hyperplasia of carotid bodies regress under these circumstances.

PULMONARY VENOUS HYPERTENSION

Surgical correction of mitral valve disease usually produces an immediate decrease of pulmonary vascular resistance and pressure (Dalen et al., 1967). Often the sys-

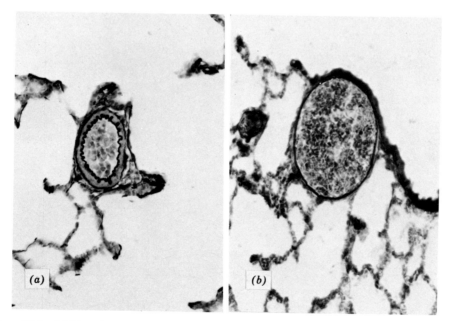

Figure 15-6. (*a*) Muscular pulmonary artery in a rat subjected to hypoxia for 14 days. There is distinct medial hypertrophy. (*b*) Muscular pulmonary artery in a rat subjected to hypoxia for 14 days but kept subsequently in normal air for another 14 days. The media has regressed to normal (El.v.G., ×230).

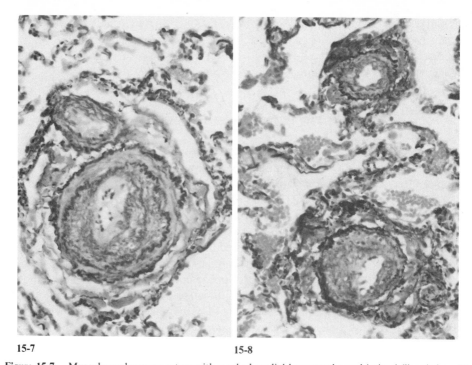

15-7   15-8

Figure 15-7. Muscular pulmonary artery with marked medial hypertrophy and intimal fibrosis in a 42-year-old man with mitral stenosis. Biopsy taken at the time of commissurotomy (El.v.G., ×230).
Figure 15-8. Pulmonary arterioles from the same patient as in Figure 15-7. There is some muscularization and severe intimal fibrosis (El.v.G., ×230).

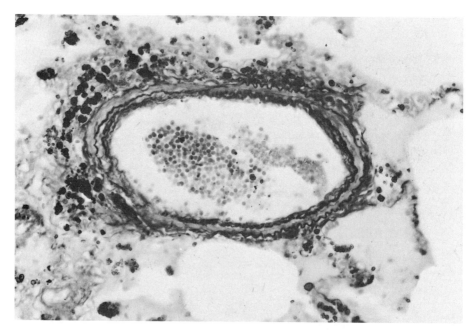

Figure 15-9. Muscular pulmonary artery with normal media and minimal intimal fibrosis from the same patient as in Figure 15-7 at the age of 52, 10 years after the previous biopsy. There was general regression of pulmonary vascular lesions (El.v.G., ×230).

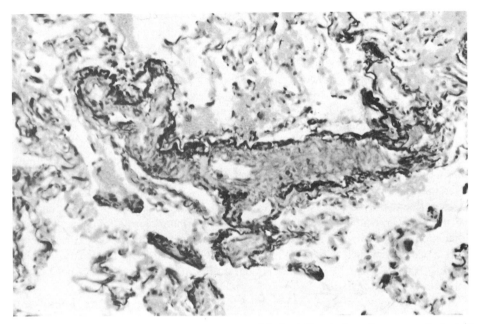

Figure 15-10. Small pulmonary vein with pronounced intimal fibrosis from the same patient as in Figure 15-7. Biopsy taken at the time of commissurotomy (El.v.G., ×230).

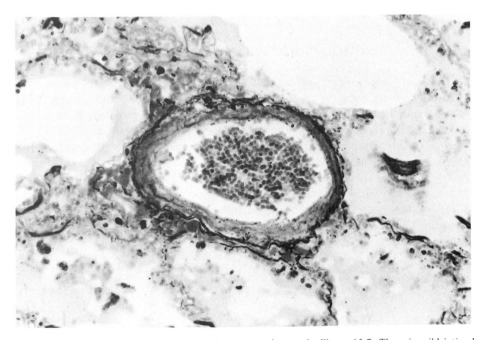

Figure 15-11. Small pulmonary vein from the same patient as in Figure 15-7. There is mild intimal fibrosis and the lumen is largely patent. Lung tissue from autopsy after accidental death, 10 years after commissurotomy (El.v.G., ×230).

tolic pulmonary arterial pressure is not restored to normal but in 27 patients with such pressures exceeding 100 mmHg, there was a fall to values in the range of 50 mmHg, according to Zener et al. (1972). Similar results were obtained by Baedeker et al. (1973). This immediate fall in pressure has been taken as a sign that vaso-constriction plays an important part in the maintenance of pulmonary vascular resistance in mitral stenosis (Goodale et al., 1955; Dalen et al., 1967).

We are not very well informed about the regression of pulmonary vascular changes in these patients. Even if lung biopsies are regularly taken at the time of a commissurotomy, there often is no chance to study lung tissue again after a prolonged interval. Normally, these patients are not operated on a second time unless there is a restenosis, but these cases are of course unsuitable for the study of reversibility of vascular changes.

Very infrequently an occasion arises to study autopsy material from a patient who did not die of mitral valve disease, while a previous lung biopsy, taken at the time of correction of mitral valve disease, was available. Ramirez et al. (1968) reported on such a case in which the original biopsy revealed medial hypertrophy and mild intimal fibrosis, while 11 years later medial thickness was restored to near normal and intimal fibrosis had disappeared.

We have seen a similar case in which a lung biopsy taken at the time of com-missurotomy showed pronounced medial hypertrophy and intimal fibrosis of pulmonary arteries (Figure 15-7) and arterioles (Figure 15-8), while almost ten years later, when the patient died as a result of an accident, the lung vessels revealed minimal medial hypertrophy and intimal fibrosis (Figure 15-9). The pulmonary veins in this case showed initially medial hypertrophy and arterialization and marked intimal fibrosis (Figure 15-10). In the autopsy material the venous walls were normal except for some residual dense intimal fibrosis (Figure 15-11).

THROMBOEMBOLIC PULMONARY HYPERTENSION

To our knowledge there are no data on the reversibility of thromboembolic pulmonary hypertension. If cardiac failure develops in patients with chronic throm-boembolism, there is little prospect of regression. Rather, progressive elevation of pressure is to be expected since the embolic process usually is recurrent.

Some information can be deduced from experimentally produced throm-boembolism particularly in rabbits. It must be realized that the embolism is in healthy animals in which recurrence of the process can be stopped at any time so that comparison with patients is hazardous. As has been described (p. 157), organi-zation of thrombi with subsequent shrinkage and recanalization may cause a revascularization of obstructed segments of the pulmonary arteries which is likely to cause a gradual fall in pressure and resistance.

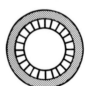

Regression of pulmonary vascular lesions: Medial hypertrophy and cellular intimal proliferation and fibrosis (*left*) may change to normal media and dense retracted intimal fibrosis (*right*).

REFERENCES

Baedeker, W., Henselmann, L., Wirtzfeld, A., and Seidenbusch, W.: Der Einfluss der Mitralkommissuro-tomie auf die reaktieve pulmonale Hypertonie. *Zschr. Kardiol.* **62**: 396, 1973.

Beck, W., Swan, H. J. C., Burchell, H. B., and Kirklin, J. W.: Pulmonary vascular resistance following closure of atrial septal defect in patients with pulmonary hypertension. *Circulation* **20**: 667, 1959.

Blank, R. H., Muller, W. H., and Dammann, J. F.: Changes in pulmonary vascular lesions after restoring normal pulmonary artery pressure. *Surg. Forum* **9**: 356, 1959.

Blank, R. H., Muller, W. H., and Dammann, J. F.: Experimental pulmonary arterial hypertension. *Amer. J. Surg.* **101**: 143, 1961.

Breckenridge, I. M., Oelert, H., Graham, G. R., Stark, J., Waterston, D. J., Bonham-Carter, R. E., and Kirklin, J. W.: Open-heart surgery in the first year of life. *J. Thorac. Cardiovasc. Surg.* **65**: 1, 58, 1973.

Burchell, H. B.: Regression of pulmonary arterial hypertension after cure of intracardiac defects. In Adams, W. A., and Veith, I., *Pulmonary Circulation.* Grune and Stratton, New York, London, 1959.

Civin, W. H., and Edwards, J. E.: Pathology of the pulmonary vascular tree. I. A comparison of the intrapulmonary arteries in the Eisenmenger complex and in stenosis of ostium infundibuli associated with biventricular origin of the aorta. *Circulation* **2**: 545, 1950.

Dalen, J. E., Matloff, J. M., Evans, G. L., Hoppin, F. G., Bhardwaj, P., Harken, D. E., and Dexter, L.: Early reduction of pulmonary vascular resistance after mitral-valve replacement. *New Engl. J. Med.* **277**: 387, 1967.

Dammann, J. F.: Congenital malformations of the heart amenable to surgery. *Bull. St. Johns Hosp. Post-grad. Assembly* **1-087**: 2, 1951.

Dammann, J. F., and Ferencz, C.: The significance of the pulmonary vascular bed in congenital heart disease. III. Defects between the ventricles or great vessels in which both increased pressure and blood flow may act upon the lungs and in which there is a common ejectile force. *Amer. Heart J.* **52**: 210, 1956.

Dammann, J. F., McEachen, J. A., Thompson, W. M., Smith, R., and Muller, W. H.: The regression of pulmonary vascular disease after the creation of pulmonary stenosis. *J. Thorac. Cardiov. Surg.* **42**: 722, 1961.

Edwards, J. E.: Functional pathology of the pulmonary vascular tree in congenital cardiac disease. *Circulation* **15**: 164, 1957.

Ferguson, D. J., Berkas, E. M., and Varco, R. L.: Process of healing in experimental pulmonary arteriosclerosis. *Proc. Soc. Exper. Biol. Med.* **89**: 492, 1955.

Geer, J. C., Glass, H. A., and Albert, H. M.: The morphogenesis and reversibility of experimental hyperkinetic pulmonary vascular lesions in the dog. *Exp. Molec. Path.* **4**: 399, 1965.

Goodale, F., Sanchez, G., Friedlich, A. L., Scannel, J. G., and Myers, G. S.: Correlation of pulmonary arteriolar resistance with pulmonary vascular changes in patients with mitral stenosis before and after valvulotomy. *New Engl. J. Med.* **252**: 979, 1955.

Grainger, R. G., Nagle, R. E., Pawidapha, C., Robertson, D. S., Taylor, D. G., Thornton, J. A., Verel, D., and Zachary, R. B.: Pulmonary artery banding for ventricular septal defect. *Brit. Heart J.* **29**: 289, 1967.

Heath, D., Helmholtz, H. F., Burchell, H. B., DuShane, J. W., Kirklin, J. W., and Edwards, J. E.: Relation between structural changes in the small pulmonary arteries and the immediate reversibility of pulmonary hypertension following closure of ventricular and atrial septal defects. *Circulation* **18**: 1167, 1958.

Kirklin, J. W.: Pulmonary arterial banding in babies with large ventricular septal defects. *Circulation* **43**: 321, 1971.

Leachmann, R. D., and Pereyo, J. A.: Decrease in pulmonary vascular resistance following surgical closure of a ventricular septal defect associated with elevated capillary wedge pressure and severe pulmonary hypertension. *Amer. Heart J.* **76**: 816, 1968.

Lucas, R. V., Adams, P., Anderson, R. C., Meyne, N. G., Lillehei, C. W., and Varco, R. L.: Natural history of isolated ventricular septal defect: A serial physiologic study. *Circulation* **24**: 1372, 1961.

Muller, W. H., and Dammann, J. F.: The treatment of certain congenital malformations of the heart by the creation of pulmonic stenosis to reduce pulmonary hypertension and excessive blood flow. *Surg. Gynec. & Obstet.* **95**: 213, 1952.

Nadas, A. S., Rudolph, A. M., and Gross, R. E.: Pulmonary arterial hypertension in congenital heart disease. *Circulation* **22**: 1041, 1960.

Ramirez, A., Grimes, E. T., and Abelmann, W. H.: Regression of pulmonary vascular changes following mitral valvuloplasty. An anatomic and physiologic case study. *Amer. J. Med.* **45**: 975, 1968.

Reeve, R., Selzer, A., Popper, R. W., Leeds, R. F., and Gerbode, F.: Reversibility of pulmonary hypertension following cardiac surgery. *Circulation* **33**: I-107, 1966.

Reid, J. M., Barclay, R. S., Coleman, E. N., Stevenson, J. G., Welsh, T. M., and McSwan, N.: Pulmonary artery banding in congenital heart disease associated with pulmonary hypertension. *Thorax* **23**: 385, 1968.

Wagenvoort, C. A., Heath, D., and Edwards, J. E.: *The Pathology of the Pulmonary Vasculature.* Charles C. Thomas, Springfield, Ill., 1964.

Wagenvoort, C. A., and Wagenvoort, N.: Pathology of the Eisenmenger syndrome and primary pulmonary hypertension. *Adv. Cardiol.* **11**: 123, 1974.

Wood, P.: The Eisenmenger syndrome, or pulmonary hypertension with reversed shunt. *Brit. Med. J.* **ii**: 755, 1958.

Zener, J. C., Hancock, E. W., Shumway, N. E., and Harrison, D. C.: Regression of extreme pulmonary hypertension after mitral valve surgery. *Amer. J. Cardiol.* **30**: 820, 1972.

Index